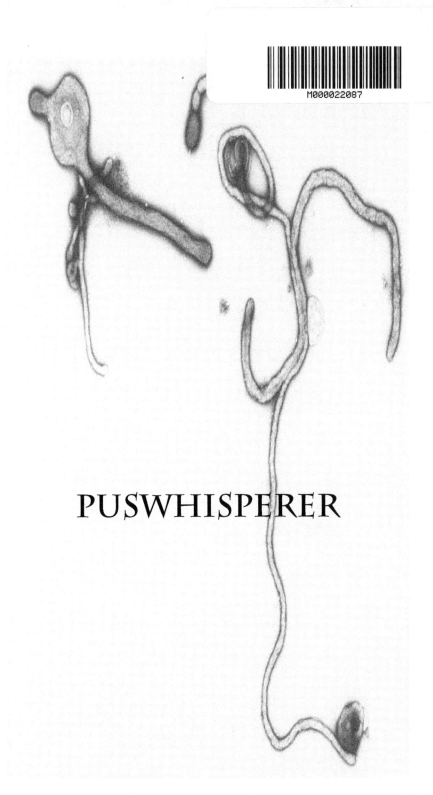

PUSWHISPERER

PUSWHISPERER:

A YEAR IN THE LIFE OF AN INFECTIOUS DISEASE DOCTOR

by Mark Crislip, MD

Bitingduck Press
Altadena, CA

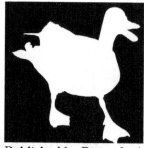

Published by Bitingduck Press
ISBN 978-1-938463-62-4
© 2014 Mark Crislip
All rights reserved
For information contact
Bitingduck Press, LLC
Montreal • Altadena
notifications@bitingduckpress.com
http://www.bitingduckpress.com
Cover art by Cary Shien
Interior image is an electron micrograph of the Ebola virus; image credit Charles Humphrey, from the CDC Public Health Image Library

Publisher's Cataloging-in-Publication data

Crislip, Mark [1957--   ]

Puswhisperer: a collection of case histories/by Mark Crislip, M.D. —1st edition
  p. cm.

Contents—Anecdotes/Case histories about infectious diseases

ISBN: 978-1-938463-62-4

[1. Medical microbiology—pathogenic microorganisms. 2. Infection--communicable diseases. 3. Tuberculosis—mycobacterial diseases. 4. Human immunodeficiency virus--vaccine 5. Bacteria, pathogenic—streptococcus.] I. Title

2014948820

To my wife, Kerry Sue Pioske

CONTENTS

Please allow me to introduce myself

Please allow me to introduce myself.
I'm a man of wealth and taste.
I've been around for a long, long year.
As an Infectious Disease doctor.
Not quite Sympathy for the Devil.

As of 2010, I have been practicing Infectious diseases (I.D.) for almost twenty-five years, if you include the fellowship.

I.D. is relentlessly cool. Everyday I see a cool case, or something unusual, or read an interesting article. I learn something new almost every day. Infectious diseases appear in history, in politics, everywhere. I have never understood why anyone would do anything else. Except, of course, if they want an income.

Why keep all this cool stuff to myself? So I started a blog, Rubor, Dolor, Calor, Tumor, first at pusware.com, then I moved over to Medscape (http://blogs.medscape.com/rdct). Included are ratholes, bad puns, and obscure references. In medical school my evaluations contained five "flips," a "flippant," and a "glib." Consider yourself warned.

The goal is simple. Every other day, depending on what I see on rounds, I write a short, referenced entry that covers one factoid. The one curious disease of the day. With emphasis on short. Just long enough to be read on the toilet, presuming no constipation. And at least one stupid attempt at humor, often repeated.

This book is a collection of my first year's blog entries, reworked, rewritten and most of the typos corrected.

Of course the entries focus on the clinical triumphs that give me the appearance of House-like infallibility.

But I guarantee (1) you will be thrilled and amazed with a year in the life of a Puswhisperer.

Disclaimer

(1) The information is not meant to diagnose, treat, cure or prevent any disease and is not intended for self-diagnosis or self-treatment of medical conditions that should be managed by a qualified health care provider.

To protect patient confidentiality, all demographic and identifying patient information was changed.

I DON'T KNOW

CALL weekends are long. I cover 2 states and 8 hospitals, and I get to see great cases, but I am glad I can go back to my mere three hospitals tomorrow. I think my nickname should be PPD, the peripatetic pus doc.

I.D. consults fall into 2 general categories:

1) How and for how long do you treat an already defined infection?

2) What the heck is this germ and what do I do with it?

3) What the hell does this patient have?

I enjoy type 3. I still cannot count. They are the most fun and offer the greatest opportunity to use those three words that increasingly define my practice:

"I don't know."

House seems to figure out each case in about an hour, although the route by which he gets to the denouement almost always gives me conniption fits. And as I always say, if the conniption fits, wear it. It's why I do not watch medical shows—they get it wrong. Except for *Scrubs*, which is closer to reality, at least my reality, of any TV show. Every year I know more and more. I read 1200 articles a year, attend 10-plus conferences a month, and each year I seem increasingly unsure about what is going on my patients. In the skeptical world they talk about the arrogance of ignorance (aka Jenny McCarthy syndrome) where the people who know the least on a topic think they are the most knowledgeable (it is really called the Dunning-Kruger effect). I have the opposite problem.

So much of the time I can't figure out what the patients have, but they get better, and I make sure I get all the credit. If things go badly, of course, I blame nursing. It is a curious phenomenon that knowledge breeds uncertainty. However, part of being a specialist is to be ignorant with panache. I have beaucoup buckets of panache.

I tell patients that as long as they are getting better, it is probably a good thing I cannot make a diagnosis. In medicine we are very good at diagnosing diseases that will kill or injure you but no good at diagnosing the trivial, self-limiting illnesses. So most of the time no diagnosis is a good diagnosis.

The problem is that when it comes to billing, I need a diagnosis and a diagnosis code. You can know a doctor by the codes she knows by heart. Here are some of mine.

S. *aureus* bacteremia: 038.11.

Fever: 780.6.

UTI: 595.

Endocarditis: 421.

There are codes for everything. Every disease. There is a code for being electrocuted in a bathtub. There is a code for being sucked into a jet engine and the follow-up. Who would have suspected being sucked into a jet engine was a survivable process? There's one for being bitten by a duck, and another for struck by a duck. There is even a code for weightlessness. I am really looking forward to the first patient that presents with that complaint.

"So, what can I do for you?"

"Doc. I'm weightless."

What I really need, and the one thing for which there is no code, is the diagnosis "I don't know."

Or maybe I just don't know it.

Rationalization

http://en.wikipedia.org/wiki/Dunning-Kruger effect

AN OUNCE OF PREVENTION: INFECTION CONTROL

Infection Control

A MONGST my many jobs (my Grandmother always said that a job is what a dog does on the carpet) is the task of infection control at my various hospitals. Infections, as many of you are aware, are an infrequent complication of hospitalization, but cause significant morbidity and mortality. I have been the Chair of our Infection Control (we now call it Infection Prevention, but for some things I am just too damn old to change) program for 19 years and have seen the continuous improvement in a variety of hospital-acquired infections, much to the detriment of my bottom line. After all, I get paid to take care of infections.

Some days I just feel like R.J. Reynolds telling people to stop smoking. The one area that has made some improvement is hand hygiene, but often it seems difficult to get people to wash their hands or to use one of the many hand sanitizers. I suspect that in their heart of hearts, people do not believe in germs. They can't see them, after all, so probably the germs are not there. Believing in things you cannot see is more the topic of the Science Based Medicine blog.

About 40% of hospital infections are due to germs carried on the hands—and probably the stethoscope and the beeper and rings and the white coat and the cell phone and the necktie, all of which have been cultured and can carry pathogens. I am starting to think rounds should be like the Greek Olympics, done naked. It could decrease the spread of infections and, as a side effect, decrease obesity. But filthy bling aside, clean hands are important. It is estimated that it takes about ten years for new medical information to be disseminated, so I have to cut people a little slack; we have only know the importance of hand washing for 160 years.

As part of my duties as Chair of Infection Control, we have made great progress at increasing compliance of hand hygiene, and have seen infections fall accordingly.

Especially beneficial is the use of the alcohol hand sanitizer, a pressurized canister that squirts out a ball of foam on your hand about the consistency of whipped cream; imagine my surprise to discover that the foam was supposed to used topically. I had been using it like Cheez Whiz. (When I was kid, to take a whiz was to urinate. Does that make anyone other than me wonder what's in the can of Cheez Whiz?)

Anyway.

Part of the campaign to increase hand hygiene is the motto, "It's OK to ask," allegedly empowering patients to ask their providers if they have washed their hands. As if. For entertainment's sake I spent a couple of hours asking patients if they understood the signs (they did) and if they would ask (they most certainly would not). When asked why, most said something to the effect they did not want to risk alienating their nurse or doctor. Not a bad policy; I wouldn't want to piss off the person who was bringing me my morphine.

I suspect that the approach to hand hygiene suggested by the "It's OK to ask" campaign is fundamentally bankrupt. The secret, if there is one, to these complicated problems is to make the default action hand washing.

Hands are not the only problem, and if push comes to shove we can always have them removed. Heh heh heh. More than hands have been associated with carrying bacterial pathogens.

Other intimate objects in the hospital that can carry bacteria include:

—public phones

"Twelve different types of bacteria were found on the surface of telephones. The level of bacterial contamination for the telephone

mouthpiece was increased to its highest point in October from its lowest value in August. It was also found that the micromouthpiece was about twice the contamination of earpiece."

—keyboards and mice

"In all 14 patients' rooms we collected a total of 1118 samples: 222 samples from keyboards and mice, 214 from infusion pumps and 174 from the ward's trolley. From the central ward 16 samples per fomites were obtained (computer keyboard and mouse at the physician's workstation and the ward's intercom and telephone receiver). Microbacterial analysis from samples in patients' rooms yielded 26 contaminated samples from keyboard and mouse (5.9%) compared with 18 positive results from other fomites within patients' rooms (3.0%; p < 0.02). At the physician's computer terminal two samples obtained from the mouse (6.3%) showed positive microbial testing."

—beepers

"Microorganisms were isolated from all pagers; 21% yielded Staphylococcus aureus, of which 14% were methicillin resistant. Cleaning with alcohol reduced the total colony count by an average of 94%."

—stethoscopes

"All but six bacterial cultures were positive (85.7%). Staphylococcal species were the most common contaminants (47.5%). One case of methicillin-resistant Staphylococcus aureus was encountered. Gram-negative organisms were isolated in nine different samples (21%) including one case of Acinetobacter baumannii in the neonatal intensive care unit."

The world is a filthier place than you can even begin to imagine. And you do not want to know what is in your mouth —if you are a germophobe you may never kiss again. In the real world it is no big deal, but in the hospital? I wish germs were the size of those creatures that were put into Chekov's ear. At least we could see them. I try to alcohol foam all my accessories, except my cell phone, even though it is piece of crap Windows mobile and I am impatiently waiting for my Verizon contract to die so I can get my iPhone.

I wonder about the touch phones, the Blackberries, the other electronic devices in our pockets that we use while sitting in the bathroom. Not me—I don't even pick my nose. But I am sure others do. I am not sure I want to douse my iPhone in alcohol. But how else to clean it? I put my iTouch in the wash by mistake and it was detrimental to its functioning, although it was temporarily cleaner.

So many contaminated surfaces, so little time to disinfect.

Rationalization

Youngster, I., et al., The stethoscope as a vector of infectious diseases in the paediatric division. Acta Paediatr, 2008. 97(9): p. 1253-5.

Tunc, K. and U. Olgun, Microbiology of public telephones. J Infect, 2006. 53(2): p. 140-3.

Hartmann, B., et al., Computer keyboard and mouse as a reservoir of pathogens in an intensive care unit. J Clin Monit Comput, 2004. 18(1): p. 7-12.

....

Changing a tire

WHEN I started practice, late last century, I wore the standard white coat. After a while, for reasons I no longer remember—but which are probably related to my wife's continued attempts to give me some style (if they ever have a male on *What not to Wear*, it should be me)—I changed to the sport coat and tie look.

Years passed, and the sport coats are looking a little ratty. They are pricey. Even at Goodwill, my preferred shopping store, a good sport coat will run 80 bucks. At Nordstrom—well, let's say you don't want to be an I.D. doc in a down economy.

So I went back to the white coat look, which my wife says is slimming (ha) and which has generated lots of comments, mostly good.

From an infection control perspective, what should one wear

in the hospital? While I am unaware of outbreaks, many routine articles of clothing have been found to carry bacteria.

Ties are the best documented carriers of bacteria, and should be abandoned. Ties are never cleaned, and when you push them out of the way so they are not dipped into the patient, they pick up whatever is on your hands. They are saturated with months of bacteria and soup. I have ties from the 90s that I do not think I have ever cleaned.

Beepers, rings, watches (very rare), phones, artificial nails and stethoscopes have all been cultured and found to contain pathogens. Probably lab coats as well, since they are not laundered very frequently, and are exposed to pus, patients, and hospital food.

So what to wear? Look professional or be relatively bacteria-free? The British have gone to the extreme of allowing nothing below the elbows (except hands) and no ties. We may be heading that way, but I need pockets and a belt to carry my electronic doodads, at least until I get that Ethernet jack in the back of my skull. Neo had the right idea.

Rationalization

Wall Street Journal, "Hospital Scrubs are a Germy, Deadly Mess" http://online.wsj.com/article/SB123137245971962641.html

Beer, D., et al., Bacterial contamination of health care workers' pagers and the efficacy of various disinfecting agents. Pediatr Infect Dis J, 2006. 25(11): p. 1074-5.

Whittington, A.M., et al., Bacterial contamination of stethoscopes on the intensive care unit. Anaesthesia, 2009. 64(6): p. 620-4.

Yildirim, I., et al., A prospective comparative study of the relationship between different types of ring and microbial hand colonization among pediatric intensive care unit nurses. Int J Nurs Stud, 2008. 45(11): p. 1572-6.

Bhusal, Y., et al., Bacterial colonization of wristwatches worn by health care personnel. Am J Infect Control, 2009. 37(6): p. 476-7.

A Budget of Dumbasses

This is updated and re-published on http://blogs.medscape.com/rdct (where these entries are born) every October.

I HAD my flu shot today. Well, my anti-flu shot. Protected me and my patients from death for another year. Whew. I wonder if you are one of those dumbasses who do not get the flu shot each year. Yes. DumbAss. Big D, big A. You may be allergic to the vaccine, you may have had Guillain-Barre, in which case I will cut you some slack. But if you don't have those conditions and you work in health care and you don't get a vaccine for one of the following reasons, you are a dumbass.

1. The vaccine gives me the flu. *Dumbass.* It is a killed vaccine. It cannot give you the influenza. It is impossible to get flu from the influenza vaccine.

2. I never get the flu, so I don't need the vaccine. *Irresponsible dumbass.* I never had a car accident, but I wear my seat belt. And you probjably don't use a condom either. So far you have been lucky, and you are a potential winner of a Darwin Award.

3. Only old people get the flu. *Selfish dumbass.* Influenza can infect anyone, and one of the groups who die of influenza are the very young. Often those most likely to die from influenza are those least able to respond to the vaccine, due to age or underlying diseases. You can help prevent your old, sickly grandmother or your newborn daughter from getting influenza and perhaps dying by getting the vaccine, so you do not get flu and pass it on to her.

4. I can prevent influenza or treat it by taking echinacea, vitamin C or Airborne. *Gullible dumbass cubed then squared.* None of these concoctions has any efficacy whatsoever against influenza. They neither prevent nor treat influenza.

5. Flu isn't all that bad a disease. *Underestimating dumbass.* Part of the problem with the term 'flu' is that it is used both as a generic term for damn near any viral illness with a fever and is also used for a severe viral pneumonia. Medical people are just as inaccurate about using the term as the general public. The influenza virus kills 30,000 people and leads to hospitalization of 200,000 in the US each year. Influenza is a nasty lung illness. And what is stomach "flu"? No such thing.

6. I am not at risk for flu. *Denying dumbass.* If your breathe, you are risk for influenza. Here are the groups of people who should not get the flu vaccine (outside of people with severe adverse reactions to the vaccine): children younger than 6 months and "completely healthy adults who have no contact with someone who isn't [healthy]." And zombies. And former President Clinton, who evidently doesn't inhale.

7. The vaccine is worse than the disease. *Dumbass AND a wimp.* What a combination. Your mother must be proud. Unless you think a sore deltoid for a day is too high a price to pay to prevent two weeks of high fevers, severe muscles aches, and intractable cough.

8. I had the vaccine last year, so I do not need it this year. *Uneducated dumbass.* Each year, new stains of influenza circulate across the world. Last year's vaccine at best provides only partial protection. Every year you need a new shot.

9. The vaccine costs too much. *Cheap dumbas*s. The vaccine costs less than a funeral, less than Tamiflu, and a lot less than a week in the hospital.

10. The government puts tracking nanobots in the vaccine and well as RFID chips as part of the mark of the beast, and the vaccine doesn't work since it is part of a big government-sponsored conspiracy to line the pockets of big Pharma and inject the American sheeple with exotic new infections. Well, that excuse is at least reasonable. *Paranoid dumbass.*

So get vaccine. Or be a dumbass. One of these days I'll let you know how I really feel about the flu vaccine.

....

Peer Pressure

ONE week I went to Employee Health and commandeered the influenza vaccine cart. We are a bit over 50% for employee flu shots, and I think it is important for as many people as possible to get the shot. It allows me to inject those government-sponsored tracking nanobots.

Then I wandered from station to station offering flu shots.

Who, I would demand loudly, dares to refuse and flu shot from the great and powerful Chief of Infectious Disease?

Most said they already had the shot, but in two hours I managed to give 13 flu shots. Actually, they are anti-flu shots. Sometimes a patient asks for something for pain, and I think, "Well, you could stub your toe." English is often imprecise.

It was fun. People were shocked that I was actually giving a shot. Several people thought I was a nurse, since a doctor giving a shot—actually doing the work instead of writing an order and walking away—is rare. Several nurses complimented me on the quality of my injection; I assume they were incredulous that I was competent to give a shot. Like a bear riding a bicycle, it is not that I do it well, but that I could do it at all.

I had the opportunity to talk to people about who should get the flu shot and about the disease. On every unit there was one person who would not make eye contact with me nor offer to get the shot. I presume they are the people who will not get the flu shot no matter what the reason but were unwilling to talk to the all-knowing Oz.

There is one nurse I still need to get. Evidently she NEVER gets the flu shot, and is proud of it, but she was off for a few days. I will not put her name on the blog, but everyone on the unit knows I am gunning for her.

If there is anyone reading this who is an I.D. doc, I suggest you put aside a couple of hours one day and to do the same thing at your hospital. It will make an impression as to the importance of the flu shot and you will have a good time.

....

Germ Theory

THE germ theory of disease is not just a theory, it's the law. For infectious disease, it is the cornerstone of the subspecialty. It should be called the germ fact. I sometimes think that there are only three causes of disease: infectious, genetic, and wear and tear. Not everyone understands the concepts of infection and contagion as a cause of disease. Some think that disease is caused by blocked meridians or blocked innate intelligence or some other kind of nonsensical magical thinking.

Fine. There is all sorts of goofy stuff in the world, and that gives fodder for blogs such as Science Based Medicine. Hint hint... (http://www.sciencebasedmedicine.org).

One would expect that if a practitioner believes that disease is caused by blocked meridians and is trying to unblock them, perhaps such a practitioner would have no truck with those pesky science based disease concepts like germs, and that perhaps such a practitioner would not be so fastidious about practicing interventions that would prevent the spread of infection.

Staphylococcus aureus is a particularly virulent organism, and it loves nothing better than finding a hole in your skin to use as a portal for invasion. Needles are good at causing holes for Staph to take advantage of. Dialysis needles. Diabetes needles. IVDA needles. And acupuncture needles.

It turns out a medical practitioner was colonized with MRSA and was sloppy with his acupuncture technique. Along with unblocking the qi, he dragged a little MRSA into his patients.

"Eight cases of invasive MRSA infection were identified. Seven cases occurred as a cluster in May 2004; another case (identified retrospectively) occurred approximately 15 months earlier in February 2003. The primary sites of infection were the neck, shoulder, lower back, and hip: 5 patients had septic arthritis and bursitis, and 3 had pyomyositis; 3 patients had bacteremia, including 1 patient with possible endocarditis. The medical practitioner was found to be colonized with the same MRSA clone [ST22-MRSA-IV (EMRSA-15)] at 2 time points: shortly after the first case of infection in March 2003 and again in May 2004. After the medical practitioner's premises and practices were audited and he himself received MRSA decolonization therapy, no further cases were identified."

If you get bored—though why would you *be bored when* you have this?—Google photos of acupuncture. There is a distinct lack of pictures of practitioners using gloves, even though they touch the skin bare-handed to locate the puncture site, and their fingers are often right next to the needle insertion. Our local acupuncture school had a photograph of the teacher and student placing needles sans gloves, sans foam, sans sterile technique, sans everything. An acupuncturist trying to generate a practice sent me a picture of herself at work, putting in a needle without gloves. I wonder if acupuncturists use contraception. Probably not condoms.

It is not all that unusual for infections to occur from quackery of all kinds. SCAM (Supplements, Complementary and Alternative Medicine) practitioners often have little to no understanding in the concepts of infections, and what understanding they do have is often erroneous.

In my career I have seen several infections, including a joint infection, due to acupuncture.

You should not be reassured by SCAM practitioners just because they call themselves doctors. The following are doctors: Dr. Demento, Dr. Doom, and Dr. Horrible. Do you suppose they know the basics of germ theory and hand hygiene? I think not. Well, the last two do wear gauntlets or gloves. You cannot expect someone who treats disease by SCAM methodologies to understand infections, or to practice good infection control techniques. It's hard enough to get real health care practitioners to wash their hands, and they understand germ theory. Or so one supposes.

Germs do not care what your theory of disease is. Modern infection control techniques are the only reliable way to prevent their spread. Ignore them at your peril, and my gain.

Rationalization

Murray, R.J., et al., Outbreak of invasive methicillin-resistant Staphylococcus aureus infection associated with acupuncture and joint injection. Infect Control Hosp Epidemiol, 2008. 29(9): p. 859-65.

Hypersensitive

WORK is slow right now. The holidays slow down as elective medical care is postponed until the new year and, therefore, the resultant infections are postponed as well.

The economy is slow, and I.D. has always been the reimbursement canary in the medical coalmine.

And finally, Portland is shut down with the worst winter storm in my memory. We get freezing rain, which is impossible to move around in. I spent three years in hell, er, I mean, Minneapolis, and they never had weather like this. Plus, we have hills, an unknown geologic feature in the Midwest. Nothing gives that feeling of "Oh crap" quite like going down a hill, hitting the brakes, and accelerating due to gravity and ice.

Anyway. I.D. wise there is not one whole heck of a lot going on to write about, so I turn to the interwebs.

The cool thing is that vaccines have the potential to prevent cancer—specifically cervical cancer due to Human Papilloma virus (HPV). The vaccine will probably prevent anal, penile and oral cancers as well, as these can be caused by HPV, although how a cervical virus makes it to the oral pharynx no one has yet explained to me. I digress.

Early on there was a report that the vaccine was associated with an increase in hypersensitivity rates, which is an uber-allergic reaction. Because of general fears about vaccines, this report did not help ease the minds of parents who were taking their daughters to get the vaccine.

However, researchers did another study and found (to quote from Medscape, published in the *British Medical Journal*)

"From the 269,680 HPV vaccine doses administered in schools, 7 cases of anaphylaxis were identified, which represents an incidence rate of 2.6 per 100,000 doses (95% confidence interval [CI], 1.0 —5.3 per 100,000), the researchers reported.

In comparison, they noted that the rate of identified anaphylaxis was 0.1 per 100,000 doses (95% CI, 0.003 —0.700) for conju-

Crislip

gated meningococcal C vaccination in a 2003 school-based program.

That report may have been an overestimate, however. The current study concludes that "true hypersensitivity" to the HPV vaccine is uncommon, and a detailed examination of case reports found only 2 cases of anaphylaxis after more than 380,000 vaccine doses."

And the association may not be causation, as kids will have other reasons for allergic reactions such as asthma and bee stings. Every week in the US there are a large number of people have a vaccine, by chance some will have a reaction after the vaccine, and blame the vaccine, when, in fact, the two are unrelated.

"They point out that 1 study estimated that if 80% of eligible American adolescent females were to receive a saline injection according to the vaccination schedule for HPV, 3 in 100,000 adolescents would require emergency care for asthma and allergy within 24 hours of vaccination (Pediatr Infect Dis J. 2007;26:979-984)."

17 of 18 girls who had a reaction to the first dose of the vaccine were skin-test negative and tolerated the re-challenge no problemo.

So it looks as if the vaccine is safe, especially in Australians. Who, I might add, are an exceptionally intelligent group of people, judging by those who listen to my podcasts.

Now if we can just figure out a way to prevent the vaccine from making them hyper-sexual. Or so the interwebs tell me. And I thought that was due to the contrails. Or was the fluoride? It is so hard to keep these things straight.

Rationalization

True Hypersensitivity to HPV Vaccine Uncommon (http://www.medscape.com/viewarticle/584651)

Doctors are not supposed to get sick

Especially Infectious Disease docs. I am punctilious about infection prevention. I wash my hands at rates that make lady Macbeth look like an amateur. But not for the same reason. I have no blood on my hands. I have been lucky that way. I got my flu vaccine the day after it came out.

My mistake was taking vitamin C and echinacea. Whenever I do, I always get a virus.

I had three days of fevers, bad headache, achy eyes, and a slight cough. Just an occasional cough. Barely anything, but a deep, raspy, painful cough when it hit. It was gone in three days and transitioned into a stuffy nose with continued sneezing.

Was it flu? I cannot get the flu. It would be like the Pope getting AIDS. Just should not happen since I do not participate in risk behaviors and do all the appropriate prophylactics.

Problem is, I may have had an attenuated clinical course because, yet again, they picked the wrong strain for the vaccine.

The vaccine contains both A and B influenza, and the vaccine makers pick the strains in the vaccine from circulating viruses from the year before. They do that because it takes a long time to manufacture each vaccine dose. One flu shot is grown in one chicken egg, and it takes that one poor chicken a long time to lay all those eggs. She sure walks funny at the end of the flu season.

There are two major lineages of type B flu: B Victoria and B Yamagata. Last year, they put the Victoria lineage in the vaccine and 98% of type B flu was due to the Yamagata lineage.

Crap.

So this year, they made the vaccine protective against Yamagata, but now two-thirds of the type B flu in circulation is from the Victoria lineage. Unfortunately, not the Victoria's secret lineage.

Double crap.

So perhaps I had the flu, shortened and attenuated by last year's vaccine. Or perhaps I had another virus. Either way, I stayed home and got caught up on the Sara Conner Chronicles.

The triple crap is flu season is peaking right about now.

So wash your hands and don't inhale.

Rationalization

The CDC provides a weekly influenza surveillance report. It can be found here: http://www.cdc.gov/flu/weekly/

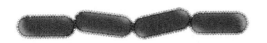

THE STAPH OF LIFE

If you only learn one thing

MY goal for each chapter is one factoid or cool infectious disease issue. Just one. If I can offer one new piece of information per day, then I figure that at the end of a year my readers will have had the opportunity to forget almost 365 facts. It is not often you can have the opportunity to forget so much information so effortlessly.

It was a call weekend. Blah. Call means lots of phone calls from lots of docs with a quick curbside.

The curbside is where they ask you a question but do not want a formal consult, which is just as well on the weekend as my tux is at the cleaners, making a formal consult difficult. The term curbside, or curbstone as some call it, evidently comes from stock advice given on Wall Street by investors who could not afford an office. From the looks of things, the past is becoming the future. How that got translated to medicine, I don't know. And who takes financial advice from someone who sits curbside?

So I got a phone call about *S. aureus* in the bloodstream of a patient, probably from a catheter infection, and I told the consulting docs to have the catheter pulled and to place the person on vancomycin pending the results of the sensitivity. The the doc said, "Then give 10 days or so of oral antibiotics, right?"

Now here is the one thing I want you to learn from this book—sear it into your brain such that when you are a drooling, mindless, demented patient in the ICU at age 102 and the medical student asks you, "How long do you treat catheter related *S. aureus* bacteremia?" even in your addled state you reply:

"The minimum minimum minimum duration of IV therapy

for *S. aureus* bacteremia from a line is two weeks of intravenous antibiotics," then lapse back into your confused dementia.

Got that? Two weeks IV. Minimum. If diabetic, prolonged fever, MRSA, and a variety of other confounding issues you go 4 or 6 weeks of IV. But the MINIMUM duration of IV is 2 weeks. (I hate pronouncing it mursa. Sounds like a Texan trying to say thanks in French. It's Em-Ar-Ess-Ay).

I suggested that they get a formal I.D. consult on after the susceptibility testing came back.

As a self-serving aside, I.D. consults for *S. aureus* bacteremia are in the patient's benefit. Not just my saying so, see:

Jenkins, T.C., et al., Impact of routine infectious diseases service consultation on the evaluation, management, and outcomes of Staphylococcus aureus bacteremia. Clin Infect Dis, 2008. 46(7): p. 1000-8

Background. Staphylococcus aureus bacteremia causes considerable morbidity and mortality, and strategies to improve management and outcomes of this disease are needed.

Methods. Routine consultation with an infectious diseases specialist for cases of S. aureus bacteremia was mandated at our institution in May 2005. We compared the evaluation, management, and outcomes of cases before and after this policy change. All comparisons are by period (i.e., before or after initiation of the policy of routine consultation).

Results. In the year before and the year after the implementation of routine consultation, 134 and 100 cases of S. aureus bacteremia, respectively, were evaluated. Consultation rates increased from 53% of cases before to 90% of cases after the policy change (P < .001). Echocardiography (57% vs. 73%; P =.01) and radiographic studies (81% vs. 91%; P =.04) were used more frequently during the period of routine consultation, and infective endocarditis or metastatic infections were diagnosed more frequently (33% vs. 46%; P =.04). All 4 standards of care (removal of intravascular foci of infection, obtaining follow-up blood culture samples, use *of parenteral B-lactam therapy when possible, and administration of, 28 days of therapy for complicated infections) were adhered to more frequently with routine consultation (40% vs. 74%; P <.001). Treatment failure (microbiological failure, recurrent bacteremia, late metastatic infection, or death) occurred less often during the intervention year (17% vs. 12%), but this difference was not statistically significant (P =.27).*

Conclusions. *A policy of routine consultation with an infectious diseases specialist for patients with S. aureus bacteremia resulted in more-detailed evaluation, more-frequent detection of endocarditis and metastatic infection, and improved adherence to standards of care.*

Of course, the study was done by I.D. docs, so the results may be biased, but the results have been confirmed in several other studies. Also done by I.D. docs. We have to look after our own.

As one last warning, note the two 'n's in annals. If you are looking for a reference on the wards and forget the second 'n', be prepared to do some 'splainin. At one time it was an adult site. I though the .org was for philanthropic organizations, and that the hospital firewall blocked access to NSFW sites. I can't log on to Facebook, but anals.org is OK? Who knew.

So three things learned today, one of which you can never, ever, never ever forget.

1) Give a minimum of two weeks IV therapy for catheter related line *S. aureus* bacteremia.

2) Get an I.D. consult for *S. aureus* bacteremia.

3) Annals has two 'n's.

Rationalization

The review of short-course therapy for *S. aureus* bacteremia may be found here:

Jernigan, J.A. and B.M. Farr, Short-course therapy of catheter-related Staphylococcus aureus bacteremia: a meta-analysis. Ann Intern Med, 1993. 119(4): p. 304-11.

The New Pig Pen

INFECTIONS are somewhat inevitable. Surgery is not a sterile procedure, since the skin cannot be sterilized. Surgery is just very very very clean. That's three verys, so you know it is clean. All people have bacteria in and on them, but some have more than others.

Infected artificial hips are no fun for the patient, and if due to *S. aureus*, often result in a need to remove the hip for several months while we attempt to eradicate the staph, such as occurred with today's consult.

But why the staph infection?

The answer lies on the skin, where the patient has a moderate case of psoriasis. Normal skin does not have much, if any, *S. aureus* on it. But if you have any kind of skin disease—eczema, psoriasis, atopic dermatitis, or use needles, which damage the skin—your *S. aureus* carriage rate goes from zero to almost 100 %.

If you have lots of skin disease, you have lots of *S. aureus*. The problem is that if you are heavily colonized with *S. aureus*, the is little if anything that can be done to get rid of all the bacteria. Think Pig Pen from Charlie Brown, except instead of dirt, the patient is in a haze of bacteria. Once the surgery is over, what *S. aureus* the sterilization procedures might have beaten down rapidly grows back.

Staph just love to take advantage of breaks in the skin and invade.

I had one poor lady who had recurrent boils due to MRSA and her 3-year-old daughter had horrible skin disease. There was no way to get MRSA out of the family.

If you need to operate on someone with bad skin disease, it is probably reasonable to give the patient a chlorhexidine shower before going to the OR. This is in fact what we did with this patient, but it didn't help. Don't be surprised when the person gets an infection. There is just so much we can do to prevent infections and when they occur, of course, Medicare will not pay for it, even though not every hospital acquired infection is necessarily our fault.

Rationalization

Gong, J.Q., et al., Skin colonization by Staphylococcus aureus in patients with eczema and atopic dermatitis and relevant combined topical therapy: a double-blind multicentre randomized controlled trial. Br J Dermatol, 2006. 155(4): p. 680-7.

....

Lemierre's syndrome

THIS respiratory virus I have is hanging on like Norm Coleman, it will not admit defeat. I just want to reach down my bronchus and scratch scratch scratch.

The French dominated infectious diseases for years, and you can tell that long tradition in many of the eponyms for infectious diseases. Many contain the name of the famous Frenchman who first described the disease, or at least were able to get it into print.

Take Andre Lemierre. He doesn't seem to warrant an internet biography, even if he does have a street named after him in Paris. In 1936 in *The Lancet* he described a series of patients with sepsis from infected clot in the neck. Occurring after a sore throat (angina means neck pain in the ancient language, for those spell casters in Alagaesia), it was called post-anginal sepsis and was due to *Fusobacterium necrophorum*, a mouth anaerobe. Part of the disease complication is that bits of infected clot break off and travel to the lung to cause multiple lung abscesses.

I see a case of this every couple of years in a person with poor dentition and no insurance. The latter is important since the patient cannot afford a doctor to prescribe the antibiotics that would, perhaps, prevent it.

However, to have anaerobes in the mouth you have to have teeth, and the patient today is sans teeth. So what is the cause of the clot in the neck and multiple lung abscesses?

Our friend, the *Staphylococcus aureus*. It isn't called coagulase positive staph for nothing, and this organism knows how to clot blood. This is the second Lemierre's I have seen due to *S. aureus*, so I almost have a series; that would require three.

There are 5 Staphylococcal Lemierre's cases reported in PubMed. I bet there are more cases out there. I have said for years that we need a searchable, online "cool ID case" site where these cases can be reported. No one listens to me. And why should they?

Rationalization

Bomke, A.K., S. Steiner, and A. Podbielski, [Multiple peritonsillar abscesses caused by Arcanobacterium haemolyticum in a young female]. Dtsch Med Wochenschr, 2009. 134(3): p. 75-8.

Fong, S.M. and M. Watson, Lemierre syndrome due to non-multiresistant methicillin-resistant Staphylococcus aureus. J Paediatr Child Health, 2002. 38(3): p. 305-7.

Gokce Ceylan, B., et al., Lemierre syndrome: a case of a rarely isolated microorganism, Staphylococcus auerus. Med Sci Monit, 2009. 15(3): p. CS58-61.

Boga, C., et al., Lemierre syndrome variant: Staphylococcus aureus associated with thrombosis of both the right internal jugular vein and the splenic vein after the exploration of a river cave. J Thromb Thrombolysis, 2007. 23(2): p. 151-4.

Puymirat, E., et al., A Lemierre syndrome variant caused by Staphylococcus aureus. Am J Emerg Med, 2008. 26(3): p. 380 e5-7.

....

S. aureus pays my mortgage

ALL but two of my consults this week were due to *S. aureus*. If it weren't for *S. aureus* I would be standing at a freeway off-ramp with a sign that says *Will do I.D. for Food*.

Sustained bacteremia is always an important clinical finding as it usually means an endovascular infection. Only an infection whose focus is in the vascular tree will have a sustained bacteremia. And sustained can be for days. It usually means endocarditis, but not always. It could be due to infection of a central line—an implanted catheter in a vein. It could be an infection elsewhere.

When I was an intern, my attending diagnosed an infected aneurysm as a result of a splenectomy. The stump of the vascular supply to the spleen had been tied off and an arteriovenous malformation had formed, which was subsequently seeded with Staph. He had heard a bruit over where the spleen had been, a physical finding missed by everyone else. No way would I make that diagnosis without finding it accidentally on a CT.

I.D. docs love to know if round purple things in the blood are transient or sustained in the bloodstream, and nothing gripes my cookies more than when one set of blood cultures are growing a gram positive bacterium and antibiotics are started without repeating the blood cultures first.

Always always always repeat blood cultures before treating gram positive bacteria in the blood. Always. It will decrease the aggravation in your I.D. doc no end. And really, there is nothing more important than making your I.D. doc, i.e. me, happy.

The patient on Friday is a dialysis patient who came in with fevers, as do most of my patients, and *S. aureus* in the blood. His catheter was pulled and he still had persistent fevers, positive blood cultures and neck pain and chest pain. ECHO did not show a vegetation, but CT showed both a big clot in the internal jugular vein and a peripheral cavitating lesion in the lung.

What he has is a nosocomial Lemmier's—septic thrombophlebitis of the internal jugular, with septic emboli to the lung. Antibiotics and anticoagulation are usually curative, as was the case in this patient.

It is curious how rarely I see septic thrombophlebitis given how common both clot and *S. aureus* are in the bloodstream.

In a study of 1275 surgical ICU patients who were evaluated for DVT, more clot was found in the upper extremity veins than the lower:

"DVT was confirmed in 39 patients. The incidence of upper-extremity DVT was higher than that of lower-extremity DVT (17% vs 11%; P = .11). Four-extremity scans diagnosed more DVT than 2-extremity scans (33% vs 7%; P < .001).

> *There was a significantly higher incidence of upper-extremity DVT in patients with sepsis or central lines. They had higher APACHE III scores on admission to the ICU, longer hospital stays, and higher in-hospital mortality rates than patients with DVTs.*
>
> *Sepsis was present in 72% of patients with upper-extremity DVT, compared with 53% of patients with lower-extremity DVT (P < 0.001), and 86% of upper-extremity DVT was associated with central venous catheters."*

I get a fair number of ultrasounds looking for clot associated with line infections; this study suggests I should get more.

Rationalization

Upper-Extremity DVT in ICP Patients: http://www.medscape.com/viewarticle/587835. Society of Critical Care Medicine (SCCM) 38th Critical Care Congress: Abstract 305. Presented February 2, 2009.

Half time

NBA playoff time and, here in PDX, the Blazers are it. If we lose, it's oh-va. So it's quickie pearl time here in Rip City.

I saw a young IV meth user who had had three days of severe low back and thigh pain. Rather than heroin, he took enough aspirin to get a level of 300 mg/L, and it was the ringing in the ears from salicylate overdose that brought him to the hospital. An MRI of the back was negative.

All the blood cultures grew *S. aureus*.

The clinical pearl?

About 30% of *S. aureus* bacteremias will present as severe musculoskeletal, especially low back, pain.

That is it. I have a game to watch.

At least it is not called Pansy Fever

IT is summer in Oregon, and people are going from floating-corpse white to freshly boiled lobster. However, you are not supposed to get a sunburn where the sun don't shine, unless, of course, you have been to Rooster Rock, the local clothing-optional beach. And in Oregon, clothing should always be the option. The glare off the large expanses of glistening white skin can damage vision and is a more common cause of blindness in the Northwest than hiking on glaciers without sunglasses.

The patient came in after a cardiac arrest and developed bilateral pneumonia as seen on chest x-ray. Two days into the hospitalization, as she started reperfusing her ischemic tissues, she got a sunburn. Her body turned bright cherry red, including her buttocks, palms and soles.

There was, interestingly, sparing around the eyes and lips, her conjunctivae were injected and, unfortunately, I couldn't see the tongue well due to various support tubes. I think it was normal.

What was the causing the erythroderma? I hate making rash decisions. Not many things cause a sunburn rash that involves the palms and the soles. It could be sunburn, but she had been in the ICU for two days. Syphilis? Maybe, but the VDRL was negative. If it could be lues, don't touch the rash, as cutaneous syphilis is a sea of wiggling spirochetes. I don't think your spouse will be reassured when you say you got the Great Pox from touching a patient. It will just sound wrong.

It looks like a toxic shock rash, but she is not toxic or shocky: blood pressure and kidney function are within normal operating parameters.

There is no skin fragility (Nikolsky sign: stroking of the skin causes the it to separate at the epidermis) so I do not think it is staphlococcal scalded skin syndrome—a disease of children, usually, although I have seen one case in an old man.

Scarlet fever? That is streptococcal, and she is growing staph. The rash does not feel like sandpaper to me, which is what the skin of scarlet fever is supposed to feel like. But *Staphylococcus* can cause a scarlet fever-like rash. According to the pediatrics texts, Staph causes neither circumoral pallor (which she had) nor strawberry tongue (which I could not see clearly).

She has yet to exfoliate, which will probably make the diagnosis of Staph pneumonia with a scarlet fever rash.

Rationalization

Schlievert, P.M., Staphylococcal scarlet fever: role of pyrogenic exotoxins. Infect Immun, 1981. 31(2): p. 732-6.

Postscript

She did exfoliate, so the rash was probably from the *Staphylococcus.*

....

Ignorance with Style

I GNORANCE with style. That is what being an I.D. doc is all about. So often there is an infection and I know what the patient has, but not why. I can almost always come up with a plausible reason, based on anatomy, physiology and microbiology about why this particular infection occurred in this particular patient. But plausible doesn't mean it is true. Sometimes it feels as if I am making up "just so" stories to explain what is going on—all sound and fury, signifying nothing. And sometimes I got nothing.

For you meat fans, the iliopsoas muscle is the pork loin in pigs. Mmmmm. Pork loin. Especially grilled.

In humans the ileopsoas usually gets infected after a groin pull, which has no resemblance to what they do to make taffy. Someone dives for a loose ball, or lifts a heavy object, or twists funny. Not ha ha funny, although when I do the twist it is ha ha funny. The last time I danced they called the paramedics since they thought I was seizing. The presumption is the trauma leads to a little bleeding into the meat, er, muscle, and it is seeded by the blood, usually with *S. aureus.* It is hard to infect muscle without trauma. The rabbit model of pyomyositis, I have been told, involves hitting a rabbit leg with a hammer, for without the trauma infection never occurs. A wittle bunny wabbit? I am glad I do not do animal research.

Iliopsoas infections are usually unilateral unless the infection originates from the low back. A low back infection, especially with TB, can cause bilateral disease as the ileopsoas inserts at the spine. The infection tracks down the muscle from the spine.

So, to define the usual ileopsoas abscess I see in the U.S.: Male, prior trauma, unilateral disease, acutely ill, *S. aureus.*

So today I had a female, bilateral iliopsoas abscesses, big as softballs, sub-acutely ill. These abscess were so large they had obstructed both ureters. At least they grew *S. aureus.* And did I mention no trauma? There was hardware in the back, but no radiographic changes or clinical history to suggest that the back was infected or the source of infection. As best I can tell from PubMed, bilateral ileopsoas abscesses from *S. aureus* are almost unreported.

And odder still: the *S. aureus* was penicillin sensitive; this century only a few percent of Staph can still be killed with penicillin.

How to put it all together? I can't. It has to be from the spine, but I can't prove it. I'll just have to kill it. Better than pork loin is a penicillin sensitive *S. aureus.* There is great pleasure "To crush yoah *S. aureus,* see dem driven befoah you, and to hear de lammentation of de vimmin!" (Arnold from Conan)

If there is karma, and you generate bad karma from killing living things, I am toast. Another billion organisms soon to die at my order.

Rationalization

Navarro Lopez, V., et al., Microbiology and outcome of iliopsoas abscess in 124 patients. Medicine (Baltimore), 2009. 88(2): p. 120-30.

Bang, M.S. and S.H. Lim, Paraplegia caused by spinal infection after acupuncture. Spinal Cord, 2006. 44(4): p. 258-9.

Coincidence? I don't think so

I DO a lot of driving for my job. I am the only I.D. doc at four hospitals, and I can spend several hours a day going from place to place in slow traffic. To while away the time, I listen to books on tape (well, books on mp3) or podcasts. It is amazing how often

I hear a word on the iPod then simultaneously see that word on a billboard or street sign. Someone must be sending me a message; it cannot just be random serendipity. It is too weird not to have an underlying meaning. Someone must be trying to tell me something. But what?

Another odd thing is how often I read an article and then see the disease I read about in the subsequent few weeks. Like today. I saw a patient who was admitted with community-acquired *Staphylococcus lugdunensis* bacteremia. *S. lugdunensis* is a skin staph, one of many coagulase negative Staphylococci that make up our normal flora (not to be confused with *S. aureus*, which is the coagulase positive *Staphylococcus*).

Just two weeks ago I read "*Significance of Staphylococcus lugdunensis bacteremia: report of 28 cases and review of the literature*" as part of the quasi-random literature reading I do for the Puscast. And, as so often happens, I then see a case of *Staphylococcus lugdunensis* bacteremia.

Coincidence? I don't think so.

Community acquired *Staphylococcus lugdunensis* bacteremia is often due to endocarditis (heart valve infection) so, although I heard no murmur, as I was writing my progress note, I made a special point of accosting the person outside of the room of the patient next door. It was the echocardiography tech, with his machine, getting ready to take a look at the heart of the patient next door. Co inky dink? No way. I told him I wanted an ECHO on my patient to look for endocarditis.

"A total of 28 patients with S. lugdunensis bacteremia were identified. Of the 13 patients with endocarditis, all were community acquired."

He called me an hour later to tell me the patient had endocarditis, as there was a big vegetation on the patient's tricuspid valve. This is the truth. When he called me I was in the drive-though of the Jack in the Box ordering a chicken bowl—first time; the rice is odd tasting—and looking at the picture of the bowl that has vegetables in it. Whoa.

And yesterday my son was playing NBA live on the Playstation, and in the video game Brandon Roy pulled a hamstring. And what happened in the Boston game last night? We got crushed. And Brandon pulled his hamstring. Too many coincidences. Someone, somewhere is trying to tell me something. Spooky, man.

Of course, it's all just a touch of confirmation bias—the tendency for humans to remember hits and forget misses. I hear thousands of words and read dozens of articles so I was bound, just by chance, to see or hear an unexpected correlation. If I were prone to finding meaning in random events, today would be full of portents. But I don't believe there is a hidden underlying meaning, so I would not go camping in portents.

What I really need to read is an article about an infectious disease physician winning Powerball.

Rationalization

Zinkernagel, A.S., et al., Significance of Staphylococcus lugdunensis bacteremia: report of 28 cases and review of the literature. Infection, 2008. 36(4): p. 314-21.

Infections in Asterix

I AM on call this weekend. Whine whine whine cry cry cry. Boo and hoo. Poor me. Call is the one downside of being a doc. But at least I get to see some good cases.

You are a tropical rain forest. Really. You have a complex ecosystem in and on you. There are 10 to 100 times more bacterial cells in and on you than there are cells of you. You may think you are a hotshot I.D. doc (I certainly do), but in reality you are a sentient transport system for bacteria, and in the end you will be consumed by the bacteria you spent a lifetime killing. Unless, I suppose, you are at ground zero of a thermonuclear weapon.

Today I saw a patient with an infected knee after two taps for gout.

It grew *Staphylococcus lugdunensis*. This century the lab has started to speciate some of the coagulase negative staphylococci, and *lugdunensis* has been popping up in the occasional cultures. Blood, a knee here, an abscess there. It may be more common than appreciated, as a recent study suggests it is not an uncommon isolate in soft tissue infections. Studies from 2002 suggest it is a cause of abscesses in the pelvic girdle. Clinically it seems to like to cause disease below the belly button, especially the toes. And that may be for good reason.

Like many bacteria, *S. lugdunensis* has a niche in your body. You are not covered in a schmear of bacteria—rather, each bug has its own area where it prefers to live. Location location location are the top three selling characteristics of real estate, but somehow the nailbed of the first toe doesn't seem to be all that desirable a place to live, at least to me. But that is the preferred location for *S. lugdunensis*. Toe > legs > groin.

I have been informed that the characteristic smell of *S. lugdunensis* is bleach, so you will never discover an outbreak in a Clorox factory.

Treat it like a *S. aureus*. It is more virulent than the usual coagulase negative staphylococcus, and if you grow it, hey, give your local I.D. doc a call. At least you can't pick your nose with your toes and spread the organism.

BTW, from Wikipedia:

> *"Lugdunensis was a province of the Roman Empire in what is now the modern country of France, part of the Celtic territory of Gaul. It is named after its capital Lugdunum."*

Which is now Lyon, where the organism was first described. And I thought it was from lug nuts.

Someone want to send me to Lyon to investigate further?

Rationalization

Bocher, S., et al., Staphylococcus lugdunensis, a common cause of skin and soft tissue infections in the community. J Clin Microbiol, 2009. 47(4): p. 946-50.

Bieber, L. and G. Kahlmeter, Staphylococcus lugdunensis in several niches of the normal skin flora. Clin Microbiol Infect, 2010. 16(4): p. 385-8.

Do the feet smell?

MIDDLE-AGED man with athalete's feet (it's atha-lete, not athlete) who got a spontaneous foot cellulitis and maybe a touch of abscess. No risk factors, to trauma, no reason for the infection.

He didn't respond to an oral beta-lactam, but eventually got betterish on vancomycin. Cultures of the abscess grow coagulase negative *Staphylococcus*. Ignore it, right? Riiiiiiggggghhhht.

That's what I would have said last year, but not this year.

Turns out that *S. lugdunensis* is not an uncommon cause of lower extremity infections. On the rare times I have seen *lugdunensis*, it has been the etiology of endocarditis or a post-operative knee infection. Unfortunately the lab usually doesn't look for *lugdunensis* in skin infections because it is thought to be a contaminant/normal flora.

Did he smell like bleach? I don't know. Pushkin I am not, so I did not sniff the foot and the lab made no note of any odor. I do know the organism is not acquired *in utero*.

Next time you call me with a foot cellulitis, sniff the foot first. Let me know if it smells like the Y.

Rationalization

Batista, N., et al., Evaluation of methods for studying susceptibility to oxacillin and penicillin in 60 Staphylococcus lugdunensis isolates. Enferm Infecc Microbiol Clin, 2009. 27(3): p. 148-52.

Postscript

They eventually identified the organism as *S. lugdunensis*.

Punch me in the Nose

IT's been a busy week. Many consults, lots of family stuff, and the Science Based Medicine (SBM) post to write. I remain in awe of my co-conspirators, er, co-bloggers at SBM and their ability to churn out reams of quality prose in short order. But now I have time to noodle around with this chapter.

Today I saw a case of endocarditis. Nothing odd except it was a pan-sensitive coagulase negative Staphylococcus, generically referred to as coag negative staph.

Probably a healthcare associated disease, as he is on dialysis, and the use of central lines is associated with bacteremia and subsequent seeding of the heart valves.

"Healthcare associated" is the current preferred term, rather than "hospital acquired" —or "god damn it, it wasn't my fault" associated, since a lot of heathcare is now provided outside the hospital. The term they really use is nosohusia, but that sounds like some sort of nasal problem in an elephant, and I can't say nosohusial without giggling.

Healthcare associated endocarditis is a significant problem with a high death rate, and coag negative staph are a common cause of the infection. In the series referenced below,

> "Staphylococcus aureus was the most frequently isolated microorganism (28 cases; 33.7%), followed by Enterococcus species (19 cases; 22.9%) and coagulase negative staphylococci (18 cases; 21.7%)"

I don't consider acupuncture to be healthcare; that would be "quack-associated endocarditis." Quackahusia?

What is odd about the case for me is that I have taken care of this patient twice in the past: both times for infected knees. Evidently we had a bad interaction on the first go-round, as today he said that yeah, he remembers me from three years ago and he wants to punch me in the nose. I do not remember the interaction, but evidently I sent him home from clinic saying his knee was OK when in fact it was not. Hence the interest in punching me.

Still. I try to get along with my patients, so I am discomforted by his need to rearrange my nose.

Of course I apologized, but kept more than an arm's length away.

Rationalization

Fernandez-Hidalgo, N., et al., Contemporary epidemiology and prognosis of health care-associated infective endocarditis. Clin Infect Dis, 2008. 47(10): p. 1287-97.

STREP TEASE

Cellulitis

YESTERDAY was one of those inundations of consults that occur on occasion, and by the time I got home and took care of real life, it was time for bed with no spare time for writing. Life does have a way of requiring one's attention.

Today was less busy, but I had a common consult: Is it cellulitis or not?

Vasculitis is inflammation of the vascular tree.

Pneumonitis is inflammation of the lungs or *pneuma*, Greek for breath.

Hepatitis is inflammation of the liver, or hepta, some ancient word or other for liver. I prefer pâté.

Cellulitis is inflammation of the cellula, which is god knows what, but is the word from the Latin cellula, which means small cell—what this has to do with a skin infection, I have never been able to find out. It is also evidently a prostitute's cubicle and, while you can get all sorts of inflammation from that kind of cellula, it has nothing to do with the case at hand.

The 3 most dangerous words in medicine are "In my experience," especially when it comes to treatments, but I am going to delve into those three most dangerous words in medicine, because there are pearls about cellulitis that can help one distinguish infection from other causes of rubor, dolor, calor, tumor in an extremity. (I finally worked those words into a sentence—I feel as if Groucho should give me a twenty).

Here are pearls, prepare to make a necklace:

Cellulitis patients <u>always have a fever or an increased white count. Always.</u>

Cellulitis is never, ever, never never, ever ever bilateral. Never ever. Now you may say to yourself, I have seen bilateral cellulitis, Crislip is wrong. And you may ask yourself, How did I get here? And you may ask yourself, am I right? Am I wrong? My god, what have I done? And in this case you were wrong. It was a misdiagnosis. It wasn't bilateral cellulitis, you had a misdiagnosis. Live with it.

Here is a key point: the rubor, dolor, calor, tumor of cellulitis does not resolve with elevation, while the rubor, dolor, calor, tumor of stasis/edema does. I have never seen this fact in print, so if some fellow wants to do a clinical study, just give me a nod. The problem is that cellulitis leads to temporary swelling and redness in a leg from edema, and the patients go to the doctor and say, "I am not getting better, it's still red." But the doc doesn't elevate the leg higher than the heart for the examination. Instead the patients get more and more expensive (but not more powerful) antibiotics until they are all Fanny Mae from the expense, and then they are sent to me. I elevate the leg higher than the heart and the 'cellulitis' is gone in a couple of minutes.

Never evaluate a leg for cellulitis in a dependent position. You will be misled.

For every fifty pounds the patient is over the ideal body weight, it takes one day more to get better.

Cellulitis on therapy progresses for one day, stabilizes for one day, then on the third day it starts to regress. You need patience with the patient.

Group A strep cellulitis will start with severe groin pain on the affected side several hours before any rubor, dolor, calor, tumor of the leg; I presume this is from local lymphatic inflammation.

All the pearls mentioned above have, to my knowledge, not been subjected to rigorous clinical trials, so take them or leave them as you see fit. My consult today had neither fever nor leukocytosis, it was bilateral and disappeared with elevation. I stopped his antibiotics.

What is interesting is that the microbiology of acute cellulitis may be changing. It is taught that most cellulitis is due to Group

A streptococcus: *Streptococcus pyogenes*, the same bug that causes strep throat.

An interesting study in Finland looked at the microbiology of cellulitis and found

> *"Beta Hemolytic streptococci were isolated from 26 (29%) of 90 patients, 2 isolates of which were blood-culture positive for group G streptococci, and 24 patients had culture-positive skin lesions. Group G Streptococcus (Streptococcus dysgalactiae subsp. equisimilis) was found most often and was isolated from 22% of patient samples of either skin lesions or blood, followed by group A Streptococcus, which was found in 7% of patients."*

I wonder if this true in the US as well. I seem to be seeing more Group G streptococci lately, but have yet to find a resident who wants to repeat this study with our local data. One considered it, but has yet to commit. I sure hate a strep tease.

Rationalization

Siljander, T., et al., Acute bacterial, nonnecrotizing cellulitis in Finland: microbiological findings. Clin Infect Dis, 2008. 46(6): p. 855-61.

....

Bacterial artha-ritis

THE alphabet soup of streptococci. A and B and C and D and E and F and G.

Gee. Dr. Lansfield was a wonderful microbiologist, but all these letters do not help me to remember which is which. Bacteria need names. Fred. Barney. Wilma.

Group G strep is beta hemolytic, like the streptococcus of strep throat, and is found in the nasopharynx, skin, genitourinary, and gastrointestinal tract of normal people. It occasionally pops loose to cause disease.

Out of nowhere today's patient had rapid onset of rubor, dolor, calor, tumor, of his knee. Unlike most patients with an infected joint, he had no prior trauma to the knee and no risk factors for infectious artha-ritis: cancer or diabetes or alcoholic liver disease or anything. His life was as uneventful as mine.

Yet, the tap of the knee grew Group G *Streptococcus* . A little incision and drainage and some IV beta lactam antibiotics should take care of it.

So where did it come from? Just prior he had been hiking in the Mt. Hood Forest and had taken a shower in a campground. The water did not drain well and he stood in a few inches of undrained shower water, probably mixed with the effluent of prior showerers. He had some foot erythema after the exposure to the shower and just prior to the infection of his knee. So I guess the bacteria went downstream from a foot cellulitis to the knee— not, by any means, a common occurrence.

That would be an intriguing source for the Group G *Streptococcus*. Not much in PubMed to suggest this was the right explanation. But there are articles from the developing world and from olden days to suggest that streptococci are often found in swimming pools with less-than-adequate maintenance.

An article from 1927 suggests that microorganisms besides *B. coli* (this is old. *B. coli* is now *E. coli*) which are commonly found in pools are *Staphylococcus* and streptococci, which were undoubtedly introduced into the pool by the bathers. *Streptococcus* was found in four pools studied. Practically every sample of water that was polluted with *B. coli* contained *Streptococcus*... Ick.

Streptococci are constant indicators of intestinal pollution and the number found in the pool parallels the amount of pollution as indicated by the number of bathers.

Ick again. I don't want to swim no more. Pools are like sausages. You do not what to know what is in them. The fetid shower water is, perhaps, the equivalent of a swimming pool and would be an intriguing source for the *Streptococcus*.

Rationalization

Mallmann, W.L., Streptococcus as an Indicator of Swimming Pool Pollution. Am J Public Health Nations Health, 1928. 18(6): p. 771-6.

Dubost, J.J., et al., Streptococcal septic arthritis in adults. A study of

55 cases with a literature review. Joint Bone Spine, 2004. 71(4): p. 303-11.

Lin, A.N., et al., Group G streptococcal arthritis. J Rheumatol, 1982. 9(3): p. 424-7.

....

Popcorn and Abscesses

Not all streptococci are the same. Most do not cause abscesses, but the *S. anginosus* group can and often does.

S. anginosus (old name *S. milleri*. Microbiologists love to get together, get drunk, and change the names of bugs. Keeps them employed, I suppose) is part of the normal flora of the mouth. If it gains access to the blood, it can go to the liver or brain or spine and cause an abscess. If it is accidentally inhaled into the lung, it will cause a lung abscess.

And, like the patient today, it somehow manages to get into the soft tissues of the neck, it gives rise to a retropharyngeal (behind the throat) abscess. The neck has numerous tissue planes down which Streptococci can invade, so these tend to be big abscesses that dissect down into the chest and, in the process, cut off the airway. I do not know yet why this patient has a *S. anginosus* abscess—he cannot talk due to a tracheostomy—but relatively minor trauma is often all that is needed. The most curious case I had was someone who, while a wee bit drunk, failed to chew his nacho chip sufficiently and it cut clean through his esophagus when he swallowed it.

The curious thing about *S. anginosus* is not the diseases it causes, or the drugs used to treat it. It is the smell. It smells like buttered popcorn. I have never smelled it (the bacteria. I have smelled buttered popcorn). For some reason I cannot bring myself to smell a culture plate. When I was a fellow, one of my colleagues ran down to the lab to smell a plate and it turned out to be *Coccidioidomycosis*. Turns out *Coccidioidomycosis* is very infectious under these conditions (it wasn't known that it was *Coccidioidomycosis* when it was smelled), and one is not supposed to smell it. That person is the only living human who knows what *Coccidioidomycosis* smells like. And it ain't Teen Spirit.

Why does *S. anginosus* smell like popcorn? It makes diacetyl. Lots of diacetyl.

> *"The caramel odor associated with the "Streptococcus milleri" group was shown to be attributable to the formation of the metabolite diacetyl. Levels of diacetyl in the 22—to 200-mg/liter range were produced by 68 strains of the 'S. milleri' group."*

What is cool is that the reason it smells like buttered popcorn is that diacetyl is one of the compounds that gives butter that butter smell. Next time you have that fake butter spread, think to yourself, "I can't believe it's not *S. anginosus*™."

Small amounts of diacetyl are found in beer and wine from the yeast fermentation, and this is what gives beer and wine a slipperiness. Or so says Wikipedia, which also says

> *"Concentrations from 0.005 mg/L to 1.7 mg/L were measured in Chardonnay wines, and the amount needed for the flavor to be noticed is at least 0.2 mg/L."*

So the bacteria make 10 to 100 times (I know, sloppy math) the amount of diacetyl found in wine. Why they make so much daacetyl, I cannot discover.

Oregon beers are many things (best anywhere), but slippery is not one of them. Makers of Chardonnay try to maximize the amount of diacetyl to give the wine that buttery taste and slipperiness. Or maybe it's really pureed slugs. A new smoothie flavor for the local Jamba Juice? Give me a good Bordeaux any day.

So next time you have that microwave popcorn and a glass of Chardonnay, remember that the buttery richness is also is the smell of abscesses.

Bon appétit.

Rationalization

Chew, T.A. and J.M. Smith, Detection of diacetyl (caramel odor) in presumptive identification of the "Streptococcus milleri" group. J Clin Microbiol, 1992. 30(11): p. 3028-9.

Also see the entry: http://en.wikipedia.org/wiki/Diacetyl

....

Strawberries

O REGON is the best place to live on earth. Period. But don't tell anyone, it will be our little secret. One of the delights are the strawberries, which are not the fibrous, only slightly sweet posers that come from California. Oregon strawberries are luscious, but do not travel, going bad in less than 48 hours after picking. The season usually doesn't begin till June, but for me the season started early.

Fevers, hypotension, acute renal failure, altered mental status, a diffuse erythroderma that included the palms and soles, red conjunctivae, and the tongue. The tongue was cool. It looked like a strawberry. Not the best I have seen, that being in a case of postpartum toxic shock syndrome (yes, it was a case of Staphylococcal toxic shock syndrome) where the tongue looked like a big Hood River strawberry. Didn't taste like it, though. (Just joking).

Strawberry tongue has a limited differential: Toxic shock syndrome (TSS), both staphylococcal and streptococcal, scarlet fever, and Kawasaki's disease—an autoimmune vasculitis found in children under 5.

There is also, evidently, a recurrent familial form. And there can be a white strawberry and a red strawberry, but not a chocolate-covered strawberry tongue. Well, I guess there could be, if a Kawasaki's patient ate a Hershey bar, but not as a clinical sign.

I cannot find why TSS causes a strawberry tongue or any reports of a tongue biopsy. I also cannot find out why Kawasaki's causes the same physical finding. What does Kawasaki's have in common with TSS? Got me.

But I did find Baboon syndrome, where you get a rash that looks like a baboon butt. Cool. It can be due to the same toxin that causes scarlet fever, so there is a link.

The patient had streptococcal toxic shock syndrome from a cellulitis, but no necrotizing soft tissue infection and improved with penicillin, clindamycin and IVIG. But that tongue was neat.

Rationalization

Handisurya, A., G. Stingl, and S. Wohrl, SDRIFE (baboon syndrome) induced by penicillin. Clin Exp Dermatol, 2009. 34(3): p. 355-7.

Ichimiya, M., Y. Hamamoto, and M. Muto, A case of baboon syndrome associated with group a streptococcal infection. J Dermatol, 2003. 30(1): p. 69-71.

Drunken Microbiologists

H ERE's my theory, completely unsupported by facts. Each year all the microbiologists meet somewhere nice, get really really drunk and then, to hoots and giggles, change the names and classification of organisms. And they do it just to bug me.

Today was a patient with an infection in a facet joint of her thoracic spine. Odd place to get an infection. I have seen a pair of these that I can remember, both of whom had had radiation in the area and both of whom grew a viridans Streptococcus.

Today's patient had no such prior trauma, but the MRI showed osteomyelitis and a fluid collection. At my behest they stuck a needle in it and it grew...

Streptococcus infantarius. Sounds like a Palestinian uprising. But I had never heard of the bug. PubMed tells me it is the bacteria formally known as *S. bovis.* That I know.

Here is a simplified table showing which group D Streptococcus is which:

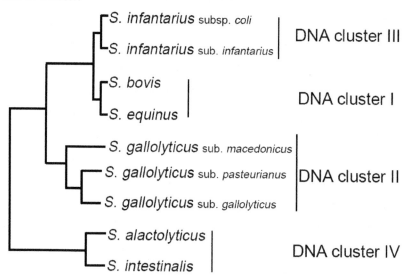

Simplified phylogenetic tree of group D streptococci based on comparative analysis of 16S rDNA

Note they call it "simplified." Yeah, right.

For those of you dying to know the biochemicals, see the table on the next page. Still, like the formally all-encompassing *S. bo-vis, Streptococcus infantarius* is associated with bowel cancer, so at some point the patient will need a colonoscopy.

It also may be associated with non-colonic GI cancers. Part of the problem is that all of the epidemiological studies are going to have to be repeated with the new classification to see which group D streptococci are associated with which cancers, if any.

See what happens when microbiologists get drunk? We all suffer.

At least I can kill *Streptococcus infantarius*, and kill it I will.

Rationalization

Bouvet, A., et al., Streptococcus infantarius sp. nov. related to Streptococcus bovis and Streptococcus equinus. Adv Exp Med Biol, 1997. 418: p. 393-5.

Corredoira, J., et al., Association between Streptococcus infantarius (formerly S. bovis II/1) bacteremia and noncolonic cancer. J Clin Microbiol, 2008. 46(4): p. 1570.

Differential biochemical characteristics of group D streptococcal strains

	S. equinus/ S. bovis	S. gallolyticus subsp.			S. infantarius subsp.		S. alactolyticus
		gallolyticus	pasteurianus	macedonicus	infantarius	coli	
No. of strains	n = 9 + 8	n = 13	n = 21	n = 5	n = 10	n = 14	n = 4
Hydrolysis of							
Aesculine	+	+	+	-	V	+	+
Gallate	-	+	-	-	-	-	-
Production of							
β-glucosidase	+	+	+	-	V	+	+
β-glucuronidase	-/+	-	+	-	-	-	-
α-galactosidase	-/+	+	V	V	+	+	+
β-galactosidase (β-GAR)	-	-	-	+	-	-	-
β-galactosidase (β-GAL)	-	-	+	V	-	-	-
β-mannosidase	-	V	+	-	-	-	-
Acidification of							
Starch	-/+	+	-	+	+	V	-
Glycogen	-/+	+	-	-	+	-	-
Inulin	-/+	+	-	-	-	-	-
Lactose	-/+	+	+	+	+	+	-
Mannitol	-	+	-	-	-	-	-
Meth-β-D-glucopyranoside	+	+	+	-	+	+	-
Raffinose	-/+	+	V	-	-	+	V
Trehalose	V	+	+	-	+	-	-

Bovis, part one

Back when I was a resident, there were Group D Streptococci angd they were divided into enterococcal and non-enterococcal streptococcus.

Easy. You only had to remember two things.

The problem with modernity is they have increasingly sophisticated ways of analyzing bacteria and separating them into different groups.

There also used to be *S. bovis*, a non-enterococcal Group D streptococcus. <u>S. bovis</u> in the blood means bowel cancer, and the patient needs a colonoscopy to look for GI pathology to account for the bloodstream infection. Not only is this a practical piece of information, but it is the kind of thing they like to ask on the boards, so make note of it. I would hate to have you miss a question because you were not paying attention.

The patient was found down, how long we do not know. It is my clinical impression (aka I am probably wrong and the victim of confirmation bias) that transient bacteremia is common in people found down for prolonged periods of time. Normal skin organisms leak into the bloodstream and cause a transient bacteremia. However, that tidbit is unsupported by any literature I can find, so someone get to work and generate a paper that verifies my insightful observation.

The patient was a heavy alcoholic and not particularly well kept, so when he was found down and febrile, he had blood cultures. These grew *S. gallolyticus*, a subtype of *S. bovis*. *S. bovis* is a bowel bug, not a skin bug, but perhaps it leaked from the skin—to judge from the smell, fecal flora may not have been confined to just his GI tract. The bug was only in one of three sets of cultures, so he did not have endocarditis, but still needed a colonoscopy. It was negative for malignancy, but he did have cirrhosis with varices and maybe that was why he has bacteremia.

<u>Liver disease may also be a risk factor for</u> *S. bovis* bacteremia.

Not all bacteria are equal in the ability to cause disease and the better they are identified, the better you can evaluate the patient.

Rationalization

Gonzlez-Quintela, A., et al., Prevalence of liver disease in patients with Streptococcus bovis bacteraemia. J Infect, 2001. 42(2): p. 116-9.

Vaska, V.L. and J.L. Faoagali, Streptococcus bovis bacteraemia: identification within organism complex and association with endocarditis and colonic malignancy. Pathology, 2009. 41(2): p. 183-6.

Bovis, yet again

A N elderly male with a new diagnosis of inflammatory bowel disease early this year.

He has had a progressively painful hip since the diagnosis of IBS, along with failure to thrive. He was admitted after suffering a transient ischemic attack. Blood cultures grew two of two streptococcus. He had a known flail mitral valve.

Positive blood cultures, abnormal valve, emboli—sounds like endocarditis to me.

He had one blood culture on a prior admission that had both a coagulase negative *Staphylococcus* and a *S. alactolyticus*, yet another group D *Streptococcus* in the bovis family. It was dismissed as contaminant, which was not unreasonable as there are no cases of any disease outside of cavities in humans. He had had some dental work, but haven't we all? This bug is also common in pigs and chickens, with which he has no contact.

There are no reported cases of endocarditis yet with this organism. I got the first one. Lets hear it, more me.

But the more interesting feature of the case was that his systemic symptoms started around the time he was diagnosed with Crohn's. IBD is associated with endocarditis, so maybe that was why he has endocarditis. And we still have to determine if the hip is infected as well. Then I also have the first case of septic arthritis with this organism.

Rationalization

Kreuzpaintner, G., et al., Increased risk of bacterial endocarditis in inflammatory bowel disease. Am J Med, 1992. 92(4): p. 391-5.

Kreuzpaintner, G., et al., An increased incidence of bacterial endocarditis in chronic inflammatory bowel diseases. Z Gastroenterol, 1992. 30(6): p. 397-402.

Unexpecting

I GAVE the residents their I.D. bored review today. Spelled correctly. I love to see their eyes glaze over as I go over the pearls they need to pass the boreds, drool flowing from the corners of their mouths.

I will probably go to internal medicine hell for this, but I don't find the physical exam all that helpful. Do NOT let Steve Jones know I said this. The physical can be fun, and occasionally you will pick up a finding that makes the diagnosis. But for me, the three important parts to making a diagnosis are history, history, and history. Cultures, labs, and X-rays should only confirm what you figured out after talking to the patient. It is why it always fries my bacon a little when patients tell me to read the chart instead of asking questions and taking a history.

There are exceptions: endocarditis, heart failure, and cellulitis are diseases where the exam is of help. As is pelvic pain.

Today's patient was a middled-aged female with group B streptococcus (GBS) in her blood for no reason except diabetes, which is probably reason enough. Most group B strep bacteremia I see is without a source and is almost never due to endocarditis. While she had a long history of joint pain, now she couldn't get out of bed due to the severe back pain.

Usually exam will elicit exactly where the pain is coming from: hip, bursa, iliopsoas, paraspinous, spine, sacroiliac (SI) joint. Simple maneuvers can quickly tell where the infection is, since new pain in a bacteremic patient is usually pus under pressure.

I thought, by exam, that she had an sacroiliac joint infection—

in part by the location of the pain, in part by all the negative findings on exam, and in part by the predilection for GBS to go to joints in the elderly (or at least a pseudo-joint in the case of the sacroiliac).

The bone scan was negative in the sacroiliac, but lit up in the L 3-4 paraspinous area.

The heck. GBS is not a cause of myositis or abscess as a rule, so I got an MRI.

I hate the phrase "expect the unexpected." If you expect it, it is no longer unexpected, and to say expect the expected is a lame tautology. Unexpect the unexpected? Naw.

MRI showed an L 3-4 epidural and paraspinous abscess.

Now THAT was unexpected. This is not, as a rule, what GBS does in adults. Even more odd was no discitis or osteomyelitis that is nearly always the proximate cause of epidural abscesses.

How commonly does Group B *Streptococcus* cause an epidural abscess? Rare as a fair election in Iran. Or Florida for that matter. It is nice to see we have been successful in bringing our form of government to at least one country in the Mideast.

A grand total of five or so GBS epidural abscesses are reported on PubMed. It looks like most cases started with a facet joint infection, which my patient did not have, though how they could tell it started in the facet joint I cannot say.

Take home: I can't trust the exam for pelvic pain either.

Rationalization

Okada, F., et al., Lumbar facet joint infection associated with epidural and paraspinal abscess: a case report with review of the literature. J Spinal Disord Tech, 2005. 18(5): p. 458-61.

Edwards, M.S. and C.J. Baker, Group B streptococcal infections in elderly adults. Clin Infect Dis, 2005. 41(6): p. 839-47.

....

Shock

SHOCK.
Septic? Toxic? Cardiogenic? Hemorrhagic? Electrical?

Marilyn Manson?

So many ways to go into shock.

A middle-aged patient was admitted in what looked like septic shock: multi-organ system failure, disseminated intravascular coagulation, platelets of 30 (one-fifth normal), blood pressure that fell to dangerous levels unless pressor drugs were given.

Exam, labs and X-rays revealed none of the big three usual causes of infection: pneumonia, urinary tract infection, or soft tissue infection, which has the nice acronym PUS.

Not a lot of things cause non-focal rapid onset sepsis: Meningococcus, plague, Group A Streptococcus, maybe *S. aureus* lead the list, but the patient had no reason for any of the above.

So we treated for everything and next day all the cultures were negative.

Talking with the family revealed that the patient had had axillary pain before admission that was thought to be due to minor trauma. Looking at the armpit was initially unimpressive, but perhaps disgusting, as all armpits lack a certain aesthetic appeal. As his blood pressure improved, cellulitis became evident in the axilla as well as a faint, diffuse erythroderma that involved the palms and soles. I suppose his blood pressure was so low he could not perfuse his tissue enough to get red in either the infected armpit or what looked like a toxic shock rash.

He was whisked off to the OR for debridement (pronounced duh breed, not dee bride. Dee bride is dee woman who walks down dee aisle of dee church). Streptococci were seen in the tissues that were edematous, but there was no necrotizing fasciitis. So far cultures are negative.

It was an odd case of both septic shock (but the blood cultures were negative) and toxic shock (TSS) (but no strawberry tongue, necrotizing cellulitis and only a brief erythroderma). And the signs of TSS occurred in slow motion, over three or four days, and manifested late in the course of the disease. But the patient is slowly getting better.

There was an interesting recent case of Streptococcal TSS jumping from patient to a health care worker, so remember the

droplet and contact isolation. My specialty is called INFEC-
TIOUS diseases for a reason.

Rationalization

Lacy, M.D. and K. Horn, Nosocomial transmission of invasive group a streptococcus from patient to health care worker. Clin Infect Dis, 2009. 49(3): p. 354-7.

Rare Bug, Rare Disease, Bad Outcome

NECROTIZING fasciitis is not all that common and is often rapidly fatal. It comes in many flavors, metaphorically speaking. Taste is one of the sensory modalities I try to avoid using in evaluating infections. Usually nec fasc, as we call it in the biz, is due to Group A *Streptococcus*. It can also be a mixed synergistic necrotizing fasciitis, a polymicrobial infection that behaves, or misbehaves, like gas gangrene. Gas gangrene, the disease that most people fear, was brought to the public consciousness by World War I. It is rare nowadays except in skin poppers——heroin users who run out of veins and inject directly into the skin.

I have seen a variety of gram negative rods cause necrotizing fasciitis over the years: *Serratia, Yersinia, Vibrio*.

MRSA is increasing as a cause of necrotizing fasciitis, arguably due to strains that make the Panton-Valentine Leukocidin (PVL), a protein that dissolves tissues the way water does the Wicked Witch of the West.

The PVL can turn meat into liquid, and is part of the reason the current strain of MRSA makes abscesses so commonly. I wonder if it would make a good meat tenderizer.

So when a patient came in with a rapidly progressive purple leg, septic shock, and multi-organ system failure, I expected one of the above from cultures.

He was in end stage liver disease and yellow, and the surgeons whisked him off to the OR and amputated his leg in an attempt to save his life. Post-op he developed new areas of necrotizing fasciitis on his abdomen and his other leg, and within 24 hours he was dead.

All the cultures grew *Streptococcus pneumoniae*. Very odd. There are less than a dozen reported cases of necrotizing fasciitis due to *Streptococcus pneumoniae* in the medical literature, most associated with some sort of immunodeficiency. The organism was sensitive to all antibiotics, as if they did any good.

The other interesting feature about the case reports is the mention of prior use of NSAIDS, like ibuprofen. There has long been an association between necrotizing fasciitis due to group A streptococci and NSAIDS. The drugs, being anti-inflammatory, probably help tilt the balance of power in favor of the bacteria. This patient was too sick to answer questions, so we will never know if we can point the finger at an NSAID or not. The severity of his disease can probably be attributed to his liver failure.

Rationalization

Frick, S. and A. Cerny, Necrotizing fasciitis due to Streptococcus pneumoniae after intramuscular injection of nonsteroidal anti-inflammatory drugs: report of 2 cases and review. Clin Infect Dis, 2001. 33(5): p. 740-4.

Unintended Goodness

I ACTUALLY got out of the house today. And there was work! The joy of a good infection. I sometimes feel a titch guilty over how much fun I have at work, since part of enjoyment is derived from the fact some poor unfortunate has to get a disease odd enough or interesting enough to warrant an infectious disease consultation.

Today was something I have not seen for a while: a *S. pneumoniae* pneumonia. What was odd about it was the organism was intermediate to penicillin.

Resistance in the pneumococcus has two flavors: intermediate (MIC [mean inhibitory concentration] to penicillin between 0.1 and 1 micrograms per ml) and resistant with MIC >= 2.

These forms of resistance have different mechanisms. The intermediate strains have DNA point mutations that have led to single amino acid substitutions at one of the three binding sites of penicillin, which results in a slight increase in the MIC to penicillin. The more point mutations, the higher the MIC. It is why the mean MIC to penicillin of *S. pneumoniae* has been slowly increasing since the discovery of penicillin.

Resistant strains have acquired a new chunk of DNA from another bacterial species that leads to complete resistance to penicillin, as well as to several other common antibiotics. Which is a story for another day. Suffice it to say I wish I could acquire the hair gene from another human with equal ease, since I am tired of my scalp getting sunburned every summer.

Here is yet another cool thing, in an endless list of cool things, in I.D.

There are 82 + serotypes of *S. pneumoniae.* The most common disease-causing strains tend to be the resistant strains. The old pneumococcal vaccine is not all that great a vaccine, it does not so much prevent disease as prevent you from dying if you get the disease, which is not that bad an outcome. There is a newer pneumococcal vaccine that is given to children and targets the 7 most common invasive pneumococcal strains, which are also the strains most likely to be resistant to penicillin. The new vaccine is excellent and prevents disease in kids, as well as decreasing the number of kids who carry the bug.

The use of this vaccine in children has resulted in invasive disease plummeting in kids and, as a side effect, disease due to these strains has decreased in adults. It appears that kids are the vectors that serve as a source of pneumococcal infection in adults.

> *"The rate of antibiotic-resistant invasive pneumococcal infections decreased in young children and older persons after the introduction of the conjugate vaccine. There was an increase in infections caused by serotypes not included in the vaccine..."*

and

> *"...the introduction of a pneumococcal conjugate vaccine for children has reduced the population rate of adult pneumococcal bacteremia due to vaccine serotypes and is associated with a reduced risk*

of bacteremic pneumococcal pneumonia for adults with children in the home."

One cannot, however, autoclave your kids to prevent infection.

Giving the vaccine to kids has resulted in a decrease in disease in adults and overall decrease in disease from resistant strains. Which is a nice change, as usually when you try something new you worry about unintended bad consequences. No good deed ever goes unpunished in medicine.

It is why I have not seen a resistant S. *pneumoniae* for a while. But this relief will be short lived. The ecological niche is being filled by strains not covered by the vaccine and resistance is not futile, but inevitable. See the last reference for a complete explanation.

For a short period of time we have had a vacation from *S. pneumoniae*. All vacations end. And I want to go to Hawaii.

Rationalization

Metlay, J.P., et al., Impact of pediatric vaccination with pneumococcal conjugate vaccine on the risk of bacteremic pneumococcal pneumonia in adults. Vaccine, 2006. 24(4): p. 468-75.

Kyaw, M.H., et al., Effect of introduction of the pneumococcal conjugate vaccine on drug-resistant Streptococcus pneumoniae. N Engl J Med, 2006. 354(14): p. 1455-63.

On the Origin of Species by Means of Natural Selection. Darwin, Charles.

....

True True and Related?

G ROUP B streptococcus bacteremia is not all that uncommon, at least in my world.

But in my world every surgery gets infected; I have a skewed outlook on the medical world. Usually Group B occurs in babies and moms around the time of delivery, or in older diabetics and alcoholics for no damn good reason. Group B strep is also known as *Streptococcus agalactiae*. When I took my internship boards I missed a question about *Streptococcus agalactiae*, which I had never heard of. I did know all about Group B strep, but did not know they were one and the same. Bastards.

The presumed pathophysiology is new gastrointestinal colonization by a strain to which the patient has no antibodies, and it manages to sneak into the bloodstream. Often, in the older patient, the organism then seeds a joint or two.

This patient I saw today was not old, nor immunoincompetent, nor peripartum, but still had group B streptococcus in the blood.

Again my usual question: why? What is a good question, but I want to know why.

When the patient developed bacteremia, she was taking a course of metronidazole for *Clostridium difficile* colitis. Could they be related? I don't know. Her colon was inflamed and filled with bacteria. It could be that she had the misfortune of being colonized (no pun intended for the first and only time in this book) at the same time she developed colitis, and had the resultant bacteremia from the organisms leaking into her bloodstream from the inflamed colon.

To make it even more unusual, the patient developed endocarditis that, while cured microbiologically, required valve repair. There are fewer than 200 reported cases of endocarditis due to *Streptococcus agalactiae* (did I mention *Streptococcus agalactiae* is also called Group B strep? I would hate to miss a test question because I didn't know that. Bitter much? Ask me about neuroanatomy in med school if you want a real rant), accounting for < 2% of causes of endocarditis. Weirdness squared. Someone owes this patient a string of good luck.

Is *C. difficile* associated with endocarditis? Nope. Not that I can find. But chronic bowel inflammation is. And there is a well known association between *Streptococcus bovis* endocarditis and bowel cancer; well-known to me, at least, but if you are going to be taking your medicine boards, don't say I didn't tell you.

My hypothesis is that the patient seeded her heart valve as a complication of the *C. difficile* colitis. If so, it is the first case ever. You heard it here first. Since I am first, we will name it after me. And about time, too.

Rationalization

Kreuzpaintner, G., et al., Increased risk of bacterial endocarditis in inflammatory bowel disease. Am J Med, 1992. 92(4): p. 391-5.

Sambola, A., et al., Streptococcus agalactiae infective endocarditis: analysis of 30 cases and review of the literature, 1962-1998. Clin Infect Dis, 2002. 34(12): p. 1576-84.

....

Shazam!

K EEPING healthy is not necessarily a process filled with comfort and dignity. Women have to endure the pelvic exam when they are young. Men get the prostate exam as they age. Note the word is prostate. Not prostrate. Although sometimes you have to be the latter to get the former evaluated. If you have problems peeing from prostate obstruction and the urine gets infected, those bacteria have to go somewhere. If not into the urinal, they will get into the bloodstream.

There is a vascular connection between the bladder/prostate and the spine, called Batson's plexus, named after Billy Batson, aka Captain Marvel. It is a set of valveless veins that go from the bladder kto the lumbar spine. This can be a highway to the spinal cord for bacteria, as the patient this week demonstrated. He, and it is always a he as it is the rare female who gets bladder outlet obstruction from an enlarged prostate, had progressive difficulty urinating, then got infected. Eventually he developed back pain which was found to be due to discitis and a spinal epidural abscess.

Most of the infections that occur for this reason have *E. coli* as the cause, since *E. coli* is the most common cause of urinary tract infections. Not so in this case, as the epidural abscess and the urine grew out *Streptococcus agalactiae*, aka Group B streptococcus.

Odd, as there are a whopping three cases in adults in the literature of this organism causing epidural abscesses. As a cause of urinary tract infection in non-pregnant females, it is also uncommon, and even more unusual in non-pregnant men. I cannot find data on pregnant men, of which we currently have one in Oregon.

Now that the abscess is drained, I expect a cure with a long course of antibiotics. At least I can still kill a Group B strep.

It is good to pee.

Rationalization

Hernaiz, C., et al., Clinical significance of Streptococcus agalactiae isolation from urine samples of outpatients from health care centers. Enferm Infecc Microbiol Clin, 2004. 22(2): p. 89-91.

....

The Joint Ain't Jumpin'

EVERY organism can grow in any space. That is what makes I.D. endlessly entertaining and interesting.

Most septic prosthetic joints are due to staph of one sort or another, and early infections after joint replacement tend to be coagulase negative staph or *P. acnes*.

Five months after a new knee, a patient developed sudden on-set of, can you guess what?

Rubor, dolor, calor, tumor in the knee. Where have I heard those words before? It is odd to see an infected knee 5 or 6 months in, and often it is a peculiar organism.

A tap shows some white blood cells, and a few days later she grew *Streptococcus intermedius* from the cultures.

I thought, Huh, that's odd. But *S. intermedius* is part of mouth flora, and people are bacteremic all the time, so why not?

Back last century I would have had to plow though the *Index Medicus* to find how often this bug has been reported in a joint. Quick PubMed and... the heck. Only one case in the literature, and that in a normal joint. So here is the first case ever of *S. intermedius* in a prosthetic knee. We shall henceforth call it Crislip's Disease. Let the call go out.

Part of the problem with *S. intermedius* is that while it can be cultured, it did not grow well enough to get antibiotic sensitivities.

As part of the human mouth, the *milleri* group—of which *intermedius* is part—have been exposed to beaucoup antibiotics. Showing intermediate resistance to penicillin is not uncommon. Makes me nervous, but in attempt to salvage the knee without taking it out, I decided to give ceftriaxone for 6 weeks.

Rationalization

Houston, B.D., M.E. Crouch, and R.G. Finch, Streptococcus MG-intermedius (Streptococcus milleri) septic arthritis in a patient with rheumatoid arthritis. J Rheumatol, 1980. 7(1): p. 89-92.

Yamamoto, N., et al., Trends in antimicrobial susceptibility of the Streptococcus milleri group. J Infect Chemother, 2002. 8(2): p. 134-7.

Postscript

It worked. Knee salvaged.

Inside Out or Outside In?

ELDERLY patient with progressive shoulder pain. It was on the side where he had decreased movement secondary to a stroke, but over several weeks his range of motion was further decreased due to pain in the shoulder. He was seen in the ER, the shoulder had no pathology, so he was treated for muscle strain. He had no other symptoms.

Then, about two weeks in, he developed increased pleuritic chest pain, i.e. pain with breathing.

Still no other symptoms, including cough or shortness of breath.

This lead to a CT, which showed a paraspinous mass infiltrating into the pleural space near the apex of the lung. He had been a smoker, so I thought of a Pancoast tumor—an eponym for a lung cancer that grows in the lung's apex, found almost exclusively in smokers.

So a biopsy was arranged, but only five days later, before it could be performed (like music, in medicine procedures are performed) he developed a huge lung abscess, had his first fever, and his blood groew *Streptococcus anginosis*—part of the milleri group of strep that are found in the mouth.

His teeth were fine, and he had no loss of consciousness nor infiltrate to suggest that he had pneumonia, so here is my hypothesis.

He had primary pyomyositis of the paraspinous muscles that eroded into this pleural space and then into the lung.

This is bass ackwards (lysdexics untied!) of the usual order of events, but the history suggested I was right, as did the CT scan. The CT showed osteomyelitis of the rib, which is more likely with a longstanding muscle infection than with a primary pulmonary infection. I will admit that rib osteo is rare as hen's teeth.

It alll started as a paraspinous phlegmon—then five days later, man oh man.

A huge abscess formed in five days. Impressive. Then he had a fever as it ruptured into the lung and he started to have a productive cough.

Arguing against this hypothesis is that there is only one report of *S. anginosis* pyomyositis in the literature. In my favor is the fact that I never let reality get in the way of a great diagnosis. I have seen a smattering of spontaneous pyomyositisesi (what is the pleural of pyomyositis?) due to *S. milleri*.

That's two *Strep milleri* group infections in two days. Will tomorrow be three? I am not going to say. You could call that a strep tease.

Rationalization

Fam, A.G., J. Rubenstein, and F. Saibil, Pyomyositis: early detection and treatment. J Rheumatol, 1993. 20(3): p. 521-4.

OTHER COCCI

Rash decisions

FEVER and a rash. A common infectious disease problem. Most rashes are often neither diagnostic nor important, a curious epiphenomenon of the underlying infection.

There is one rash that makes me nervous: petechiae. The patient this morning had sudden onset of fevers and rigors shortly followed by a progressive petechial rash.

Cue the music from Jaws, as the issue of *Neisseria meningitidis* rears its ugly pili. Nasty bug, it can kill almost as fast as a great white. I have seen people go from normal to dead in less than 8 hours from this organism.

There are curious epidemiologic features around *Neisseria meningitidis*. The main disease causing serotypes are A,B,C, W-135, and Y. What happened in the lab for D though V and W-1 to 134, I have never discovered. Wolverine, beware, there is a new strain of meningococcus, X, that in 1992 accounted for over half of the cases in Niger; it had been considered a relatively non-virulent strain in the past. Does Speed Racer suspect?

The vaccine does not cover group B meningococcus. Cuba had an outbreak with group B and they developed a vaccine that has some efficacy. For reasons I cannot discover, Cuba has been unwilling to share the vaccine with the US. Go figure. Molecular epidemiology suggests Cuba did share the organism with the US. Outbreaks of group B meningococcus in Florida are thought to have reached the US with Cuban immigrants. Another failure of immigration officials. Never would have happened in Arizona.

Group B is thought to have started in Europe in the 1970s, then to Cuba, to South America (thanks, Che) and then to my own state of Oregon, where we had an outbreak in 1992. We continue to have issues with group B disease.

Fortunately this bug is still easy to kill. Antibiotic resistance is reported, but is rare.

The other curiosity is there is a wide variety of reasons people can get ill with meningococcus: complement deficiencies, alterations in Toll-like receptors, but my favorite is variations in snot. If you have the wrong kind of snot, you are more likely to get meningococcus and die:

"Meningococcal disease occurs after colonization of the nasopharynx with Neisseria meningitidis. Surfactant protein (SP)-A and SP-D are pattern-recognition molecules of the respiratory tract that activate inflammatory and phagocytic defences after binding to microbial sugars. Variation in the genes of the surfactant proteins affects the expression and function of these molecules. METHODS: Allele frequencies of SP-A1, SP-A2, and SP-D were determined by polymerase chain reaction in 303 patients with microbiologically proven meningococcal disease, including 18 patients who died, and 222 healthy control subjects. RESULTS: Homozygosity of allele 1A1 of SP-A2 increased the risk of meningococcal disease (odds ratio [OR], 7.4; 95% confidence interval [CI], 1.3-42.4); carriage of 1A5 reduced the risk (OR, 0.3; 95% CI, 0.1-0.97). An analysis of the multiple single-nucleotide polymorphisms in SP-A demonstrated that homozygosity for alleles encoding lysine (in 1A1) rather than glutamine (in 1A5) at amino acid 223 in the carbohydrate recognition domain was associated with an increased risk of meningococcal disease (OR, 6.7; 95% CI, 1.4-31.5). Carriage of alleles encoding lysine at residue 223 was found in 61% of patients who died, compared with 35% of those who survived (OR adjusted for age, 2.9; 95% CI, 1.1-7.7). Genetic variation of SP-A1 and SP-D was not associated with meningococcal disease.

CONCLUSIONS: Gene polymorphism resulting in the substitution of glutamine with lysine at residue 223 in the carbohydrate recognition domain of SP-A2 increases susceptibility to meningo-

coccal disease, as well as the risk of death ."

Life and death often hinges on little things like a glutamine instead of a lysine in your mucous.

The patient today is fine thanks to prompt diagnosis and antibiotics. I will never know about his snot.

Rationalization

CDC, Serogroup B meningococcal disease—Oregon, 1994. MMWR Morb Mortal Wkly Rep, 1995. 44(7): p. 121-4.

Boisier, P., et al., Meningococcal meningitis: unprecedented incidence of serogroup X-related cases in 2006 in Niger. Clin Infect Dis, 2007. 44(5): p. 657-63.

Jack, D.L., et al., Genetic polymorphism of the binding domain of surfactant protein-A2 increases susceptibility to meningococcal disease. Clin Infect Dis, 2006. 43(11): p. 1426-33.

....

Prophylaxis?

Few diseases freak the ER out more than a case of meningococcal meningitis. The reason is not only the rapid, horrible death of the patient, but also the fact that that this is one of the few diseases where casual contact with the index case, aka the patients, increases your risk of getting the disease yourself. Then you get to have a rapid, horrible death, too.

If you are a household contact with a case of meningococcal meningitis, your risk of getting the disease is 500 to 800 times that of the general population.

Because of this, it is recommended that anyone who has been in a room for 4 or more hours with a person with meningococcus without a mask, or anyone who has contact with a patient's spit, needs chemoprophylaxis: rifampin or ciprofloxacin or ceftriaxone.

It is also recommended that those who have sat next to an index case on an airplane receive prophylaxis as well, not that there has been a case of meningococcus spread this way, although there has been spread of TB. It is a recurrent theme of this book: just do not inhale. It only gets you in trouble.

No doctor has EVER spent 4 hours in a room with a patient, although we do get exposed to the odd bit o' spittle now and then, mouth-to-mouth resuscitation being the classic exposure. So it is rare that a doc needs prophylaxis, and most other health care providers do not need prophylaxis either, especially if they are wearing masks. However, if there is a case of meningitis, many of the providers are in panic mode before the cultures are back, running to the ER looking for an antibiotic.

The family of the case mentioned in the previous chapter ended up in the ER asking for prophylaxis, which they did not need as the meningitis was not due to meningococcus.

The interesting question that arises with the need for prophylaxis is whether family members need prophylaxis not because the strain causing the meningitis is more virulent, but because the hosts are more susceptible.

There are several genetic variations in the immune system, aka polymorphisms, that predispose patients to developing meningococcal meningitis. My favorite, as I have mentioned before, is alterations in snot, or as the more scientific among us call it, surfactant protein-A2. It I ever get a parrot I am going to teach it to say "Polly want a morphism." Just as if I ever get a monochromatic dog, it will be named Spot.

The reason we get sick and die is often in our genes. I have a vial of MRSA in my Calvin Kleins. For homeland security, if you are reading this, that was meant to be a joke.

It may be that the health care professional, as well as the talented amateur, does not need the prophylaxis. Perhaps a genetic predisposition in families is the reason why families have an increased risk of disease, and not the exposure in and of itself. Perhaps we are inappropriately extrapolating family data to health care workers who screw up on basic infection control procedures.

On the other hand, I had a patient with meningococcus whose only exposure was sharing a beer three week prior with his friend who subsequently had meningococcus. As is often the case, the answer in not clear-cut, although the take-home message here may be to not drink from a friend's longneck.

Rationalization

CDC, Exposure to patients with meningococcal disease on aircrafts—United States, 1999-2001. MMWR Morb Mortal Wkly Rep, 2001. 50(23): p. 485-9.

van der Pol, W.L., et al., Relevance of Fcgamma receptor and interleukin-10 polymorphisms for meningococcal disease. J Infect Dis, 2001. 184(12): p. 1548-55.

....

A new personal record

I TELL my older patients that for each day they are in bed with a fever, it is three days to get their strength back. It isn't supposed to apply to me. I am young—yes I am, only 357 in dog years. Everyday I hit a wall at about 3 and need a nap, which I get on the drive home. But at least, thanks to the swimming-in molasses-speed at which I am moving at this week, I hit that wall slowly.

Today I saw an elderly male with classic meningitis, and the spinal fluid grew *Neisseria meningitidis*. Old people get *Streptococcus pneumoniae*; the oldest patient in whom I have seen *N. meningitidis* cause meningitis is about 45. It is rare in folks my age, with an attack rate of 0.1/100,000 in the elderly.

He had no immunosuppression and no good exposure or travel history (sub-Saharan Africa and the Hajj are popular ways to acquire meningococcus). So I guess this fell under the title: fecal matter occurs.

I bet it will be type B, the strain that predominates here in the Northwest, and the strain not covered by the vaccine. Other parts of the world have other strains, and sub-Saharan Africa is having an issue with type X. Perhaps that type will not been seen in people under 21 or only be available on hotel cable.

When there is an exposure to an index case of meningococcus, the exposed needs to take an antibiotic to prevent disease. The problem is that the current prophylaxis is ciprofloxacin, and there are now two reported cases of ciprofloxacin resistance.

In one case, the ciprofloxacin resistance was due to a point mutation in the binding site of the antibiotic. The other case the Meningococcus went and got new genes from a *Neisseria lactima* to become resistant. I hates it when they get new genes.

I still have the beta-lactams, so I will be able to kill this bug for a while yet.

Rationalization

Boisier, P., et al., Meningococcal meningitis: unprecedented incidence of serogroup X-related cases in 2006 in Niger. Clin Infect Dis, 2007. 44(5): p. 657-63.

Wu, H.M., et al., Emergence of ciprofloxacin-resistant Neisseria meningitidis in North America. N Engl J Med, 2009. 360(9): p. 886-92

....

A surprise

MY elderly (well, greater than 50 is often considered elderly, so I fit) patient with the *Neisseria meningiditis* meningitis awoke, but then had elbow pain and swelling.

The state (lab) told me the serotype was B, which is the most common *Neisseria* serotype in Oregon. The big four serotypes being A, B, C, and, after skipping D though V and 1 through 134, W-135. B is also the serotype not covered by the vaccine.

We (meaning someone else. I don't do anything that requires a needle) tapped his painful elbow, and there were 92,000 white cells and no crystals. He had an infected joint. How often does that occur with meningococcus? Rarely in kids, and less often in adults. Meningococcus is a rare cause of disease in adults, and a septic joint is a rare complication of the disease, so this is rare squared.

Curiously, some strains of meningococcus have an increased propensity for seeding joints, mostly W-135. Why? One of the many mysteries in medicine.

For those of you taking medicine boreds, remember: the underlying immunologic defect in patients with recurrent meningococcus is terminal complement deficiency.

Rationalization

Vienne, P., et al., The role of particular strains of Neisseria meningitidis in meningococcal arthritis, pericarditis, and pneumonia. Clin Infect Dis, 2003. 37(12): p. 1639-42.

....

Sine qua non

STILL the clinging brain fog of post-viral recovery. Good thing I am a professional and can fake it as needed. It makes the typing slllllloooooooowwwwwwwwwwwww. Tell me about the rabbits, George.

I like that phase. *Sine qua non* is a Latin legal term for "that without which it could not be."

There are symptoms or tests that define an illness. For an endovascular infection, the *sine qua non* is sustained bacteremia. Most infections result in intermittent bacteremia, but if the infection is in the bloodstream, then it seeds the blood continuously and the blood cultures are positive day after day, hour after hour.

Blood cultures two week apart for the same organism, *Enterococcus* in this case, means an endovascular infection, which usually means a heart valve infection. Today's patient had a pacemaker, so maybe that would be the source of bacteremia.

You tend to see enterococcal endocarditis in old men, which is probably the gift of an enlarging prostate. Prostate enlargement leads to urinary obstruction which may push the bug into the blood, and hence to the valve. It is my understanding that the womenfolk don't have a prostrate, and I have seen only one case of enterococcal endocarditis in a female.

There are two ways to give a rabbit endocarditis. One, make it a heroin addict. As Hef knows, nothing sadder than a junkie bunny. Two, put a wire across a valve and give the rabbit an intravenous bolus of bacteria. The valve, whacking against the wire 130+ times a minute (remember, it's a bunny), gets a little rough. This results in platelet-thrombin deposition, a place for the bug to grab a hold, and then endocarditis.

Pacers give that roughened valve, but most patients don't get a bolus of bacteria. Unless they have that pesky prostate. That reminds me, I need to have mine removed to be safe. I no longer need it. Or is that oversharing?

On transesophageal ECHO, the patient had an infection on the tricuspid valve, right where the valve bumped uglies with the pacer wire.

Now I can occasionally salvage an infected catheter, prosthetic joint, or artificial valve. But for whatever reason, the literature suggests you just can't save an infected pacer system. I have always failed when asked to try, no matter what magic cocktail of antibiotics I used.

Early in my career I had a patient with an infected pacer with *Serratia* and cardiology told me, "No way can we take it out without killing the patient." In a flash of genius, I thought: the problem is that the pacer wire is covered with clot. If I can strip off the clot with tissue plasminogen activator (tPA), then I can cure the infection. A serine protease enzyme, tPA is used in almost all cases of myocardial infarct to dissolve the clot. It's also used, more controversially, in ischemic stroke—the controversy being that an ischemic stroke that becomes a hemorrhagic stroke is a very, very bad thing. I hadn't read of any reports of using tPA to clean off pacer wires, but I tried it anyway.

Bad idea.

Not only did I strip off clot, the bacteria followed and he got "a touch septic," as I said afterwards with deliberate understatement. It did cure the infection, so he had the pacer pulled and did just fine, as they always do. I have since learned that, despite their protestations that they will kill the patient, cardiologists are actually quite incompetent at the task and have never followed through on the promise.

Rationalization

Friedberg, H.D. and G.F. D'Cunha, Adhesions of pacing catheter to tricuspid valve: adhesive endocarditis. Thorax, 1969. 24(4): p. 498-9.

Utili, R., E. Durante-Mangoni, and M.F. Tripodi, Infection of intravascular prostheses: how to treat other than surgery. Int J Antimicrob Agents, 2007. 30 Suppl 1: p. S42-50.

Postscript

The pacer came out with no complications.

....

Not a bacteria for a 'real' man

THE patient has known valvular heart disease and part of the evaluation as an outpatient is an echocardiogram, just called ECHO.

It shows a small vegetation on the aortic valve, confirmed on a transesophageal ECHO.

Years ago, in my L.A. days, I was called about what to do because the surgeon had worn her mask around her neck during lunch, and in the middle of the case a broccoli floret fell onto the heart. Largest vegetation I've ever seen.

In this case, the history and exam did not really support a heart valve infection, but it was hard to deny the reality of a floppy vegetation.

For four days the blood cultures were negative. Damn. The patient had no risk factors for the odd organisms that cause culture-negative endocarditis. Then, suddenly, there were gram positive cocci in clusters. Coagulase negative staph? Maybe, but then it turns out to be *Micrococcus*.

Huh. *Micrococcus* is a gram positive coccus that forms tetrads, which makes it sound like some sort of Ninja. *Micrococcus* is found in soil, water, beer (Oh. My. God.), marine sediments, dry Italian sausages, miso, and Spanish dry-cured ham. Pretty much my favorite dinner. Mostly a part of the human skin and mouth, it is what causes the smell in a stinking foot. The organism responsible for the Scholl's fortune.

Endocarditis from *Micrococcus* is unusual: 17 cases or so in the literature. And I suppose it could be a contaminant, but I will treat it.

Rationalization

Seifert, H., M. Kaltheuner, and F. Perdreau-Remington, Micrococcus luteus endocarditis: case report and review of the literature. Zentralbl Bakteriol, 1995. 282(4): p. 431-5.

Postscript:

He was cured with antibiotics. Whether he would have been cured without them, we shall never know.

TALES OF RESISTANCE

Chicken Feed

THE last call of the day yesterday, before I turned off my beeper for a weekend of kids' soccer and *Saccharomyces*, concerned a bad case of colitis. An elderly man had been admitted to the hospital with a case of bloody diarrhea, so bad they were worried he had bowel ischemia. He was placed on ciprofloxacin and metronidazole, didn't get better, then had a CAT scan that demonstrated a severe pan-colitis. After a couple of days his stool cultures grew *Campylobacter jejuni*. No big deal, case closed. The patient had a relatively common cause of bacillary diarrhea.

What is interesting is that the organism is resistant to ciprofloxacin, and what is even more interesting is the why. Ciprofloxacin is a quinolone, a class of synthetic broad-spectrum antibiotics.

Antibiotic resistance can occur from many mechanisms. Most of our antibiotics are derived from molecules that exist in bacteria and their ilk. Microbes are in constant competition with each other, and some compete by producing antibiotics that kill off the competition. The drug companies modify these natural antibiotics so that they have better pharmacologic properties. But as a defense in the wild, other organisms make molecules that destroy the antibiotics so they are not killed by the antibiotics made by other organisms or by the antibiotics they themselves make. There is an ongoing low grade battle in the dirt and in your colon between the production of antibiotics and anti-antibiotics.

Articles in *Science* suggest that the number of potential resistance genes seen clinically pales in comparison to the number of resistance genes available in the wild. Bacterial species can fairly easily acquire genes from other species and put them to use, so there is a large reservoir of resistance genes just waiting to jump into human pathogens given the right opportunity. Infectious disease is nothing if not applied evolution.

The other way we breed resistance is to induce new mutations in organisms by exposing them to low levels of antibiotics. In the microbial world, what doesn't kill you truly makes you stronger. Low levels of antibiotics can lead to a variety of mutations that make antibiotics less active, a mechanism independent of new gene acquisition.

The Borg were wrong: resistance is not futile, it is inevitable. And because the bacteria out—multiply us, they have an evolutionary advantage over any antibiotic we can throw at them. We intensify this battle by adding huge amounts of antibiotics into the world, some in people, but even more in agriculture. In the US, 70% (yep, seventy, seven-zero percent) of antibiotics are used in agriculture. Low levels of antibiotics in chicken feed (and other animal and vegetable feed) lead to bigger, healthier (someone will argue this point) animals that go to slaughter sooner. Your cheap 8 lb. fryer at Safeway gets that way in part because there have been small amounts of antibiotics in the chicken feed.

And that leads back to the *Campylobacter*. When quinolones are used in chicken feed, resistance develops from a simple amino acid substitution at the antibiotic binding site which occurs in days and lasts for weeks, even after the antibiotics are stopped. Resistant organisms can be found in the chicken at the time of slaughter. Some studies have found resistance *Campylobacter* in grocery chickens approaching 50% of chickens tested.

The agricultural industry has long argued that there is no proven connection between animal antibiotics and human pathogen resistance, and fought for years any attempt to restrict the use of antibiotics in farm animals. Go, Bayer. But the data were clear enough that the *Campylobacter* resistance seen in human disease was from use of quinolones in animal feed that the use of these antibiotics was banned in 2005.

This ban is a good thing. Many of the bacterial causes of diarrhea (*Campylobacter*, *Salmonella*) are found in the colons of the animals we love to eat and to whom we give tons of antibiotics, breeding further resistance. I always bear in mind that everything we eat has a fine film of human and/or animal stool on it. The last act of every animal when it dies, including you, is to release its bowels, and if the animal is to be eaten, some part of the final BM ends up in the food. Bon appétit.

One hopes that without the ongoing pressure of quinolones in the chicken feed, *Campylobacter* will revert to susceptible again, since resistance is costly to the organisms. It helped in Australia. Maybe not—but that is the topic of a future essay.

Rationalization

D'Costa, V.M., et al., Sampling the antibiotic resistome. Science, 2006. 311(5759): p. 374-7.

Martinez, J.L., Antibiotics and antibiotic resistance genes in natural environments. Science, 2008. 321(5887): p. 365-7.

Powerful Antibiotics

B IG Gun.
  Strong.
Powerful.

These are adjectives that are often used to describe antibiotics. There are few things in medicine that are 100%, but any physician who uses the above adjectives to describe an antibiotic doesn't know a burro from a burrow (1). It is 100% sensitive and 100% specific that the speaker is a moron when it comes to antibiotic use, is a sucker for drug company commercials, and/or is blowing smoke up your butt.

These are advertising terms. Antibiotics have no intrinsic power. They are marketed that way to fool clinicians into thinking they are doing right by their patients. My patient has what appears to be a serious infection. Should I have give a strong, powerful, big gun, and heavily detailed antibiotic? Like Cipro, whose web site says "19 years of Power and Confidence"? Or Zosyn, which features a lightening bolt, presumptively from the gods, hitting an agar plate? Can't get stronger than a lightening bolt. Or Ertap-enem, whose motto is the "Power of One." Me? I thought one was the loneliest number I ever knew. It is my considered opinion that two can be as sad as one, it's the loneliest number since the number one. Ohhhh. Of course I'll give one of those antibiotics. They have POWER.

The question is rather, what is the best antibiotic that will op-timally kill an organism in a given body space? It may well be one of those antibiotics. It may not. It depends, curiously enough, not on some mystical "power," but whether a given organism is sus-ceptible to being killed by the antibiotic and whether that antibi-otic achieves killing levels where the infection is. And you know that from the local microbiology and the pharmacokinetics of an antibiotic, not a marketing slogan.

Antibiotics are also sometimes considered strong not because of marketing, but due to a mistaken tradition. Vancomycin is be-lieved, incorrectly, to be a strong antibiotic. Now, if I had neu-rosyphilis—and there may be those readers who, after reading a few chapters, think that I do—treatment with vancomycin would have zero effect. Nothing strong about vancomycin when it comes to syphilis.

Sometimes, because of resistance, all we have to offer is a half-assed antibiotic. Vancomycin is an archetype of a lousy an-tibiotic: toxic, poor pharmacokinetics, bacteriostatic, and, when compared against a penicillin, always inferior. Over the last de-cade the use of vancomycin has increased because it is one of the few drugs we have to treat methicillin-resistant *Staphylococcus aureus*, the dread MRSA.

Vancomycin's lack of reliable efficacy is demonstrated in a re-cent retrospective study (one of many):

"Two-hundred and fifteen cases were included. Vancomy-cin monotherapy was given in 73%. Failure rates by infection site were as follows: osteomyelitis 37/81 (46%), epidural ab-scess five/18 (28%), surgical wound four/15 (27%), pneumonia eight/45 (18%), endocarditis five/32 (16%), bloodstream five/42 (12%), joint 1/23 (4%), and meningitis 0/1 (0%)."

As a treatment for infection, those response rates stink on ice. So much for a strong, powerful, big gun antibiotic. Instead, give the appropriate antibiotic.

Rationalization

(1) Burro = ass, burrow= hole in the ground.

Dombrowski, J.C. and L.G. Winston, Clinical failures of appropriately-treated methicillin-resistant Staphylococcus aureus infections. J Infect, 2008. 57(2): p. 110-5.

....

MRSA Questions

ONE definition of an expert is someone who knows more and more about less and less until she knows everything about nothing.

For me, it is the opposite. I seem to know less and less about more and more until one day I will know nothing about everything.

Take MRSA. Please.

Today was another day of community acquired methicillin resistant *Staphylococcus aureus* infections. No big deal; it is our plague of toads for the 21st century. Resistant bacteria are no surprise. Antibiotics are used, the organisms mutate or acquire new genes to compensate, they become resistant. Simple intellig,..... I mean evolution.

But here is what I do not understand.

Resistance is costly for the organisms. It takes more energy to reproduce a genome encoding resistance genes, and it takes energy to make the resistance proteins, so resistant organisms often multiply slower. As a rule, in an antibiotic-free environment, MRSA should be out-competed by sensitive strains and should not survive in the community. Hospitals, yes. Nursing homes, yes. Pig farms, yes. These are antibiotic-rich environments and should select for MRSA.

But the community? Not only is MRSA surviving in the community, it is apparently supplanting the sensitive strains. MRSA infections are on the rise and here in StumpTown, 80% of community acquired Staphylococcal infections are MRSA. The community-acquired MRSA is a new strain as well, called the USA 300 strain.

USA. USA. USA. Hmm. Maybe the wrong time to be jingoistic. The USA strain had not been reported prior to 2000. Hmmm. The real Y2k bug?

So why is it that a resistant organism (and MRSA is resistant to many antibiotics besides methicillin) is so easily out-competing the wild type strains? New virulence genes? New ecologic niche? Lack of herd immunity to a new strain? I don't know. Probably all of the above.

And that leads me to another question.

I had a 78-year-old male who had broken his leg playing football when he was 16. Sixty years later the *S. aureus*, which had been hibernating all these years, finally cut loose and became symptomatic. Not a real surprise—sixty years between trauma and symptomatic infection is not even close to the reported record.

I knew it was probably a sixty-year-old Staphylococcus as it was susceptible to all antibiotics, including penicillin. It was like looking in the backyard and seeing a Neanderthal wander by.

Having *S. aureus* reactivate after 60 years is my personal record, but isn't going to win me any awards. Even in the era of antibiotics we sometimes get to see a bone infection that festers for decades before becoming symptomatic.

What to do about it? Probably nothing. The only cure would be amputation, and since there is no loss of structural integrity of the bone, it is best to beat it down with a little antibiotic.

The last 50 years have seen the intense pressure of antibiotics and other medical interventions on *Staphylococcus*: better nutrition, antibiotics, etc. have all helped to make it harder for *Staphylococcus* to infect humans. Is the MRSA of today really the same *Staphylococcus* of 50 years ago? I did a back of the envelope calculation that suggests that 50 years for bacteria is about the equivalent to 6 million years of human doubling. We were a 3 foot high hominid 6 million years ago, aka Lucy. What changes have occurred in *Staphylococcus* during the 50 years of the antibiotic era?

Do we have a new species? Is it still the same *S. aureus* as 50 years ago, or has there been enough change in the DNA of the organism that we should declare a new species? Have we missed the evolution of a new species? Is the new MRSA the equivalent of *H. sapiens* pushing out Neanderthals? Have I had one IPA too many? Enquiring minds want to know.

I have asked many a microbiologist these questions and all I get is a "What the hell are you talking about?" look.

Rationalization

Tenover, F.C. and R.V. Goering, Methicillin-resistant Staphylococcus aureus strain USA300: origin and epidemiology. J Antimicrob Chemother, 2009. 64(3): p. 441-6.

Donati, L., P. Quadri, and M. Reiner, Reactivation of osteomyelitis caused by Staphylococcus aureus after 50 years. J Am Geriatr Soc, 1999. 47(8): p. 1035-7.

Sarfati, F., et al., Chronic osteomyelitis caused by Klebsiella pneumoniae with a 50 year course. Medicosurgical management. J Chir (Paris), 1995. 132(8-9): p. 342-5.

Donati, L., P. Quadri, and M. Reiner, Reactivation of osteomyelitis caused by Staphylococcus aureus after 50 years. J Am Geriatr Soc, 1999. 47(8): p. 1035-7.

Gallie, W.E., First recurrence of osteomyelitis eighty years after infection. J Bone Joint Surg Br, 1951. 33-B(1): p. 110-1.

Here's the math

Bacteria divide every hour (approximate)

50 years x 365 days x 24 hours in a day = 438000 generations in 50 years.

18 years for humans to double ie reproduce. The legal lower end, at least outside of the South.

To get 438000 generations would take

438000 x 18 = 7, 884,000 years.

....

Incurable

LONG day, short chapter.
I had a consult today for something that used to never happen, but which I am seeing with increasing frequency: a staphylococcal infection I cannot cure.

The problem is MRSA. Some strains are resistant to damn near everything and when combined with a poor host (immunologically, not financially) and allergies, treatment options are limited.

I have a patient with an infection of her arm bone, the humerus (no joke here) with an MRSA that is sensitive to vancomycin, linezolid and daptomycin only. She developed an allergic reaction to vancomycin that shut down her kidneys, a rash to linezolid, and has relapsed after a 6 week course of daptomycin. A problem with daptomycin is that resistance can develop on therapy, so I am less than sanguine that I will still have that antibiotic when testing comes back. I really do not want to amputate her arm to cure her.

The reason that *S. aureus* is resistant to methicillin (the M in MRSA) is an alteration in the binding site on the surface of the bacteria where the antibiotic sticks. Instead of the normal cell wall protein, PBP, MRSA has a variant called PBP-2a (short for Penicillin Binding Protein Two aaaaaa; named by the Fonz). So no beta-lactam works. Not a cephalosporin, not a penicillin, not a carbapenem. All of these antibiotics function by attaching to PBPs and inhibiting cell wall biosythesis. In the 2a variant, the beta-lactam ring molecules bind weakly or not at all.

All the remaining antibiotics are equally lousy for treating MRSA and have higher failure rates than beta-lactams. There are new cephalosporins coming down the pike that are designed to bind to PBP-2a. I really hope these antibiotics are as good for

MRSA as cefazolin is for MSSA. Ceftobiprole is one of a class of agents that I am sure will be heavily detailed when it is released. As a rule, new antibiotics are rarely as good as they companies say they are—they almost never live up to the hype. No one can hype a piece of crap better than a drug rep, but I so badly need a drug that will kill MRSA that I am hoping that for once I am wrong, and that ceftobiprole or its equivalent will be all I need it to be. I want to be able to kill again.

You watch. It is going to cost a fortune. It will not be as active against MRSA as touted. I am sure to have my heart broken. Again.

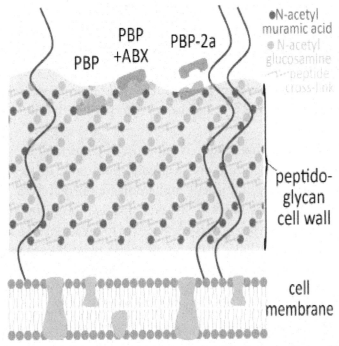

Schematic of antibiotic resistance in Gram positives. Penicillin-binding proteins (PBPs) catalyse transglycosylation and transpeptidation, resulting in cross-linking of the cell wall into its typical peptidoglycan structure. Beta-lactam antibiotics (ABS) inhibit wild-type PBPs, resulting in lack of polymerization and eventual cell death. The PBP-2a variant, encoded by the mecA gene, does not bind beta-lactams, rendering the organisms resistant.

The Continued MRSA Brouhahahahahahaha

THERE is a slow but continued pressure to do something about MRSA.

No doubt that MRSA is a problem. I cannot reliably kill it with the current antibiotics and it is becoming resistant to alternative agents.

Just this month there was an outbreak of linezolid resistant MRSA that killed half the patients who developed it. Not a surprise. Linezolid resistance should be easy enough for the organism to develop.

So we have to do something. But what?

Check patients for MRSA and isolate them when they are admitted? To adequately check each patient for MRSA, you would have to culture nose, throat, rectum and skin. Four cultures. And if you were to use one swab to obtain 4 specimens, in what order do you do the collecting? The CDC guidelines say once an MRSA, always an MRSA, and isolate the patient. Unlike love, MRSA is forever.

The problem is that Staph is more or less normal flora. It comes and goes depending on local conditions, and in the end it will be futile to try and isolate and eradicate normal flora. The patient who is MRSA negative today is positive tomorrow from a visitor. The doctor who is MRSA negative today is positive next week from the handshake from his psoriatic neighbor. Staph is everywhere you don't want it to be, the anti-VISA card.

Isolation of patients is not without its dangers. Patients who are in isolation get less care and have more complications and falls. No good deed ever goes unpunished.

The problem is not MRSA, which is probably a sentinel chicken of bad infection control practices. If there is transmission of pathogens in the hospital then the problem is not the pathogens, but the health care providers. We probably markedly under-appreciate the number of organisms spread in the hospital, because it is expensive and time-consuming to type organisms to look for relatedness in outbreaks.

The key to control of MRSA is proper infection control. Like hand washing.

If you have a problem with MRSA in your institution, the problem isn't the bug. Look in the mirror. Someone isn't serious about infection control.

Rationalization

"Outbreak of Linezolid-Resistant Staphylococcus aureus in Intensive Care." ICAAC—IDSA 2008; Abstract C2-1835a.

....

Failure

I HATE failure. Even though I should expect it, the annoying thing about medicine is that you can do everything correctly and fail.

Eight weeks ago a patient came in with sustained staphylo-coccal bacteremia. Sustained bacteremia is the *sine qua non* of endocarditis, and it was the dread MRSA. Worse than the dread Pirate Roberts.

He was treated with a 6-week course of vancomycin, and now he is back with another case of sustained bacteremia. Crap. To quote the dread poet Robert, "The best laid schemes of mice and men / Gang aft a-gley." Could not have said it better myself, although I try not to drink when I write poetry.

The problem with vancomycin is that all susceptible organisms are not the same.

The MIC (mean inhibitory concentration in micrograms per milliliter) for a susceptible *S. aureus* can be 0.5, 1.0, 1.5 and 2.0. As the MIC increases, the treatment success rates fall. His MRSA had an MIC of >= 1.0. Should have been fine by the vancomycin. It wasn't. It could be that heterogeneity of vancomycin resistance was a factor. Staph, like humans, can be a sloppy reproducer. By kicking out mutant sub-populations that had slightly higher MICs to vancomycin, and perhaps I selected for these strains.

"Data from multiple laboratories demonstrated that the resistant subpopulations (i.e., vancomycin MICs of 8-16 mg/mL) typically

represented 1 in 15 to 1 in 10⁶ colony—forming units (CFUs)."

I hope I have not bred a vancomycin resistant staph. Shouldn't happen, but one frets.

The outcome can hinge on as little as 0.5 micrograms per milliliter of vancomycin. Vancomycin just isn't all that great a drug, and the alternatives—linezolid and daptomycin-are no better in head to head trials. As best I can tell, them what think the alternatives are better than vancomycin have drank deeply at the trough of Big Pharma.

Fortunately, we do have new drugs coming down the pike that are cephalosporins that specifically target the mutation that makes MRSA MRSA. I predict 1) it will be very expensive and 2) resistance will occur. On the bright side, I may be able to kill MRSA again, if only for a short period of time.

Rationalization

Lodise, T.P., et al., Relationship between vancomycin MIC and failure among patients with methicillin-resistant Staphylococcus aureus bacteremia treated with vancomycin. Antimicrob Agents Chemother, 2008. 52(9): p. 3315-20.

Tenover, F.C. and R.C. Moellering, Jr., The rationale for revising the Clinical and Laboratory Standards Institute vancomycin minimal inhibitory concentration interpretive criteria for Staphylococcus aureus. Clin Infect Dis, 2007. 44(9): p. 1208-15.

....

Damned if you do, Damned if you don't

WHAT do you do when all the solutions stink on ice? Do something? Do nothing? Both?

The patient had bad (as opposed to the good?) methicillin resistant Staphylococcus endocarditis (MRSA) endocarditis (yet another) with a large vegetation on the mitral valve and emboli everywhere. Also, he has seeded both his eyes.

His MRSA was resistant to all the standard antibiotics except vancomycin, and that with an MIC of 2.

Once the MIC to vancomycin exceeds 1.0, failure rates start

to increase and it becomes impossible to safely dose vancomycin. So do you hold? Change? I have zero confidence in linezolid for endocarditis, at least when used as monotherapy, so I reasoned that if daptomycin is noninferior to vancomycin when the MIC to vancomycin ain't so bad, it should be better if the MIC to vancomycin is higher.

All men die. Socrates was a man. All dead men are Socrates. So much for reasoning. Daptomycin has no indication for left sided endocarditis either, but then none of the newer agents do. New antibiotics are usually approved for skin and soft tissue infections, which an antibiotic shampoo would probably cure.

So with trepidation I changed him to daptomycin. Whether or not it was the change (I do not think it was) he progressed his endocarditis, destroyed his valve and remained bacteremic.

He was, for a variety of reasons, a horrible surgical candidate. So now what?

Clinical Infectious Diseases suggests the best option is linezolid with a carbapenem for salvage, and he responded to that therapy. I had a similar patient with refractory MRSA endocarditis whom I cured with linezolid and ertapenem. Not my first choice, but I suppose reasonable if the patient is failing. Better than daptomycin? Eh.

I want the new MRSA cephalosporins, so called fifth generation (and I can always use fifth), to come out yesterday. I know they are going to charge an arm, leg and kidney for them (someone has to pay for that pizza at conference), but to be able to kill MRSA. Ah 'tis a consummation devoutly to be wished.

Rationalization

Jang, H.C., et al., Salvage treatment for persistent methicillin-resistant Staphylococcus aureus bacteremia: efficacy of linezolid with or without carbapenem. Clin Infect Dis, 2009. 49(3): p. 395-401.

Postscript

He was cured with a combination of linezolid and ertapenem,

and there are in vitro data to suggest the combination is synergistic. Two cures. I could say that in "in case after case" the combination is effective. If I can get three, I have a series.

....

Zoe Sin

THE holidays are over, so it is back to reality.

The Intensive Care Unit fellow said to me, "So, I hear you do not think much of Zosyn."

True story. I can count on one finger, probably the middle one, the number of times I have prescribed Zosyn, aka piperacillin/tazobactam.

I don't trust it, or any of the other penicillin/beta-lactamase inhibitors—Timentin (ticarcillin/clavulanate) or Unisin (my spelling for ampicillin/clavulanate).

Why? you might ask. Because the beta-lactamase inhibitor once said there were WMDs, and when I looked, well, no WMDs. So I can't trust them. As our soon to be ex said so eloquently "There's an old saying in Tennessee, I know it's in Texas, probably in Tennessee, that says, fool me once, shame on, shame on you. Fool me, you can't get fooled again." He must have been thinking of The Who. Greatest rock band of all time.

For all of you who are unaware, I am talking about a class of antibiotics that contain two drugs. One, the antibiotic. One of the mechanisms by which bacteria are resistant to antibiotics is to make enzymes, called beta-lactamases, that degrade antibiotics. Makes them wear bunny suits; very degrading. The antibiotic is combined with a drug, a beta-lactamase inhibitor, that prevents the antibiotic from being degraded by inactivating the beta-lactamase. Builds its self-esteem, as it were.

My problem?

Several.

The antibiotic and the inhibitor have different pharmacokinetics, so you are always hoping that there is enough inhibitor around to allow the antibiotic to kill. Antibiotics are referred to as bullets, but that is a bad metaphor; I can kill you with one bullet, but it takes hundreds or thousands of antibiotic molecules to kill a bacterium. Rather than bullets, antibiotics are more akin to death by a thousand cuts. I worry that there is not enough inhibitor around to allow the thousand cuts needed to kill the bacteria.

If the organism makes a beta-lactamase that is not affected by the beta-lactamase inhibitor—and many beta-lactamases are not inhibited by the current beta-lactamase inhibitors—then the inhibitor actually slightly inhibits the antibiotic instead. *Pseudomonas* does not make a beta-lactamase that is inhibited by tazobactam, and as a result the combo drug is less active than piperacillin alone.

The result of this may be death. Most antibiotics are given before the cultures come back. If you delay therapy in sick patients, they have 30% higher death rates, so you give the best antibiotic you can think of for the presumed organisms.

If that infecting organism is *Pseudomonas* and you gave Zosyn, then your patient is more likely to die.

"A total of 34 bacteremia episodes were identified involving isolates with reduced susceptibility to piperacillin-tazobactam (minimum inhibitory concentration, 32 or 64 mg/L, reported as susceptible); piperacillin-tazobactam was empirically given in 7 episodes. There was no significant difference in baseline characteristics between the 2 groups. Thirty-day mortality was found to be 85.7% in the piperacillin-tazobactam group and 22.2% in the control group (P = .004). Time to hospital mortality was also found to be shorter in the piperacillin-tazobactam group (P =; .001). In the multivariate analysis, 30-day mortality was found to be associated with empirical piperacillin-tazobactam therapy (odds ratio, 220.5; 95% confidence interval, 3.8-12707.4; P = .009), after adjustment for differences in age and APACHE II score."

I recognize that when I choose my empiric antibiotic, sometimes I am literally betting my patient's life that I can choose right.

I do not like losing that bet. So I never give Zosyn, especially if I do not know what bacterium is trying to kill my patient.

Rationalization

Tam, V.H., et al., Outcomes of bacteremia due to Pseudomonas aeruginosa with reduced susceptibility to piperacillin-tazobactam: implications on the appropriateness of the resistance breakpoint. Clin Infect Dis, 2008. 46(6): p. 862-7.

Unknown unknowns

"There are known knowns. There are things we know that we know. There are known unknowns. That is to say, there are things that we now know we don't know. But there are also unknown unknowns. There are things we do not know we don't know."

~ Donald Rumsfeld

Who knew?

That's the problem with fighting terrorists abroad so that they will not attack here at home, or at least not attack us again. All those unknowns. War wounds are expected. Whatever bacteria are in the soil, or on the skin, or on the uniform, or in the water can be dragged into humans by whatever projectile is trying to kill them. Post-traumatic infections are part of trauma, although good care can keep them at a minimum.

One of the now known knowns from our most recent war—but which was a prior unknown unknown—was the fact many of these war wounds are due to a relatively unusual organism, *Acinetobacter*. In the US *Acinetobacter* is an occasional ICU acquired infection; it is not usually seen in patients from outside the hospital. Iraq is a little different. One US military hospital ship had 57 *Acinetobacter* infections occurring in 211 inpatients admitted from March through May 2003.

That's a lot of *Acinetobacter* infections. We don't see that many per decade in my hospitals. These organisms cause a wide variety of trauma-associated infections with a relatively high mortality rate and, worst of all, tend to be resistant to almost all antibiotics except carbepenems and colistin, a detergent used as an antibiotic in the 1960's. You know you are in a world of hurt if you have to recall to duty detergents that were retired in the 1970's.

The source of these wound infections seems to be field hospitals where the wounded first receive care. This organism is ubiquitous in the environment:

"Thirty-six were isolated from samples of the hospital environment, and 1 was isolated from soil surrounding the hospital. Most (68%) were collected in critical care treatment areas (11 from intensive care units, 7 from operating rooms, and 7 from emergency departments). In patient care areas, ABC isolates were recovered from operating room equipment (anesthesia machine [n = 2], operating room table [n = 1] and light [n = 1], unspecified locations in the operating room [n = 2], environmental control units [i.e., heaters and air conditioners; n = 2], patient beds [n = 12], sinks [n = 8], and tent walls [n = 2]). ABC isolates were also recovered from other locations, including an environmental control unit (n = 1), environmental control unit drip lines or soil bags (n = 4), a drinking water source (n = 1), and soil outside a field hospital nutrition care section (n = 1). No ABC organisms were re covered from the 31 archived soil samples. Twenty-Five (20%) of the 125 environmental samples collected from the Dogwood, Mosul, Tikrit, and Balad hospital locations yielded ABC isolates."

With so much *Acinetobacter* in the environment, it is not surprising that there were wound and other infections. Organisms such as *Acinetobacter* do love to take advantage of traumatized flesh. There was one case where *Acinetobacter* was spread from an infected soldier to a healthy nurse.

Antibiotic resistance is also a worry, some isolates being resistant to all antibiotics.

"A. baumannii strain AYE exhibits an 86-kb genomic region termed a resistance island, the largest identified to date, in which 45 resistance genes are clustered. At the homologous location, the SDF strain exhibits a 20 kb-genomic island flanked by transposases but devoid of resistance markers. Such a switching genomic structure might be a hotspot that could explain the rapid acquisi-

tion of resistance markers under antimicrobial pressure. Sequence similarity and phylogenetic analyses confirm that most of the resistance genes found in the A. baumannii strain AYE have been recently acquired from bacteria of the genera Pseudomonas, Salmonella, or Escherichia."

45 resistance genes. Holy cannoli. That is a lot of resistance genes. It is a chest-pain-inducing number of resistance genes. If I were prone to anxiety, this would make me anxious. The thorazine does keep me calmer, and the voices a little softer.

If you see the words "resistance islands," think plate tectonics. These islands will drift to other places or, to mangle yet a another metaphor, explode like Krakatoa. Bacterial genes do not stay put. Bacteria can easily exchange resistance genes, and these organisms could be a source for future antibiotic resistance in other bacteria. Why Iraq has bred such resistant organisms is a mystery at the time this essay was published. Subsequently it was found to come from English hospitals.

Resistance is costly for organisms; resistance does not develop without a reason. I wonder, half seriously, if the *Acinetobacter* was the result of Iraqi genetic engineering gone bad. *Acinetobacter* would be a poor choice for a biological weapon, but accidents do happen when people are less than fastidious about their technique. But science prevails over paranoid conspiracy theories. Never attribute to malice that which is adequately explained by stupidity. It was probably a natural occurrence:

"Genomic islands are unstable regions and hotspots for the successive integration of resistance determinants in Salmonella spp., Escherichia coli, or Streptococcus thermophilus. We can safely assume that the mosaic-like structure of the AbaR1 island is the result of successive acquisitions of DNA fragments from different hosts, mainly Pseudomonas spp., Salmonella spp., and E. coli. "

The world is always odder than we can imagine.

Bacteria do so love to acquire other genes and use them. And pass them on. It is why we always lose the race between new antibiotics and resistance.

I wonder what bacteria lurk in the country of... never mind.

Rationalization

Scott, P., et al., An outbreak of multidrug-resistant Acinetobacter baumannii-calcoaceticus complex infection in the US military health care system associated with military operations in Iraq. Clin Infect Dis, 2007. 44(12): p. 1577-84.

Sebeny, P.J., M.S. Riddle, and K. Petersen, Acinetobacter baumannii skin and soft-tissue infection associated with war trauma. Clin Infect Dis, 2008. 47(4): p. 444-9.

Fournier, P.E., et al., Comparative genomics of multidrug resistance in Acinetobacter baumannii. PLoS Genet, 2006. 2(1): p. e7.

Wired, "The Invisible Enemy," Issue 15.02 (February 2007). http://archive.wired.com/wired/archive/15.02/enemy.html

Belt and Suspenders

A RESIDENT hit me up for a curbside after Grand Rounds. A curbside is where a doc asks you a question about a case, but does not want a formal consult. I like that term, formal consult. Like I should wear a tux. It is a way of giving me liability without remuneration, but is an important way that physicians learn.

He had a patient with a case of MRSA and gave the patient two antibiotics because he wanted to "double cover" the staph. Was that the right choice? Maybe. An enduring medical myth, that you need to give two antibiotics for infections.

I think this evolved from tuberculosis therapy, where it is critical to give at least two antibiotics to prevent the emergence of resistant organisms. Or perhaps from the early cancer chemotherapy era, when we had lousy drugs for *Pseudomonas* and two antibiotics were given. The mechanisms for prevention of resistance in TB do not apply to the treatment of most bacteria. In TB there are already preexisting resistant strains that are selected for by the antibiotic, while generally (and there are always exceptions) this is not true for most bacterial infections.

There are occasional bacterial infections that require two antibiotics: prosthetic valve endocarditis, prosthetic joint infections, toxic shock syndrome, and some kinds of streptococcal native valve endocarditis come to mind. But for routine staphylococcal and other infections, there is no reason to give more than one antibiotic once you know the susceptibility. If you don't know the susceptibility of the organisms as they are still growing in the lab, and there is a high probability that the organism is resistant to one of the empiric antibiotics, it is reasonable to give two antibiotics to CYA, or CYPA. In infected people, chose the wrong antibiotic up front and the patient has a much higher chance of dying.

You gotta double cover *Pseudomonas*. No, you don't. It's a myth. Most of the time one drug (as long as it is not Zosyn), if the organism is susceptible, is sufficient. Combination therapy does not increase cure rates or prevent the emergence of resistance. Double coverage does increase toxicity and expense, and is only of benefit in sepsis from gram negative rods.

The more intense the environmental pressure, the faster organisms will evolve to survive. Some bacteria have mechanisms that increase their mutation rates in the face of environmental stress. Antibiotics are an environmental stressor for bacteria. Combining antibiotics can lead to four different results in killing bacteria: the combination has no extra killing (it has no more killing than one antibiotic (1+1 = 1)); the combination can have additive killing (1+1 = 2); the combination can have synergistic killing (1+1 = 5); or the combination can be antagonistic (1+1 = 0).

It turns out, at least in *E. coli*, that combination antibiotic therapy leads to faster development of resistance compared to single antibiotic therapy. I had always thought the main way to get resistant organisms was to give a little amount of antibiotic for a long time, the application of the dictum "What doesn't kill you makes you stronger."

In a recent study, a group discovered that the more effective a combination of antibiotics was at killing bacteria, the faster the bacteria developed resistance. The better antibiotics are at killing bacteria, the faster they push the evolution of resistance. Bummer.

"We found a correlation between synergy and the rate of adaptation, whereby evolution in more synergistic drug combinations, typically preferred in clinical settings, is faster than evolution in antagonistic combinations. We also found that resistance to some synergistic combinations evolves faster than resistance to individual drugs."

Not only does double coverage not increase efficacy or decrease the development of resistance, in *E. coli* it accelerates the development of resistance. There are times when the evidence demands the use of combination therapy to improve outcomes. Outside of those conditions, monotherapy should suffice, and it has less impact on the local microbial resistance. As we slowly slide into the post-antibiotic era, avoiding combination antibiotics when they are not needed may help prevent the emergence of resistant bacteria.

It is always the rule in medicine: No good deed ever goes unpunished. The sooner you understand that little pearl, the less harm you will do.

Rationalization

Hegreness, M., et al., Accelerated evolution of resistance in multidrug environments. Proc Natl Acad Sci U S A, 2008. 105(37): p. 13977-81.

CYA: cover your ass

CYPA: cover your patient's ass

GANGRENE

....

Clostridia

WHEN I was a kid, I thought that the most horrible scene in the movies was the one in *Gone with the Wind* where the doc lops off the soldier's gangrenous leg without anesthesia and Miss Scarlett goes running out of the hospital in a panic.

I do not blame Miss Scarlett from running away from the sight, smell, and sound of a gangrenous leg amputated without anesthesia. Eew. And I certainly never wanted to know nothin' about birthin' babies.

Gas Gangrene is usually due to *Clostridium perfringens*, and *Clostridium perfringens* is an odd bug. Either it causes a rapidly progressive necrotizing infection with an equally rapid progression to death, or it is nothing important.

But when people get *C. perfringens* in a culture, it results in a quasi-urgent call to your friendly neighborhood I.D. doc.

The patient on Friday had a hip wound that, thanks to some bad post-operative diarrhea, became infected. So the surgeon cleaned it out and the cultures grew stool organisms, including *C. perfringens*.

The patient was fine. No necrosis, not sepsis, no gas in the tissues.

Under these circumstances, the *C. perfringens* was just sitting there, doing nothing, like a teenager on a Saturday afternoon, and was not pathogenic, unlike a teenager. It is estimated that half of *C. perfringens* isolates are colonization/contaminants. *C. perfringens* is part of the normal GI flora, and will show up as a fellow traveler in wounds, gallbladders and the blood, especially post-delivery. It has been found in every soil sample except, evidently, the Sahara desert. So it is not surprising that after a gunshot wound and a fall into the dirt, gangrene was a frequent complication of war wounds like the poor sod in Gone With the Wind. It kills impressively fast; I have seen skin poppers (when heroin users run out of veins they "pop" heroin under the skin and the heroin, especially the black tar kind, is rich in *C. perfringens*) go from fine to dead in less than a day.

Gas gangrene can also occur from *C. septicum* when the organism invades into bowel cancer. Since the infection starts internally and burrows out, it is hard to diagnose early, and is the source of the one and only post-mortem consult I have ever had. The patient came in multi-organ system failure from septic shock and died in about an hour after reaching the ICU. As they were preparing the body for transport, he developed a spreading, necrotic infection over his right hip and the pathologists called me, worried that something communicable was happening. It turned out that the patient had had *C. septicum* of the right colon that burrowed out through the hip. A quick gram strain showed the boxcar-shaped gram positive rods, and I could reassure the nurses they had nothing to worry about. Well, nothing so far as acquiring an infection from this patient was concerned, at least.

Over the years I have seen a handful of patients with lymphoma of the gut get chemo, which killed the lymphoma in the gut wall, offering the Clostridium a colon hold and allowing *C. perfringens* or *C. septicum* a chance to cut loose. One patient refused antibiotics and wanted to be given comfort care. And he survived. It was like falling out of an airplane without a parachute and surviving because you landed in swamp mud. In Nevada. Amazing.

The other *Clostridium* that kills you quickly, and which I hope never to see, is *Clostridium sordellii;* it causes sepsis after medical abortion using mifepristone and intravaginal misoprostol.

Those darn Clostridia, lurking everywhere, just waiting to kill us.

Oh yeah. Go Ducks. The Gang Green.

Rationalization

CDC, Clostridium sordellii toxic shock syndrome after medical abortion with mifepristone and intravaginal misoprostol—United States and Canada, 2001-2005. MMWR Morb Mortal Wkly Rep, 2005. 54(29): p. 724.

Garcia-Suarez, J., et al., Spontaneous gas gangrene in malignant lymphoma: an underreported complication? Am J Hematol, 2002. 70(2): p. 145-8.

Krautter, U., et al., Fatal Clostridium septicum infection in a patient with non-Hodgkin's lymphoma undergoing multimodal oncologic therapy. Onkologie, 2009. 32(3): p. 115-8.

....

French Eponym

THE French dominated infectious diseases for decades because of the head start afforded by Louis Pasteur, whose name is immortalized in the song Louie Louie, a little ditty recorded by the Kingston Trio in Portland, Oregon. The lyrics have a history of being obscure, and perhaps obscene, but I think the song is about the sterilization of food to prevent acute diarrhea.

"Louie Louie, oh no. Me gotta go. Aye-yi-yi-yi, I said. Louie Louie, oh baby. Me gotta go."

The application of Pasteurization has made food-borne gastroenteritis less of a problem, but the downside has been fewer Top 40 hits with obscure, perhaps obscene, lyrics.

There are numerous eponyms for infectious diseases that carry the names of French physicians and they are all bad. The diseases, not the French physicians.

Today was one of the dreaded eponyms, Fournier's gangrene. Gangrene is bad enough, but add a dead French physician to it and you have disaster.

Fournier's is also called "mixed synergistic necrotizing fasciitis."

Mixed, because it is due to multiple organisms.

Synergistic, as the organisms work together in a supportive

environment to self-actualize and cause more damage than any single organism could. Usually it is a mixture of *E .coli*, streptococci, and anaerobes.

Necrotizing, meaning it dissolves tissues.

Fasciitis, referring to a deep, burrowing infection of the fascia, the connective tissue between the muscle and the skin.

Fournier's usually occurs in diabetics and in the perineum, the area you use to sit on a bicycle seat. It is one of many infections that liquefy soft tissues. It is what accounts, I believe, for the death of Elphaba Thropp, aka the Wicked Witch of the West.

Antibiotics are all well and good, but the real treatment is widespread debridement. The first case I saw was a young male that required removal of most of the soft tissue of his thighs and abdomen, including his scrotum. His testicles were resting on a damp towel; I cringe and curl up as I type this. All forms of gangrene require extensive and disfiguring surgery to cure the infection. But the only other alternative is rapid death. (Thanks to the magic of plastic surgery, this patient eventually had a pretty good cosmetic result).

Today's patient had his debridement and is doing well, albeit with a cantaloupe-sized chunk of flesh gone. It is important to make all metaphors in medicine related to food in some way.

It is the unstated goal of every doctor to become immortalized with an eponym, although in fairness it should be named after the patient rather than the doctor.

What, I wonder, will be Crislip's syndrome. Ideas?

Rationalization

A terrific site with medical eponyms for all platforms:

http://eponyms.net/

....

Cringe Worthy

B EFORE penicillin, a chance to cut was a chance to cure. As resistance is slowly increasing in all the major pathogens, I expect I may have to relearn how to scrub into a case. Ick.

Fournier has a sign, a tibia, and a gangrene named after him—not bad for a lifetime studying syphilis.

Fournier's gangrene is usually a little strep, a little gram negative rod (usually *E. coli*) and a lot of anaerobes. There have been an increasing number of cases of MRSA causing necrotizing fasciitis, but only few Fournier's.

The patient came in with rapidly progressive necrotizing infection and was treated rapidly with aggressive debridement and broad-spectrum antibiotics. Much to my surprise, all the cultures grew methicillin sensitive *Staphylococcus aureus* (MSSA). Not the typical organism. The key for patient survival is rapid and extensive debridement. And they found "frank pus." What the hell is frank pus? There is frank bleeding, which is contrasted with occult bleeding. But there is not occult pus, so there is no reason to ever append the adjective "frank" to the noun "pus."

MSSA is reported in a smattering of cases of Fournier's, but is my first causing this disease.

There are three reported cases of Fournier's after vasectomy, although with vasectomy they report the more typical of group A strep post-op necrotizing fasciitis than the classic mixed microbiology.

Still. Hardly seem like a good trade-off to be sterile.

Rationalization

Viddeleer, A.C. and G.A. Lycklama a Nijeholt, Lethal Fournier's gangrene following vasectomy. J Urol, 1992. 147(6): p. 1613-4.

....

It's a gas

B UT while all that glitters is not gold, all that is gas is not *Clostridium*.

Today I saw a young female who twisted her ankle and 24 hours later had an abrupt onset of marked rubor, dolor, calor, tumor of her leg from ankle to knee. And lots of pain. She was seen in the ER and X-rays showed gas. A CT scan was obtained, showing even more gas, all up and down her calf. The patient was surprisingly non-toxic and had no underlying medical problems, but was whisked off to the OR for fasciotomies. No gas gangrene, the tissues looked fine and the gram stain had gram positive cocci. I am betting group A strep (which it was).

Gas in tissues is always worrisome, but is not always clostridial. With gas gangrene, by the time you see the gas it is probably too late—it is a late finding of the disease and you better call the coroner. I have seen much larger volumes of gas over the years for *S. aureus*, Group A *Streptococcus* and *Candida* than I ever have from *C. perfringens*. I have seen one other case of acute cellulitis with lots of gas in a cook who stabbed his hand.

It would appear from PubMed that gas with cellulitis but no necrosis is infrequency reported, but in emphysematous pyelonephritis there is lots of gas produced from a wide variety of organisms. And often there is gas in abscesses, presumably from the infecting organisms.

Gas bad. But sometimes maybe not all that bad; only a vigorous bacterial farting.

FUNGI

Yeast in the Urine

THERE are diseases that are difficult to treat. *Candida* in the bladder is probably self-limited, but upper urinary tract disease is problematic and there are no satisfactory therapies, especially for non-*albicans Candida* (Can da da, not can DEE da).

If you have a diabetic with kidney stones and post-obstructive pyelonephritis due to *C. tropicalis*, like today's consult, what do you treat the patient with? Which preposition is best to end a sentence? First, of course, relieve the obstruction. But which antifungal?

Non-*albicans Candida* are relatively resistant to fluconazole.

The echinocandins are a class of drugs often called the "penicillin of antifungals," since they inhibit fungal cell wall synthesis by non-competitive inhibition of the enzyme that makes glucan. These drugs are great—everywhere but the urine, where they get no urinary levels. Capsofungin is the echinocandin usually used against *Candida*. But for a urinary tract infection, it is a piss poor drug. Wha wha wha wha.

Amphotericin B is great for killing *Candida*, but it can also kill the kidney. I am not a fan of calling it amphoterrible, since most of the time bad side effects can be avoided if you know what you are doing and are judicious in your use of the drug. Most of the time. If I have a 90-year-old with diabetic nephropathy in his one transplanted kidney, and who's on cyclosporin—well, maybe there is not much you can do to protect the three remaining nephrons.

Decisions. Decisions.

Perhaps I could get away with caspofungin, as there was a series of cases reported in *Clinical Infectious Diseases* of caspofungin used successfully in *Candida* cystitis. On the other hand, it was by Merck minions and the lead author got many dollars from Merck.

"Manuscript preparation. Merck initially submitted case record forms of patients with candiduria to J.D.S. but had no role in selection of the patients described. Potential conflicts of interest. J.D.S. has received recent funding support from Pfizer, Merck Research Laboratories, and Astellas Pharmaceuticals, has previously participated in multicenter clinical research with and studies funded by Merck, and has served as a consultant to and is on the speakers, bureau for Merck. S.K.B., C.J.L., and N.A.K. are all employees of Merck Research Laboratories."

It did not inspire confidence as a study free of bias.

The best bet is probably amphotericin B, and if I give a small amount (0.3 mg/kg a day) using constant infusion, I may avoid the nephrotoxicity.

I am not that big a fan of lipid-complexed amphotericin. It costs a mint (about 400 dollars a dose. Yes, $400. How else is that "free" pizza paid for at conference?), is not more effective agaisnt *Candida*, and for most cases only somewhat less toxic. If I am treating a kidney infection, I WANT my ampho in the kidney where it can kill some yeast, rather than complexed to fat and taken up by the reticuloendothelial system instead. I prefer regular amphotericin if the patients can tolerate it, and with constant infusion they often do.

Rationalization

Sobel, J.D., et al., Caspofungin in the treatment of symptomatic candiduria. Clin Infect Dis, 2007. 44(5): p. e46-9.

Imhof, A., R.B. Walter, and A. Schaffner, Continuous infusion of escalated doses of amphotericin B deoxycholate: an open-label observational study. Clin Infect Dis, 2003. 36(8): p. 943-51.

I.D. man. Pronounced eye-dee, not id, like the Freudian dealy-bob.

Like Superman, I have powers. Special powers. Not like special education.

I am the only doctor who can stop an antibiotic. I am the only doctor who can ignore cultures.

Today, I had the opportunity to do both. While I was gone this weekend, one of my patients had a bronchoscopy and the cultures grew *Candida tropicalis*. The patient was started on caspofungin. I stopped the caspofungin with my superhuman powers. Next up is leaping over a tall building.

Candida in the sputum can virtually always be ignored.

My wife likes to garden. More, I think, than anything else. Her favorite garden tool is the chipper-shredder and she can spend hours stuffing plants into it, making mulch. It worries me that her favorite movie is *Fargo*, and she says it is due to the fact she is a Minnesotan. I am not so sure, and I keep my distance when she is chipper-shreddin'.

Now if I were to be involved with a tragic chipper-shredder accident and lose all but both thumbs, I could easily count the number of true *Candida* pneumonias I have seen in my 25 or so years as a superhuman infectious disease physician.

One was a massive aspiration in a patient with severe *Candida* esophagitis, and there was *Candida* in the alveoli at autopsy. The other was what I thought was an *Aspergillus* fungus ball, but when it was resected it was a big ball o' *Candida*.

Candida just almost never ever causes a lung infection in mostly normal patients. Well, sometimes it will infect the hematologic malignancy patients, especially if they have profound neutropenia. But these patients can grow anything in any site.

If you grow *Candida* in a sputum of a normal patient, pay no attention to it. Especially do not go starting caspofungin. That stuff runs 2 to 3 hundred dollars a dose.

Be my sidekick. I.D. lad, ignore the *Candida*.

Rationalization

Meersseman, W., et al., Significance of the isolation of Candida species from airway samples in critically ill patients: a prospective, autopsy study. Intensive Care Med, 2009. 35(9): p. 1526-31.

Haron, E., et al., Primary Candida pneumonia. Experience at a large cancer center and review of the literature. Medicine (Baltimore), 1993. 72(3): p. 137-42.

....

Leukemoid

THE higher the white count, the more you fret. This patient was admitted with a WBC of 1800 thanks to the magic of chemotherapy—a bit low, but not bad for a cancer patient. She also had *C. difficile* diarrhea thanks to the magic of antibiotics. Within four days her white count had jumped to ten times normal—106,000—with a nasty differential. Myelocytes and metamyelocytes and I have never metamyelocyte I liked. Thank you, Will Rogers. These are immature neutrophils, and in a normal blood smear, all neutrophils should be mature. The presence of immature neutrophils is called a "left shift," and usually indicates a bacterial infection.

One would think she was heading to have her colon removed due to severe colitis, at least to judge from her white count. And yet. She was stable. No fevers, no hypotension; her belly was slightly distended and moderately tender. The flat plate showed no toxic megacolon. Should she go to the OR? If she was heading for perforation, the sooner the colectomy, the better. But what might be happening instead is that she has a form of IRIS—Immune reconstitution inflammatory syndrome, first described in AIDS when patients would become symptomatic with preexisting infections as their immune systems returned on anti-retroviral therapy. As the T cells came back, they started to recognize pre-existing pathogens, causing symptoms of infection.

IRIS has been described in cancer patients who have *Aspergillus* lung disease. As the immune system returns after chemotherapy, there is clinical and radiological worsening of the lung disease. Interestingly, getting sicker as the white cells return is a good prognostic sign. IRIS has also been described postpartum, since pregnancy is an immunosuppressive state. Could IRIS be occurring in this patient's colon? If so, she needed time, not an operation. There was a real disconnect between the highest non-leukemia white count of my career and how clinically good she looked. Time to nervously drum my fingers on the table.

And time, that wounder of all heels, worked yet again. The patient did fine: like this sentence she has a colon.

Rationalization

Miceli, M.H., et al., Immune reconstitution inflammatory syndrome in cancer patients with pulmonary aspergillosis recovering from neutropenia: Proof of principle, description, and clinical and research implications. Cancer, 2007. 110(1): p. 112-20.

Singh, N. and J.R. Perfect, Immune reconstitution syndrome and exacerbation of infections after pregnancy. Clin Infect Dis, 2007. 45(9): p. 1192-9.

Never Heard of It

ALMOST a quarter of a century. That's how long I have been an MD. I realized that there is only one other doc older than me in the Department of Medicine at Good Samaritan, and he is my boss. I now get to complain in a querulous old voice about how much better it was back in the day.

But even after all this time I am still called upon to kill things I have never heard of.

Another urinary obstruction. I seem to have a run on these, with yeast in the nephrostomy tubes and acute renal failure.

I expect some sort of *Candida* or other, but after 5 days the lab said it was..

Cue up the dramatic prairie dog…

Trichosporon asahii.

Never heard of it. Well, I have, evidently, as it is in the Compendium, but I will be damned if I remember writing about it.

PubMed is not of much use, although evidently it is a common yeast in Japan, I have never seen a case in the US. Is there a genetic or environmental reason for the disease in Japan? Or is it found in the Japanese beer? And no, not Kirin. Asahi means "morning sun" in Japanese, in case you wanted to know. So I assume it is the rising sun *Trichosporon*.

In Japan, T. asahii acts like Candida, causing a variety of infections in patients with poor immunity, but I can't find much on therapy.

Thank goodness for Dr. Fungus (http://www.doctorfungus.org/). If you have a weird-ass fungus (or a weird ass-fungus) and no clue as to what to do, search Dr. Fungus.

Voriconazole is evidently the best of breed and amphotericin cannot be trusted.

So voriconazole it is.

But don't forget Dr. Fungus, even if it sounds like one of Spiderman's rogues.

Candida parapsilosis

THERE are a bunch of *Candida* out there.

When I was a young whippersnapper, all clinical isolates of *Candida* were *C. albicans*, but there has been a slow shift away from *C. albicans* to non-albicans *Candida* causing disease. Like the patient I saw today, who was in the ICU leaking bile into his peritoneum. He was growing *C. parapsilosis* and had had a fever and increased white count, so it was probably the real deal.

But what to treat him with?

C. parapsilosis has higher minimum inhibitory concentrations (MICs) to fluconazole, so I get nervous with that agent in general. This patient would probably be just fine if I used it, though, given that he had no other issues with his immune system.

The echinocandidins are a good bet, and as a rule all the *Candida* are sensitive—except, it turns out, some *C. parapsilosis*, which isn't your father's *C. parapsilosis*.

C. parapsilosis is actually three in one, a trinity of *Candida*: *C. parapsilosis sensu stricto, Candida orthopsilosis,* and *Candida metapsilosis.* My lab can't tell the difference, but depending on which one it really is, there are different susceptibilities to the various antifungals.

Voriconazole or posaconazole may be good choices, but are pricey, and like so many patients, he is not uninsured. I hate to add cost to a patients care without good reason.

Decisions decisions, and the problem is no clinical trials, just *in vitro* susceptibility, to guide therapy. I think I will call a psychic to guide my decision. The first five minutes are free.

Rationalization

Tay, S.T., S.L. Na, and J. Chong, Molecular differentiation and antifungal susceptibilities of Candida parapsilosis isolated from patients with bloodstream infections. J Med Microbiol, 2009. 58(Pt 2): p. 185-91.

van Asbeck, E., et al., Significant differences in drug susceptibility among species in the Candida parapsilosis group. Diagn Microbiol Infect Dis, 2008. 62(1): p. 106-9.

Postscript

The patient did fine on high dose fluconazole. The benefits of a normal immune system and draining the pus.

Answer these questions three

THREE questions. Not name, quest and favorite color. Every infection comes with three questions that I should try to answer:
* What is the bug?
* How best to kill it?
* How did it get there?

The last is often the more interesting question. The name of the bug often will be the hint as to where it came from. Infections have patterns.

Years ago I was called by the nurse to see a patient in the ICU.

"He has *Candida* in his chest tube drainage," she told me.

"I'm on my way in. In the meantime have him drink methylene blue."

When I walked into the Unit, a quick glance at the chest tube output revealed that all the pleural fluid was blue. He had an esophageal-pleural fistula and the blue water he drank went down the esophagus and into the pleural space

"Oh," said the nurse. "That's why his chest tube output went up every time he had a glass of water."

If you get *Candida* in a pleural space, it is due to a bronchopleural fistula. *Candida* pneumonia is rare as hen's teeth, so it is odd to see it reach the pleural space by way of the lung. A hole connecting the esophagus and pleural space, an esophageal-pleural fistula, is just about the only reliable way *Candida* can get to the pleural space.

This month I have seen two patients in the ICU with *Candida* empyemas—pus in the chest cavity. One was a *C. tropicalis* due to an esophageal leak after removal of an esophageal cancer. The fluid also grew lactobacillus. Radiographic studies only confirmed what the microbiology suggested must be present. The patient had upper and lower dentures, which are often heavily colonized with *Candida*. Perhaps the source?

The other was more unusual: *C. albicans* that occurred after an aspiration lung abscess ruptured into the pleural space. In the space of five days he went from a clear chest x-ray, to large round fluid density, to big pleural collection. At video assisted thoracoscopy the surgeon said he had a lung abscess that had perforated into the pleura. The patient, not the surgeon. *Candida* is not a common cause of aspiration lung abscess (maybe 8 reported cases), but he had upper dentures and lower poor dentition. I bet the *Candida* came from his dentures as well. Not that there is much literature to confirm my hypothesis. Anyway, that's my story and I am sticking to it.

Rationalization

Lotfi-Kamran, M.H., et al., Candida Colonization on the Denture of Diabetic and Non-diabetic Patients. Dent Res J (Isfahan), 2009. 6(1): p. 23-7.

Ko, S.C., et al., Fungal empyema thoracis: an emerging clinical entity. Chest, 2000. 117(6): p. 1672-8.

....

More yeast

Today's patient presented three weeks ago with *S. aureus* bacteremia from heroin use. No surprise. She had a vegetation on the mitral valve, so the diagnosis was not in doubt. Endocarditis.

She was sent to the nursing home for treatment of endocarditis, but came in three weeks later with *Candida albicans* in her blood. Still, surprisingly, using heroin. Who would have figured? Presumptively the Candida is from using her central catheter line to inject drugs; heroin often has Candida in it. So we pulled the line, waited a day, and repeated the blood cultures. At day 3 they popped positive. This was a bad sign, because it meant there was still a source of fungi somewhere in her body, seeding her bloodstream. Repeated ECHO showed no new or changed vegetation on the mitral vale, but now she had clot in her jugular vein.

Probable fungal septic thrombophlebitis. Crap. Evidently there are less than 20 cases ever reported on PubMed.

The take-home is that sustained positive blood cultures over time means some sort of endovascular infection, usually endocarditis or a catheter infection. But the vascular tree is big and sometimes you have to look around to find the source.

Some coumadin and antifungals and, one hopes, no more heroin, and the patient will get better.

Rationalization

Block, A.A., et al., Thrombolytic therapy for management of complicated catheter-related Candida albicans thrombophlebitis. Intern

Med J, 2009. 39(1): p. 61-3.

Benoit, D., et al., Management of candidal thrombophlebitis of the central veins: case report and review. Clin Infect Dis, 1998. 26(2): p. 393-7.

Postscript

She did. Get better.

....

Cryptococcus

Growing Lung Nodule

BACK from four days at the Oregon Coast with my youngest. No infections for four days. No broadband for four days. Very odd to be on dial-up, but we always have a good time together. Now the party is over and it's back to work.

Today's patient had an odd lymphoma for which he was getting chemotherapy. As part of his followup, he was supposed to get a CT scan every few months, and the previous one showed a small round nodule in his lung. Now, a few months later, it had grown bigger. What was it? The only way to know is to put a needle into it. So I did, and it grew *Cryptococcus neoformans*. This is not an uncommon cause of a round lesion in chest CT, and I have seen at least one lung removed thinking the fungus was a tumor.

Unlike lung cancer, *Cryptococcus* is curable, at least most of the time. The literature suggests that pulmonary *Cryptococcus* is unusual in immunocompetent people, although I bet that what this actually means is that symptomatic disease is uncommon in people with intact immune systems. If the fungus is in the environment, then I bet a lot of people get asymptomatic infections—such as this patient, who had no pulmonary or infectioous symptoms whatsoever, and who would have gone undiagnosed if it weren't for his regular scans.

Normal people, if such a thing exists, probably need no therapy, but in the immunocompromised the yeast can disseminate to cause meningitis. Because of his history of lymphoma, we checked this patient's blood and spinal fluid. They were negative, so he only needed a course of oral fluconazole.

4 A's or 5?

When I started in practice, my father, a cardiologist, told me the 4 A's of being a consultant: Appearance, Affability, Ability and Availability. Three out of four ain't bad. If you are going to be an I.D. doc, the 5th A is Amaze them.

Doctors tend to blather on and on about the possible diseases a patient could have. If you can, on minimal information, before the diagnosis is given, blurt out the answer. If you are right, it will impress people to no end, and if you are wrong—well, hell, you are always wrong at the beginning. It is why we blather on and on and order a boatload of tests.

I was scheduled to see a patient in clinic Friday who had had a headache and fevers of a month or so duration. The primary care physician had asked me about the case on the phone, and at that time I had no good ideas.

But the patient got sicker and went to the ER, and I got a call from the ER doc. He ran through the same history I already knew, and then said, "We did a spinal tap, and there are 240 white cells, mostly monocytes and lymphocytes, the glucose is 15 and the protein is 226, and the gram stain..."

Here is where you butt in.

"It showed yeast," I said.

He was flabbergasted. He asked if I was looking at the labs on the computer.

Nope.

Then how did I know?

I said it is what I.D. docs do. The lumbar puncture was typical of a chronic granulomatous meningitis (fungal or tubercular) and the only organism in the great Pacific Northwest to do that is Cryptococcus. Elementary, my dear Watson.

Who needs false modesty, right?

Patient has Cryptococcal pneumonia with meningitis.

I try to do this about once a week and I succeed one a year. But everyone remembers when Babe Ruth pointed to left field, and then went and had a candy bar.

I.D. is perhaps unique in the opportunity to come up with an odd diagnosis with a few facts and an educated lucky guess. It is the medical equivalent of a cold reading.

When John Edwards does it, he makes millions talking to the dead. When I do it, I get the medicare discount rate.

But if you can get the diagnosis on minimal data occasionally, it will impress everyone.

Where did he get the yeast? Maybe a horse barn; he had extensive exposure to horse barns whose bark dust comes from Vancouver, BC. Maybe not. *Cryptococcus* is one of the endemic fungi in the Pacific NW, imported from Vancouver. But pigeon poo and barns are not uncommonly a source for *Cryptococcus*.

Rationalization

Denton, J.F. and A.F. Di Salvo, The prevalence of Cryptococcus neoformans in various natural habitats. Sabouraudia, 1968. 6(3): p. 213-7.

Werchniak, A.E. and R.D. Baughman, Primary cutaneous cryptococcosis in an elderly man. Clin Exp Dermatol, 2004. 29(2): p. 159-60.

It's coming

No, not flu. Well, maybe. It's too soon to tell whether the swine flu is going to be a pandemic disaster that kills millions or fizzles. I hope the latter. But concrete information about the swine flu is rare, and the reports on the TV define histrionic. However, I am dining primarily on pork. Ribs and loin and chops and bacon.

No swine, no swine flu, so I am doing my part.

No, something wicked this way comes, and it isn't, yet, a virus.

Today I saw a very old male with a right lung filled with something. It was a near total white-out but, while short of breath, he was surprisingly non-toxic. His bronchoscopy showed a heavy growth of *Cryptococcus*. That's two cases of *Cryptococcus* I've seen in less than two weeks.

Since 1999, *C. neoformans* has been newly established on Vancouver Island and causing disease in Canadians. Thanks to a strong show of force by Homeland Security, it has not been a problem in the U.S. Until now. The prevailing winds and the local environment are carrying the yeast our, meaning my, way. This may be the start of something bad.

Here are the cases:

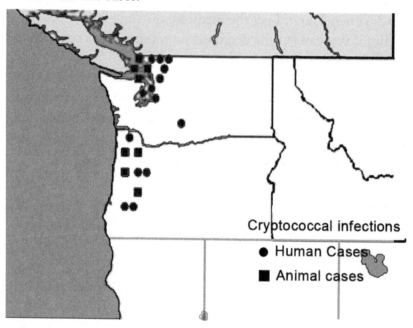

And how they got here:

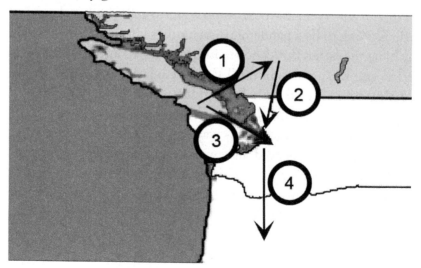

I wish border patrol were a bit more selective in what it lets through. I expect the Northwest will become endemic for *Cryptococcus* unless we get lucky and global warming turns the area into a desert. Take that, *Cryptococcus*.

Rationalization

Byrnes, E.J., 3rd, et al., Molecular evidence that the range of the Vancouver Island outbreak of Cryptococcus gattii infection has expanded into the Pacific Northwest in the United States. J Infect Dis, 2009. 199(7): p. 1081-6.

Right again

I no longer remember why I became a doctor; it was too long ago and I barely remember yesterday anymore. But I do remember why I remain one, and it is because being an ID doc is so cool. Not cool, like what my kids consider cool, since as a human I am the antithesis of cool. Cool as in fun and interesting.

It is nice to make people better and talk with them and help them, don't get me wrong. But the fun, what really bakes my potato, is figuring out the diagnosis before the cultures pop positive.

Like the patient today. Old heart transplant, as an outpatient he had a new temporal headache. He was given a biopsy of the temporal artery to check for temporal arteritis, a granulomatous inflammation of the external carotid artery that produces mononuclear cell infiltrates with a characteristic histology in the vessel wall. Unfortunately, the biopsies have a high false negative rate, and the disease is difficult to diagnose with confidence. So when his biopsy was negative, he was put on high dose prednisone just in case he actually had the disease—which can cause catastrophic, irreversible vision loss if not treated.

He got sicker, had hemoptysis, developed a nodular upper lobe infiltrate on CT scan and petechiae on his legs.

He was admitted, his blood cultures grew a yeast, and he was transferred to my hospital.

I am far more often wrong than I am right, and it is always

annoying how often reality gets in the way of a good diagnosis. I wish I were an alternative medicine provider and did not have to worry about reality.

I said that it would be *Cryptococcus*, that this was the ONLY diagnosis possible, and by gosh and by golly his serum cryptococcal antigen was > 1:2048. CNS evaluation is in process.

It always impresses people when you hit one out the ballpark.

In my mind there are two take-homes from this case.

One. And I can't prove this by any data that I can find, but my local rheumatologist agrees. If you are on transplant medications, you cannot develop a vasculitis. I wonder if the "temporal arteritis" was, in fact, early cryptococcal disease.

B. Disseminated *Cryptococcus* causes petechiae. I didn't know that. Red bumps and molluscum contagiosum-like lesions are the most common skin manifestations of *Cryptococcus*. Ulcers and cellulitis are rarer, and while I cannot find petechaie on PubMed, doing the Google on the interwebs finds all sorts of references.

III. 3 out of 2 people do not understand arithmetic, but everyone seemed to worry it might be *Candida*. *Candida* does not get into the bloodstream unless there is a intravascular catheter, which he did not have. Just because he had a heart transplant doesn't mean he was equally at risk for all fungi. *Candida* just ain't on the list.

That is now four cases of *Cryptococcus*, three in less than a month.

This will be the year of *Cryptococcus* and West Nile in Oregon. Something wicked this way comes.

Cue up the music from *Jaws*.

Rationalization

Murakawa, G.J., R. Kerschmann, and T. Berger, Cutaneous Cryptococcus infection and AIDS. Report of 12 cases and review of the literature. Arch Dermatol, 1996. 132(5): p. 545-8.

Postscript

As of June 2014, we still lack West Nile in Oregon.

Cross Reaction

I spent the day watching my son in the state golf tournament. He did OK. First time to State. No infections on the golf course.

My latest *Cryptococcus* case? Doing great, thanks to amphotericin B and flucytosine.

When the patient first came in, he had nodules on his chest CT scan and was coughing up blood. In the differential was *Aspergillus* infection, so the pulmonologist sent off cultures for both *Aspergillus* and *Cryptococcus* as well as a serum *Aspergillus* galactomannan assay.

The galactomannan assay is a reasonable way to determine if a patient has invasive *Aspergillus*. Galactomannan is one of the fungal cell wall constituents, and when the organisms get into the blood, bits of the cell wall flake off, like dandruff, and can be measured.

His assay was positive at 0.56, just above the cutoff of 0.5.

Did he have fleas and lice? Flice? Lleaes (pronounced like llama, or the way George Hrab can say yes).

Nope.

The galactomannan assay can be false positive due topiperacillin/tazobactam of all things. Sometimes a bored question. Yawn.

And it turns out the *Cryptococcus* makes glactoxylomannan, which cross-reacts with the assay—so it is not really a false positive, it is true positive for the wrong fungus.

Since the patient had a serum cryptococcal antigen titer > 1:2048, I wasnot surprised the assay was positive, or is is a true false positive? A false true positive? Something like that, if you know what I mean, and I am sure you do.

More importantly, since the patient who is at risk for *Aspergillus* is also at risk for *Cryptococcus*, a positive galactomannan assay in the right host should probably result in a serum cryptococcal antigen as well.

Rationalization

Dalle, F., et al., Cryptococcus neoformans Galactoxyloman-
nan contains an epitope(s) that is cross-reactive with Aspergillus Galactomannan. J Clin Microbiol, 2005. 43(6): p. 2929-31.

Sulahian, A., S. Touratier, and P. Ribaud, False positive test for aspergillus antigenemia related to concomitant administration of piperacillin and tazobactam. N Engl J Med, 2003. 349(24): p. 2366-7.

Something Wicked This Way Comes

One of the last patients I saw before vacation was an elderly female with end stage liver disease who was admitted with several
days of progressive shortness of breath. Her liver disease was due
to some autoimmune process and she had recently been started
on moderate doses of prednisone, but her bilirubin continued to
climb and was 19 mg/dL when I saw her (normal is < 1.9).

She had been on a ventilator for a few days, afebrile, but with
increasing oxygen requirements and her chest x-ray showed bilateral infiltrates that looked more like congestive heart failure
than infection.

She had no risks for odd infections (travel, etc.) and all her cultures were negative. Her bronchoscopy was growing a yeast to be
identified, but _Candida_ is common in the upper airway, and can
be ignored in the sputum of about 99.99%, or more, of patients.

I ordered diagnostic tests looking for the typical atypical organisms that cause culture negative pneumonia and left for vacation. Within the next 24 hours, the patient died.

Several days later her sputum grew not _Candida_, but _Crypto-
coccus gattii_. The docs sent some of her blood for testing, but the
serum Cryptococcal antigen was negative, so this was primary
Cryptococcal pneumonia.

The more interesting thing is the species causing her infection.
There are two forms of _Cryptococcus_: _neoformans_ and _gattii_.

C. gattii is new to the Northwest and is now endemic on Vancouver Island. It is more virulent than the *neoformans* strain and less responsive to therapy. *C. gattii* was associated with eucalyptus trees, but this strain is found in the fir trees of the Northwest and is perhaps one of the infections associated with global warming. It has found a new ecological niche to fill, and has now caused hundreds of cases in British Columbia in humans and many more in animals. Visitors to the Island need to be careful to not inhale.

One would think that Koala bears, which subsist entirely in eucalyptus leaves, would be immune, but *Cryptococcus* is the number two killer of this animal. Also, and I am uncertain why I find this delightful, but the strain in Vancouver is the result of same-sex mating (how? See reference). I will let you come to your own conclusion as to what, if any, significance that fact has.

Recent reports in *Emerging Infection Diseases* suggest that *C. gattii* is increasingly common in Washington and Oregon (you can tell when someone is not from around these parts as they call it Washington State not Washington. The capital is Washington DC. And there is no 'r' in Washington). Unlike *neoformans*, *C. gattii* likes to infect normal people as well as the immunocompromised and is also more refractory to treatment. A bad combination.

Looks like after years of being relatively dull, Oregon may be perking up with odd infections. Just don't tell any potential tourists. The joke used to be "What is the difference between Oregon and yogurt? Yogurt has culture." No longer.

Rationalization

Datta, K., et al., Spread of Cryptococcus gattii into Pacific Northwest region of the United States. Emerg Infect Dis, 2009. 15(8): p. 1185-91.

Fraser, J.A., et al., Same-sex mating and the origin of the Vancouver Island Cryptococcus gattii outbreak. Nature, 2005. 437(7063): p. 1360-4.

Lindberg, J., et al., Cryptococcus gattii risk for tourists visiting Vancouver Island, Canada. Emerg Infect Dis, 2007. 13(1): p. 178-9.

Cocci

L AST night was the first time in twenty years that I was awake at midnight for New Year's. Mr. Clark is looking pretty good, given his stroke, but the bands that played were who? Fergie, The Jonas Brothers, Taylor Swift, and the Pussycat Dolls? I am so out of touch. The reason I was up was that I had to pick up my 15-year-old from a party. After midnight. And all too soon he will be driving. And dating. What have I done?

Cocci. This is pronounced cox-e, not cox-eye. As in *Coccidioidomycosis*, or Valley fever.

An endlessly interesting disease, it is a fungus found in the soil of the American Southwest as well as in South America. The first case ever reported was a disseminated infection in a South American cowboy, Domingo Ezcurra, who eventually died of the disease. His pickled head is still available for observation, in a jar at a S. American medical school. It can be found on-line (see the references) if you want to be grossed out. What other book gives you the opportunity to see not just a pickled head, but a historically important pickled head?

My current patient is not going to be that unfortunate, but he does have chronic Cocci pneumonia with cavities, which is not responding as it should to high dose oral fluconazole. He is probably not improving because his diabetes is not under the best of control, but then the infection makes it hard to control the diabetes, so around and around we go.

But, after a good college try, it is time to declare a fluconazole failure and try intravenous amphotericin B.

There is a difference in diabetics with Cocci that makes them less responsive to medications. I wonder if this is due to differences in the Cocci rather than just to the usual worse white cell function of the diabetic. Diabetics are more likely to have mycelial forms of the disease:

"Type 2 diabetic patients with pulmonary coccidioidomycosis were four times more likely than non-diabetics to develop parasitic mycelial forms. We formulated a comprehensive definition based on

the results as follows: patients with pulmonary coccidioidomycosis with an evolution longer than 8 months, cough, hemoptysis, radiological evidence of a cavitary lesion, and type 2 diabetes mellitus, develop parasitic mycelial forms of Coccidioides spp. Based on microscopic images of patient specimens, we propose incorporating mycelial forms into the parasitic phase of Coccidioides spp. in patients with type 2 diabetes mellitus and chronic and cavitary pulmonary coccidioidomycosis."

Way back in the last century, when I was a young I.D. fellow with hair and vision, I was taught there was one Cocci, found in the New World. But that makes no sense. The Cocci of South America evolved separately from the Cocci in the San Joaquin valley, and should be different. And indeed they are. The U.S. Cocci is *Coccidioides immitis,* while that in South and Central America is *C. posadasii.* They are treated the same and are probably clinically the same. But they are not the same. Like the Patty Duke show.

This patient got his Cocci the old fashioned way: wintering in Arizona. When I go to the American Southwest I make a point of not inhaling. However, exposures to Cocci can be brief. I have seen two people get a lung resected for fear of cancer: smoking truckers with big lymph nodes on their chest on CT, weight loss, and chronic pneumonia. In both cases the bronchoscopy showed atypical cells that could be cancer, so, given the history, off to the OR to take a lung out. It was only on the deep pathology that the classic spherules of Cocci were seen. There is no Cocci here in Oregon, but these truckers drove I-5 to L.A., right through the heart of Cocci territory.

Take home message: don't take out a lung until after you have taken a good history.

Rationalization

Munoz-Hernandez, B., et al., Mycelial forms of Coccidioides spp. in the parasitic phase associated to pulmonary coccidioidomycosis with type 2 diabetes mellitus. Eur J Clin Microbiol Infect Dis, 2008. 27(9): p. 813-20.

Pickled head:

http://botit.botany.wisc.edu/toms_fungi/images/ezcurra.jpg

....

Cocci. Again

I AM not a big fan of weekend call, and as I slide into advanced decrepitude, it has less and less allure.

I know. Whine whine whine. But since I am on call, it can't be wine wine wine.

No matter how much I am not a fan of working weekends, at least I get to see interesting cases when I make it to the hospital.

The patient this Saturday had a dense pneumonia, fevers, and cough that were unresponsive to antibiotics.

History revealed that she was just back from two months in Arizona, which reminded me that *Coccidiomycosis* was a common cause of (missed) outpatient pneumonia. Cocci is also increasing in incidence, and may be one of those diseases that increases with global warming. Or not. Hard to know what to make of a three-year trend, but the incidence has been increasing in California as well.

Cocci, aka Valley Fever, is an endlessly interesting fungus found in the soil of the American Southwest. One of its manifestations is pneumonia, often associated (not in this case, although she did have a rash) with the skin disease *erythema nodosum*. Dermatologists can't use real words to describe disease, just Latin terms so they can sound infallible, a pope-y way of doing things. It just means red bumps, but you can't look smart if you tell a patient, "Yeah, you have red bumps." The patient knows that already, but does not know he has *erythema nodosum*. I had one patient with acute Cocci with about 90% of her body having red bumps.

Cocci is a self-limited disease in most normal people, and today's patient ibegan getting better with no specific anti-fungal therapy.

The motto of Arizona is *Ditat Deus*, with is Latin for "God gives you Cocci." The key thing is that if you go to Arizona, do not inhale. Ever.

And when your patients come back from wintering in the Southwest, beware of Cocci.

Rationalization

Kim, M.M., et al., Coccidioidal pneumonia, Phoenix, Arizona, USA, 2000-2004. Emerg Infect Dis, 2009. 15(3): p. 397-401.

Park, B.J., et al., An epidemic of coccidioidomycosis in Arizona associated with climatic changes, 1998-2001. J Infect Dis, 2005. 191(11): p. 1981-7.

CDC, Increase in Coccidioidomycosis—California, 2000-2007. MMWR Morb Mortal Wkly Rep, 2009. 58(5): p. 105-9.

Do you have blue mold rot?

TODAY I saw a young female who'd had months of vaginal itching and discharge; the wet prep showed yeast. *Candida* is the usual reason, so she was given fluconazole. She didn't get better, so another round of fluconazole, and still not better.

So a culture is sent, thinking maybe it is a non-albicans *Candida*, since it is full of yeast, and no germ tubes are seen. Germ tubes are mycelial outgrowths from spores that are seen when colonies from a smear are suspended in growth medium. It was discovered around the turn of the century that only *C. albicans* makes germ tubes at 39 degrees C in serum, and is a rapid was of distinguishing the species.

Maybe *C. glabrata*, I thought—a known cause of recurrent vulvovaginitis, especially in diabetics

Nope. *Cryptococcus*, and not even neoformans but *Cryptococcus laurentii*.

Where did that come from?

Cryptococcus laurentii is a soil organism, but occasionally is seen causing disease in the profoundly immunoincompetent, like AIDS and leukemia patients. Not that there are many cases of this yeast causing disease in the lit-tra-ture.

No cases of vaginitis reported with this organism, so mine

would be the first. I wonder how many firsts I have reported in these stories, not that they are considered peer-reviewed or a legitimate source for the announcement of new discoveries.

How to treat was also a problem. *Cryptococcus laurentii* has higher MICs to fluconazole than Candida, but voriconazole, to which it is more susceptible, costs an arm, a leg, and your first born's left kidney. The right kidney is reserved for linezolid.

So I went with high dose fluconazole first, which she could afford and to which she had had some response to low doses.

Oh, and if you have some blue mold rot on your apples, due to *Penicillium expansum, Cryptococcus laurentii* is an effective biological agent against blue mold rot. One never knows when one will be on Jeopardy and it will be "fruit diseases for 500."

Rationalization

Bernal-Martinez, L., et al., Susceptibility profile of clinical isolates of non-Cryptococcus neoformans/non-Cryptococcus gattii Cryptococcus species and literature review. Med Mycol, 2010. 48(1): p. 90-6.

Postscript

High dose fluconazole worked.

....

Kiss my *Aspergillus*

*A*SPERGILLUS is everywhere. It can be the mold on your bread, the mold on your cheese, and the mold on the cup of coffee that is left out for three or four weeks. My wife, and most females, have curiously never seen mold on a cup of coffee left out for weeks. Most males have. I don't know why, but when I was single I would let the dishes sit in the sink until the growth on them evolved into a life form that wanted to clean itself. I don't do that anymore.

So when *Aspergillus* is in a bronchoscopy culture, you have to ask if it is real or a contaminant, and Ella Fitzgerald can't help you with that.

The patient had had Wegener's, a kind of vasculitis, for 5 months. She was on dialysis, prednisone, and had just finished the Cytoxan that cleared up the pulmonary infiltrates on her CT scan. Now back in the hospital, she had cavitating pulmonary nodules, and the lavage fluid from the bronchoscopy grew *Aspergillus* after only three days. She was a touch short of breath, but no hemoptysis.

The gold standard for invasive *Aspergillus* is biopsy showing invasion of the organisms, but the bronchial biopsy did not show this.

Do an open lung biopsy? Treat and see what happens?

The bronchoalveolar lavage showed *Aspergillus* on staining, so the fungi must have been at fairly high concentrations, and she had no prior structural lung disease to predispose to heavy colonization. The chance that the *Aspergillus* was the real deal is about 25%.

"Organisms such as cytomegalovirus, Aspergillus, and Candida were frequently identified in BAL specimens but were eventually proved to be pathogens in only 24%, 25%, and 0% of cases, respectively."

Not good odds. But it is a compatible CT, host, and large amounts of *Aspergillus* that grew rapidly. If the galactomannan assay is positive, then the diagnosis is clinched.

So she was put on voriconazole and we shall see. Thats the royal we, not the multiple personality we. You don't want to see my goth cowgirl. Trust me.

Rationalization

Pisani, R.J. and A.J. Wright, Clinical utility of bronchoalveolar lavage in immunocompromised hosts. Mayo Clin Proc, 1992. 67(3): p. 221-7.

Postscript

The galactomannan was postive and she slowly improved on the voriconazole.

Onycomycosis gone bad

THE patient rolled his car with his dog, not seat belted, in the front seat with him. It is always a bad idea to roll your own. Something—exactly what is not certain, maybe his dog's nail as the beast was thrown into him—punctured his palm. His hand, not the PDA.

Since then he had ongoing pain and erythema on the palm of his hand and when he moved his middle finger.

I do not know about you, but I have trouble driving if I cannot fully extend my middle finger.

He received several courses of oral antibiotics without resolution, and then was sent to a hand surgeon, and then to me.

The striking feature on exam was that all his nails were heavily involved with a fungal infection. It had cleared years ago after a course of terfinibine, but relapsed almost immediately after stopping the medication. At least as immediately as a nail can grow.

The surgeon opened it up and it was a low-grade gooey mess, not typical of a bacterial infection.

I made sure that the specimens were sent for fungal cultures as well as those for acid-fast bacilli, but now the cultures are growing a *Trichophyton* species.

I bet whatever penetrated his palm (probably his nail, not the dog's) dragged in his nail mold and caused a tenosynovitis, since the most common pathogens for nail infections are the dermatophytes *Trichophyton rubrum* and *Trichophyton mentagrophytes*.

There are at best 18 references on PubMed that mention soft tissue infections with these organisms, almost all in the profoundly immunocompromised, and no cases of tenosynovitis.

The *New England Journal of Medicine* suggests the best therapy is itraconazole. In I.D. the answer to the cause of the infection is all in the exposure history. You get infected with what you are exposed to. My wife, fortunately, has an infectious smile, so I am safe for the time being.

Rationalization

de Berker, D., Clinical practice. Fungal nail disease. N Engl J Med, 2009. 360(20): p. 2108-16.

....

Why?

I SOMETIMES get asked what: What does the patient have?

Sometimes I get asked how: How to treat the patient. That was today's patient. The patient had a fever the day after a laparoscopic mesenteric biopsy, and three days later his blood cultures popped positive for *Candida glabrata,* of all things.

The surgeons asked me about the best antibiotic to use (I picked caspofungin).

But the interesting question is why.

Preop, he had no symptoms.

Past medical history included diabetes, a pacemaker placement, and obesity with chronic "diaper rash" in his skin folds. His pacer was three years old.

His exam was negative.

The classic risk factors for *Candida* in the blood are central lines, hyperalimentation, broad spectrum antibiotics, neutropenia, and a major surgery. He had none of the above.

The only reason he could have positive blood cultures is if he had seeded his pacer system from his intermittently oozy groin. Unfortunately, his echocardiogram today showed probable infection on the pacemaker wires.

Crap.

I can't cure a bacterial pacer infection, much less a *Candida* infection, medically. But if the pacer system comes out, he has no rhythm. He has no rhythm, who could ask for anything more? Me. It is why I am glad I am not a cardiologist.

There is exactly one case of *C. glabrata* pacer infection in the lit-tra-chure and a smattering of a handful of a smidgen of other *Candida* species on pacers. Like all infections of pacers, the system absolutely, positively has to be removed. Unlike prosthetic valve endocarditis, the literature suggests you are as likely to cure a pacer infection medically as you are to get an accounting of the money spent to bail out Fanny Mae.

Rationalization

Roger, P.M., et al., Medical treatment of a pacemaker endocarditis due to Candida albicans and to Candida glabrata. J Infect, 2000. 41(2): p. 176-8.

Postscript

The pacer came out without incident and the wires grew *Candida*. He did fine.

COLDS AND FLU

Cold

COLD, cold, cold. This week, in what is usually the mild Pacific Northwest, it is going to be below freezing. When I die and go to the hell that so many have promised me, it will not be fire and brimstone. It will be cold. And I will be naked. And wet. With a breeze in my face. In Chuck E. Cheese. And they will be playing country music.

Now there are those of you reading this who are calling me a wimp, but I spent my residency in Minnesota, where I learned to hate cold. But I was asked today, as I wandered the hospital stomping out illness, can you catch a cold? Nope. It's a myth. Then I was asked 'What's the data?'

Um. Er. Well.

I'll be damned. What ARE the data?

They are old data. 1958. One year younger than me. So old they don't exist in electronic form. But people claim the data say that chilling doesn't increase cold risk.

A subsequent study in the NEJM had the same result. No increased incidence of colds when chilled people are challenged with rhinovirus. When I ask my eldest what he was doing with his friends, he usually replies "Chillin'." At least he will not be catching a cold. Or will he?

But then, in one of the odder studies I found, some researchers did show that those who had their feet chilled were more likely to get cold symptoms:

*"**BACKGROUND**: There is a common folklore that chilling of the body surface causes the development of common cold symptoms,*

but previous clinical research has failed to demonstrate any effect of cold exposure on susceptibility to infection with common cold viruses.

OBJECTIVE: This study will test the hypothesis that acute cooling of the feet causes the onset of common cold symptoms.

METHODS: 180 healthy subjects were randomized to receive either a foot chill or control procedure. All subjects were asked to score common cold symptoms, before and immediately after the procedures, and twice a day for 4/5 days.

RESULTS: 13/90 subjects who were chilled reported they were suffering from a cold in the 4/5 days after the procedure compared to 5/90 control subjects (P=0.047). There was no evidence that chilling caused any acute change in symptom scores (P=0.62). Mean total symptom score for days 1-4 following chilling was 5.16 (+/-5.63 s.d. n=87) compared to a score of 2.89 (+/-3.39 s.d. n=88) in the control group (P=0.013). The subjects who reported that they developed a cold (n=18) reported that they suffered from significantly more colds each year (P=0.007) compared to those subjects who did not develop a cold (n=162).

CONCLUSION: Acute chilling of the feet causes the onset of common cold symptoms in around 10% of subjects who are chilled. Further studies are needed to determine the relationship of symptom generation to any respiratory infection."

Lack of a placebo arm makes controlling for bias impossible. I have had a lot of cold feet in my dating days, but I do not remember a subsequent infection; those followed when I didn't get cold feet. But I share too much.

I suppose I should be convinced, but the data are not compelling and not relevant to the "real world." I just got in from my evening walk and my nose was congested and my throat dry. I seem primed for upper respiratory compromise with mechanical alterations that could make it easier for a rhinovirus, or other bacteria like *Streptococcus pneumoniae*, to gain a foothold. Or a nose hold.

A good study would be to challenge people after a 3 mile trek on a below-freezing day in a 25-mile-an-hour wind as I did today. That was a cold stress. The increase of respiratory disease seen in the winter is always attributed to crowding and easier transmission, but there is some, albeit contradictory information, that physical cold does increase the risk of bacterial infections.

Whether cold causes infection depends how much stress the cold exposure causes.

"Psychological stress was associated in a dose–response manner with an increased risk of acute infectious respiratory illness, and this risk was attributable to increased rates of infection rather than to an increased frequency of symptoms after infection."

Does cold cause a cold? Maybe. I bet it does. It is too bad the other forms of temperature do not have names like beer, sex, and golf. Those might be worth catching.

Besides, "a cold in the head causes less suffering than an idea."—Jules Renard

---

Rationalization

Dowling, H.F., et al., Transmission of the common cold to volunteers under controlled conditions. III. The effect of chilling of the subjects upon susceptibility. Am J Hyg, 1958. 68(1): p. 59-65.

Johnson, C. and R. Eccles, Acute cooling of the feet and the onset of common cold symptoms. Fam Pract, 2005. 22(6): p. 608-13.

Cohen, S., D.A. Tyrrell, and A.P. Smith, Psychological stress and susceptibility to the common cold. N Engl J Med, 1991. 325(9): p. 606-12.

Douglas, R.G.J., K.M. Lindgren, and R.B. Couch, Exposure to Cold Environment and Rhinovirus Common Cold — Failure to Demonstrate Effect. N Engl J Med, 1968. 279: p. 742-747.

....

Influenza deaths

I T's flu season. Quiet so far; most states with flu have only had sporadic cases.

Got my vaccine. You?

People die of influenza, both directly from the virus and from secondary bacterial infections. Some years have more deaths than others, and in modern times nothing has surpassed the mortality of the 1918-1919 influenza pandemic, where about 1/5 of the world was infected and 50 million died worldwide, 675,000 in the US.

Should history repeat itself (which it NEVER does, right?), epidemiologists expect 2 million US deaths. What was the cause of death in the 1918 pandemic? The conventional wisdom is that since the 1918 pandemic was an avian (bird) flu, it was a primary influenza infection that killed everyone. This theory is supported in part by the fact that the reconstituted virus is particularly virulent in mice. BTW, Decon is cheaper.

But men are not mice, John Steinbeck notwithstanding.

So why did all those people die?

"In the present study, we have examined re-cut tissue specimens obtained during autopsy from 58 influenza victims in 1918-1919, and have reviewed epidemiologic, pathologic, and microbiologic data from published reports for 8398 postmortem examinations bearing on this question."

Those studies that reported the bacteriology of the patients who died almost always found pathogens: *Streptococcus pneumoniae* (24%), *Streptococcus hemolyticus* (17%), *Staphylococcus aureus* (9%), *Bacillus influenzae* (10%) and a smattering of other pathogens. Looks like those microbiologists have been changing names for over a century.

The studies also reviewed the lung specimens, which had the typical histopathological changes of bacterial pneumonia. Death from bacterial superinfection was thought to be the case at the time:

"Although the cause of influenza was disputed in 1918, there was almost universal agreement among experts that deaths were virtually never caused by the unidentified etiologic agent itself, but resulted directly from severe secondary pneumonia caused by well-known bacterial pneumopathogens, that colonized the upper respiratory tract (predominantly pneumococci, streptococci, and staphylococci)."

Good news, right? We have antibiotics, and they didn't, so we will not die. I would not be so sanguine. Antibiotic resistance continues to increase, and I continue to worry about the MRSA sweeping the world. There was a recent outbreak of linezolid resistant MRSA that killed half the patients. Resistance to daptomycin, our other MRSA drug, develops on therapy and, cannot be used for pneumonia due to poor tissue penetration. While only 10% or so of the deaths in 1918 were due to *S. aureus*, I have seen a few post-viral secondary infections due to MRSA; the rapidity with which it killed my patients, despite the best antibiotics we have, was sobering. Not to imply that I wasn't sober.

A bad influenza year and relatively widespread MRSA colonization could be a perfect storm for a marked increase in pneumonias that we can't treat and influenza deaths.

Glad I got my vaccine. You?

Rationalization

Morens, D.M., J.K. Taubenberger, and A.S. Fauci, Predominant role of bacterial pneumonia as a cause of death in pandemic influenza: implications for pandemic influenza preparedness. J Infect Dis, 2008. 198(7): p. 962-70.

Sanchez Garcia, M., et al., Clinical outbreak of linezolid-resistant Staphylococcus aureus in an intensive care unit. JAMA, 2010. 303(22): p. 2260-4.

Google the Flu

GOOGLE, as you may not know, tracks everything. Every search term, every search. They say the data can't be tracked back to you, and I trust Google. It is why I am helping my Gmail coorespondant move millions from Nigeria to my US bank account.

The home page is so cute, with the changing logo for every holiday. How could they do anything evil with their data?

Google does have a cool application of all that data collection that applies to an infectious disease.

If people get the flu, or there is flu in the community (you know, the dumbasses who didn't get the vaccine), people look for information about influenza. And the first place they go is Google.

Google keeps track of those searches, and they reported today that searches for "flu," "muscle aches," or "fever" go up dramatically when there is flu circulating in the community. The searches go up about two weeks before the usual reporting mechanisms (culture results) discover that flu is active in the community. Data going back to 2003 showed that the search terms paralleled the standard reporting data very closely. It appears that for flu, Google searches are a good early warning system for disease activity.

The data have yet to be published in a peer-reviewed journal, although the *NY Times* suggests the study's authors are looking at *Nature* for publication.

This is not the first time surrogate makers have indicated the presence of an infectious outbreak.

Over-the-counter cold remedy sales increase when there are influenza-like illnesses in the community, and sales of anti-diarrheals such as Kaopectate increase when there have been cryptosporidial outbreaks, sales of each preceding recognition of the outbreak.

I expect that clever people will discover other surrogates that can be tracked for early warning of outbreaks. As I type this it looks as though the top Google search terms are Lady Antebellum, Martina Mcbride, Miranda Lambert, Rodney Atkins, Kelly Pickler and George Strait, suggesting we are about to have an outbreak of country music. The horror, the horror. If you thought Norovirus was bad, just you wait.

Rationalization

Google Flu Trends: http://www.google.org/flutrends/

New York Times, "Google Uses Searches to Track Flu's Spread" (November 11, 2008). http://www.nytimes.com/2008/11/12/technology/internet/12flu.html.

Das, D., et al., Monitoring over-the-counter medication sales for early detection of disease outbreaks—New York City. MMWR Morb Mortal Wkly Rep, 2005. 54 Suppl: p. 41-6.

....

I can't leave even for a few days...

I HAD five days off with my youngest for his spring break, and we spent the time at the Oregon Coast. Great time. No TV, only dial-up internet, no newspaper, no contact with the real world. So I got back on Sunday and my wife told me we are in a State of Emergency.

What?

We have closed the borders with Mexico.

No way. Why?

Because of Swine Flu.

Huh? Flu season is over. Where in the hell did that come from?

Whether or not this is going to be a pandemic strain, and whether it is going to kill off 2-5% of the world like the 1919 pandemic, I can't say. It may just dribble off the court and be a false alarm. I hope so.

However, people already seem to be in panic mode. As I write this there are 40 cases in the US, no deaths. People are wearing masks around town and asking for oseltamivir. Some people are keeping their kids home from school, even though no cases have been reported in Oregon.

We are just finishing the flu season. There were about 30,000 documented cases of flu, 55 deaths documented in kids, and thousands of extra deaths in adults. And it was a slow year.

There is a Cinco de Mayo party coming up (what day is that?) and concern was expressed about having the kids attend. Maybe 30,000 people die each year in car accidents. If you really wanted to protect your kids, you would make sure they got a flu shot and not let them in a car. And don't get me started on deaths from guns.

Swine flu? We will see. "Prediction is very hard, especially when it's about the future" —Yogi Berra. Or perhaps it was "I predict the future to be full of pic-a-nic baskets,"-—Boo-Boo. Ask a psychic, not me.

I would prefer the government to over-react than under-react with infections. They (infections, not government. Or did I get it backwards?) can spread too fast and kill too quickly. Better safe than sorry. One of these days—be it avian flu, or this swine flu, or another strain—flu will come out of nowhere and kill a boatload of people. If it is going to kill lots of people, there is not much we can do for now except not inhale. Worked for President Clinton.

Postscript

An interesting bit of personal history, my first reaction to H1N1.

....

Flu for you

I HAVE been hesitant to write about the bacon, er, swine flu. So little data, so much hysteria. If you want to hear me babble on about Swine flu, listen the Skeptics' Guide to the Universe number 197 (available on iTunes). I hope Steve Novella uses his usual psychic ability and edits out all the dumbass things I say.

I have worried for most of my career about another influenza pandemic that repeats the 1919 pandemic, and, as the body count has not risen since the start of the Swine flu, I think we have maybe maybe maybe dodged a bullet.

Maybe.

As the body count has not increased (as I write, 367 cases and no deaths in the industrialized West except for a case acquired in Mexico), it would appear that—-hope hope hope—-it is not a particularly virulent strain of flu if you can get proper medical care.

Maybe.

To get a pandemic like 1919 that infected half the world and killed maybe 2 to 5% of the human population, you need a strain of flu that is both very infectious and very virulent. Looks like swine is infectious but not virulent. It causes, maybe, mostly mild flu. Flu that does not kill you.

"There are some genetic tests that have shown the virus we are dealing with right now does not have the factors that we think made the 1918 virus so bad," said Julie Gerberding, former head of the CDC, in an interview yesterday on ABC News. "But we have to be careful not to over-rely on that information, because these flu viruses always evolve."

There is a suspicion, yet to be proved, that severe, fatal flu is the exception, not the rule.

However.

Influenza is one pain in the ass, or the lung.

It has segmented DNA, so what happens is that a pig gets simultaneously infected with human, pig and, say, bird flu. Then, as it reassembles, it takes a few DNA segments from the bird, a few from the human and a few from the pig and, voilà, a new strain of flu.

So I am still nervous.

We (may) have an strain of flu, the bacon flu, that is (maybe) infectious but not virulent.

For the last several years we have had a very virulent (killed 257 of 421 cases, about a 61% death rate) avian flu wandering though the world. But the avian flu is not infectious. You have to wallow in bird flu to get infected.

Worst case: the avian and the swine and a human flu will meet in a pig somewhere and recombine like some sort of horrible transporter accident and we get the worst of both worlds: an infectious AND virulent new strain of flu.

It could happen. And if it can happen, eventually it well. In nature, if it is not forbidden to occur, it is required to occur.

So maybe maybe maybe this is the start of a huge shitstorm. I watched *I Am Legend* too many times.

EXOTICA: UNUSUAL ORGANISMS

Hanging Chad

I saw a case of the Hanging Chad Disease this week—at least that is what I call it.

What is Hanging Chad Disease?

In 2001 there was an election in Florida that was decided, in part, because of punch card ballots that (like the wardrobes of the time) malfunctioned.

Little bits of paper, chad, did not separate cleanly from the ballot and it was uncertain how to count them, at least to the Secretary of State of Florida.

So the hanging chad lead to the election being sent to the Supreme Court, who decided the election went to Bush, who decided there were weapons of mass destruction in Iraq, which lead to an invasion of a part of the world where *Leishmania* is endemic.

What I saw was a case of old world *Leishmania*, a parasite that causes, among other things, a chronic ulcer on the skin. The patient had had a half-dollar-sized ulcer on his upper arm for three months, one which had not responded to a variety of antibiotics, and then it was biopsied. Once the *Leishmania* was discovered he was sent to me.

This patient was not a soldier, but a refugee from Afghanistan by way of Iraq and Pakistan, all places where *Leishmania* thrives.

Leishmania is spread by the sand fly bite. There are three species of Old World *Leishmania*, along with many more New World species, and I am waiting for the culture at the CDC to grow to tell me which type of *Leishmania* he has before I start a course of therapy.

I anticipate he will get pentavalent antimony, which is often the treatment for *Leishmania*.

I expect we will see some cases in our returning soldiers—either soon, or in 100 years, depending on the results in November.

This is why I.D. (for this book, I.D. stands for Infectious Dis-

CRISLIP?

eases, not Intelligent Design) is the coolest of subspecialties. It has connections to everything.

Legionella: it's not just for Legionnaires any more

MY medical career started around the time of the first cases of toxic shock syndrome, HIV, and the first outbreak of Legionnaire's in Philadelphia. I am that old. Or mature. Or over-ripe. I gave a lecture at the Med School this week and there were students who were not yet born when I received my MD. At least I do not (yet) smell of mothballs.

The hotel where the first outbreak occurred (at an American Legion Convention) has been demolished; no one would stay there. Curiously my brother, on a trip to China, stayed at a hotel where there was a SARS outbreak and business was booming.

Legionella are, from a disease etiology perspective, cool. They are found in fresh water, such as lakes and streams, where the bacteria need free-living amoebas as hosts for survival and multi-plication. Neat. They need amoebas to live. *Legionella* is found not only in lakes and streams but in showerheads, decorative fountains, nuclear cooling towers, and potting soils, all of which have been implicated in transmission of the disease. I see a cooling tower, I think *Legionella*. I suppose it will kill Homer Simpson some day.

Here in the Great Pacific Northwest, despite the penchant for rain and other forms of wet, we do not have much Legionnaire's pneumonia. It is not for lack of looking; we spend thousands every year testing for *Legionella* and maybe get one case a year at the hospitals where I practice.

It turns out that out lack of *Legionella* is even odder than I had supposed, as *Legionella* is having an upswing in the rest of the USA this century:

"A total of 23,076 cases of legionellosis were reported to the Centers for Disease Control and Prevention from 1990 through 2005. The number of reported cases increased by 70% from 1310 cases in

2002 to 2223 cases in 2003, with a sustained increase to 12,000 cases per year from 2003 through 2005. The eastern United States showed most of the increases in age-adjusted incidence rates after 2002, with the mean rate in the Middle Atlantic states during 2003-2005 exceeding that during 1990-2002 by 96%."

Why is that? And why not in the Great Pacific Northwest? I think the good beers are protective. But then I always credit beer.

The other interesting thing is *when Legionella* occurs. Rates of infection increase after hot, humid weather. Thundershower weather. If you have those meteorological conditions, then 6 to 10 days later you get a spike in *Legionella* cases. Hot, wet, humid weather is not the hallmark of Oregon. Historically we get the long, cold drizzle. I remember a Ray Bradbury story about a kid who lived on a planet where it stopped raining only once every 100 years and everyone went out for the one day of sun. Except for the protagonist who was locked in a closet by his classmates. That is what Oregon winters are like—lots of rain, not being locked in a closet.

But the last two years we have had more summer days like Minnesota: hot and humid with thundershowers. I always challenge the housestaff to find me *Legionella* after a thundershower, and they usually do. And they get a Scooby Snack. Good boy. It may be due to increased surveillance for the disease, but it is a fun predictor nonetheless and gets the residents interested. Climate scientists are predicting that with global warming there will be more hot, humid, wet thundershowers here in the Great Pacific Northwest (tired of my chauvinism yet?), so I wonder if we will also see an upswing of *Legionella* in the last half of this decade. Bet we do.

How, and even if, climate change is going to increase or decrease local incidence of *Legionella* is not yet well worked out. However, this is only one of many diseases that have the potential to increase with climate change. But that will be the subject of future essays.

Rationalization

Fisman, D.N., et al., It's not the heat, it's the humidity: wet weather increases legionellosis risk in the greater Philadelphia metropolitan area. J Infect Dis, 2005. 192(12): p. 2066-73.

Neil, K. and R. Berkelman, Increasing incidence of legionellosis in the United States, 1990-2005: changing epidemiologic trends. Clin Infect Dis, 2008. 47(5): p. 591-9.

Zebras are so last century

THERE are those in medicine who love to hunt zebras. Not me. Too mundane. I prefer to hunt zebra unicorns with red and yellow stripes.

Like the consult today.

Diabetic with five days of leg cellulitis that was getting worse on vancomycin and pipercillan-tazobactam. More redness, more pain, white cell count climbing.

A leg with, well, there is no other way to say it: rubor, dolor, calor, and tumor. And today he has developed two areas of small hemorrhagic bullae on his calf and thigh.

The probable reason for the worsening symptoms was undrained pus. Common things are usually common. That's why they are commonly referred to as common.

But. But. But.

It turns out that all this occurred shortly after a hike in the Mt. Hood Wilderness, marked by time spent in the Bagby Hot Springs. Bagby Hot Springs are a series of hot tubs fed by geo-thermally heated water where hippies go to get stoned and soak neckid in the wilderness, or so I am told. I try to avoid stoned neckid hippies.

Cool hint. Or really hot. What infections do you get from hot springs? Besides sexually transmitted diseases?

Hemorrhagic bullae make an I.D. doc think of *Vibrio* infections, but they occur after saltwater exposure.

Pseudomonas causes folliculitis after hot tub use but not, as a rule, cellulitis.

Aeromonas is a cause of soft tissue infection with necrosis after fresh water exposure. But that should have responded to pipercillan-tazobactam.

So PubMed to the rescue.

Acanthamoeba, fungi I can neither spell nor pronounce, and an outbreak of a gram negative rods that could not be cultured have been reported as hot spring associated infections.

I am not surprised that the gram negative rods could not be identified. Most organisms that grow in hot water, thermophiles, have evolved to survive only at higher temperatures and probably would not grow at the lower temperatures of the micro lab.

But I did not know, until I went looking, that *Legionella* has caused cellulitis and so when you think of fresh, hot water, you should always think of *Legionella*. And tea.

So that's the red and yellow striped unicorn I went hunting today, *Legionella* cellulitis. *Legionella* studies are pending. Listen carefully. If, in a few days, you hear a triumphant shout of "Yes!" that was me.

As I am sure will happen, a great diagnosis will be ruined by the reality of the lab results.

But it is the journey, not the destination, that is fun.

That's a lie. I just want to be right.

Rationalization

Kilborn, J.A., et al., Necrotizing cellulitis caused by Legionella micdadei. Am J Med, 1992. 92(1): p. 104-6.

Lin, Y.E., et al., Environmental survey of Legionella pneumophila in hot springs in Taiwan. J Toxicol Environ Health A, 2007. 70(1): p. 84-7.

Waldor, M.K., B. Wilson, and M. Swartz, Cellulitis caused by Legionella pneumophila. Clin Infect Dis, 1993. 16(1): p. 51-3.

Follow-ups

It was not *Legionella* that caused the cellulitis. All the studies were negative. He went to the OR as there was no improvement, and there was no necrotizing disease or abscess, and all the gram stains and cultures were negative. Serology and urinary antigen for *Legionella* were also negative.

Another beautiful hypothesis killed by facts.

Could this be a non-infectious disease? I don't think so, but more esoteric thermophiles from a hot spring don't seem likely. If they can't be grown in a micro lab, why would they grow in a cool leg?

I suppose that of the other diseases that can mimic cellulitis—Sweet's—is most likely, and the pathology of the debridement is pending.

"The Sweet syndrome (acute febrile neutrophilic dermatosis) is characterized by papules that coalesce to form inflammatory plaques. These lesions are erythematous and tender; they most commonly occur on the upper extremities, face, and neck. Associated findings include fever, conjunctivitis or iridocyclitis, oral aphthae, and arthralgia or arthritis. Patients also have moderate neutrophilia and dermal infiltration by polymorphonuclear leukocytes. Sometimes the syndrome is mistaken for infectious cellulitis. Ten percent of patients with the syndrome also have an associated malignant condition, usually acute myelogenous leukemia. Immunologic disorders, such as rheumatoid arthritis and inflammatory bowel disease, have also been implicated. Corticosteroids remain the mainstay of treatment."

West Nile Virus

IT has been a slow year for West Nile Virus (WNV) and, while it is a good thing, the CDC isn't sure why.

368 severe cases, only (only? I hate referring to any death as an only) 18 deaths. Not bad compared to prior years like 2007, when there were more than 1,200 cases of severe West Nile illness with 124 deaths. The peak in cases was in 2002 and 2003, when there were 3000 severe illnesses and more than 260 deaths. Not much compared to handguns and cars, but enough.

Why the decline in cases?

It could be fewer mosquitoes. At least here in Oregon, it has been a dry summer and the kids have had far fewer bug bites this year. My children, especially the youngest, are sentinel chickens for mosquitoes. The US drought monitor suggests the US has had less rain, which would lead to fewer mosquitoes, which would lead to less West Nile. I can't see that mosquitoes are counted in the US, so perhaps this isn't true. Someone go out there and start counting mosquitoes, please.

An increase or a decrease in rainfall always leads to changes in infectious disease incidence of all kinds. Wet seasons have lead to increases in the cases of Hantavirus (more rain leads to more plants leads to more seed leads to more mice which carry the virus that were in contact with people and gave them the disease). This is only one of many examples. The changes in the seasons and the climate mean changes in infections.

It may be that the birds are not dying. Mosquitoes prefer to feed on birds and go after humans only when the birds are dead. If the remaining birds are less likely to die from WNV, as survivors of prior WNV seasons would be, then they would still be around for the mosquitoes to feed on. I don't know if this is true either.

I doubt it has anything to do with a change in the human populations. We haven't been exposed to enough WNV long enough, and we are a secondary host for the virus.

So we had a slow year. Good. Lets hope it stays slow.

Rationalization

U.S. Drought Monitor: http://droughtmonitor.unl.edu/

Housing Market

The housing market is tanking, people cannot afford their mortgage payments and are losing their homes. Abandoned homes are not cared for. In California, that means that the backyard pools are also not being cared for. No chlorine, big pools of stagnant, warm water = an ideal breeding ground for mosquitoes. And mosquitoes are a vector for all sorts of diseases.

Like West Nile Virus.

And wouldn't you know it: Bakersfield, California has a problem.

Despite the unusually dry and hot conditions, the mosquito populations in Bakersfield are booming.

The dry conditions have also lead to a decrease in house finch populations that had previously had high herd (flock?) immunity to West Nile, but a boom in the population of previously uninfected western scrub jays and house sparrows, which had no herd (flock?) immunity.

As a result, there was a West Nile epidemic in non-immune jays and sparrows, which died. Then the mosquitos, needing to eat and unable to find birds to feed on, turned to humans. At the peak of the epidemic, 19 out of every 1000 mosquitoes had West Nile, and there was a 280% increase in human West Nile cases.

At the same time, Bakersfield had a 300% increase in loan defaults, leading to pools and hot tubs not being cared for.

"An aerial photograph of a representative Bakersfield neighborhood shows the extent of the problem, with 17% of the visible 42 pools and Jacuzzis appearing green and likely producing mosquitoes."

There is also a shift in the mosquito population as the pools are left untended.

"Alarmingly, during 2008, many of these unmaintained pools previously positive for Cx. p. quinquefasciatus were now occupied by Cx. tarsalis, a more competent vector of WNV than Cx. p. quinquefasciatus."

The abbreviations and Latiny words are the names of the mosquito strains. I would guess that for every 1% loan default there is a 1% increase in West Nile.

When I was a kid I thought the show *Connections* was the

coolest series ever, and I still love how odd connections can end up in an outbreak of disease in a Suessian cascade of events. Imagine what would have happened if a bug had sneezed.

In this case it was an increase in West Nile infections because of the financial meltdown.

Rationalization

Reisen, W.K., et al., Delinquent mortgages, neglected swimming pools, and West Nile virus, California. Emerg Infect Dis, 2008. 14(11): p. 1747-9.

Tuberculosis

Hamlet Act 3, scene 1, 55

SAW a bad case of tuberculosis today. As opposed, I guess, to a good case of TB. Bad for him, good for me. Multiple involved lobes of the lung, consumption, and coughing up blood. Fortunately he is from the Western hemisphere, so I do not have to worry much about resistant TB. He should get better with antibiotics and time. Although he has no insurance, TB is one of those diseases that will be taken care of.

People always act surprised when I mention that I saw a case of active tuberculosis as they think it is a disease of the past, a killer of artists and musicians. I learned as I wrote this that WC Fields died of TB. The heck. Unfortunately, TB is alive and well in the world. It kills about 1.5 million people a year, one third of the world's population is infected with TB, and there is a person infected every second. And boy is he pissed.

The US and Western Europe do not have much TB. It has been on the decline for decades. Most of the cases of TB are in the developing and third world. But.

I think of humans as surrounded by a sea of germs, and most of our energy output is to keep these germs from consuming us— which they will do eventually. I have the unproven idea that doctors die of their subspecialty, so I am certain to die of an infection.

At least I am not an OB doc. I have told my wife to cremate me immediately upon death so the bacteria I have spent a lifetime killing do not get their chance to eat me.

And the US is like a person. We are an island of low infection rates for diseases that infect most of the world. Good nutrition, flush toilets, and public health departments across the country have kept these infections at bay. I wonder for how long. If you want to get good and anxious, read the books by Laurie Garrett (*Betrayal of Trust, The Coming Plague*). You will want to pull the covers over your head and stay in bed.

The problem with TB is that it is contagious, the method of spread is coughing, and in this country no one ever worries about covering a cough. Turn your head and cough. Why turn your head? It doesn't make it easier to find the hernia—it is so the patient doesn't cough TB (or some other infection) on you. Every couple of years we get a patient with active TB who has spent the prior months coughing on everyone he meets, spreading TB. Coughing is an efficient way to spread disease.

The other problem with TB is resistance. The way you breed resistant TB is to give intermittent and inadequate therapy for long periods of time, and that is just how TB is treated outside the West. Most US patients with infectious TB receive DOT, directly observed therapy, so we can help ensure that all the medications are taken. Not so in the rest of the world, where half of people who even get therapy for TB receive inadequate or intermittent therapy to guarantee the organisms develop resistance.

The result?

Worldwide, 20% of TB is multidrug resistant (MDRTB) and 2% of TB is extremely drug resistant (XDRTB). I expect those numbers will get worse. Most of these cases are in Korea, China and the Old Soviet Union. If you visit those countries, do not inhale.

And the bugs will come our way. They always do.

Today, at least, I can still treat TB. Even if I can't treat some MRSA and *E. coli.*

Rationalization

World Health Organization tuberculosis site: http://www.who.int/ mediacentre/factsheets/fs104/en/)

List of tuberculosis victims on Wikipedia: http://en.wikipedia.org/ wiki/List_of_tuberculosis_cases

It's all in where you come from

The history reveals all. If you ask the right questions and listen, often you will figure out the right diagnosis and sometimes even predict the organism.

An ex-nurse presented with a two-year history of a red, hot, painful, swollen knee. She didn't respond to standard therapy and didn't get better after arthroscopy. The knee continued to degenerate, so she got a new knee. No better. So the knee is revised. Still no better. At each evaluation of the knee there were a smattering of white blood cells, but routine bacterial cultures were negative, so it was passed off as degenerative joint disease.

So this time ortho calls me and says he is going in again, and do I have any ideas?

Nope.

Then he mentions that she is from the Philippines.

Two Burk You Losis.

Knee jerk reaction to the word Phillippines, in this case a chronically red, hot, painful, swollen knee jerk reaction.

If you say seizure and give me a Mexican last name, I'll say pork tapeworm faster than you can eat a strip of bacon. Mmmmmm. Bacon.

If you say fever and trip to Africa, it will be malaria.

And if you say the Philippines, it's TB. Or not TB. That is the question.

So I said, "Well, I have never seen a case of TB in a knee, much less in a prosthetic knee, but you had better send off fungal and especially acid-fast bacilli (tuberculosis) cultures, just in case. If it is infected it's from something that doesn't grow using usual techniques."

And it was TB.

I saw the patient the next day, and not only was she from the Philippines, but she had always had a positive TB test and never received therapy.

TB of artificial joints is rare—only a handful of cases have been reported. But as best I can gather from the literature, the chances that I will be able to salvage her joint are reasonable. We will see.

Ask and you will receive the diagnosis. Maybe the Secret is right after all.

Rationalization

Khater, F.J., et al., Prosthetic joint infection by Mycobacterium tuberculosis: an unusual case report with literature review. South Med J, 2007. 100(1): p. 66-9.

Addendum

As of 2012 the patient is functional, but still has a swollen, warm knee. Ortho tells me she can't get another knee, so she is on chronic antituberculosis therapy, isoniazid and rifampin.

As of 2014 she as a new knee. Her knee had been recalled and when it was removed the joint space was filled with fine, black metal shavings that may have the cause of the ongoing knee problems. Repeat cultures and pathology were negative for TB and she is no longer on TB therapy.

There is no place like Ghon

Today's case is an elderly lady with recent pleural effusions (fluid between the lung and the chest wall). Maybe pneumonia—she responded to a course of moxifloxacin, a quinolone antibiotic, on her last admission. But now she is back with more of the same.

The CT scan was interesting: large pleural effusion with a large calcified something-or-other in the right middle lobe.

Large, calcified something-or-others in the right middle lobe

(RML) are often old TB. When you first inhale TB, it most often goes to the RML and sets up the primary infection. After the immune system gets the TB under control, over time the initial infection calcifies, leaving the Ghon complex, named after Dr. Ghon. Crohn and Ghon share an 'h' that should not be there and of which I can never remember the correct location.

The patient's history is interesting. She lived her entire life in Oregon, but all the members of the family of her childhood play-mates had TB, and it (TB, not the playmates) evidently killed a couple of them.

She tells me she has always had this bit of calcium in her lungs. Even though the Ghon complex is calcified, there are probably still live organisms in the center. Unlike love, TB is forever.

The pleural fluid is midway between exudate and transudate, and has 30% eosinophils. More than 10% is considered eosin-ophilia, which is certainly consistent with TB, although this is a nonspecific finding that can also be seen in malignancy, other infections, and asbestosis.

Some pleural effusions from TB occur when an old pleural granuloma ruptures into the pleural space causing an intense al-lergic response, not unlike the swelling seen on a positive skin test for TB. The result is recurrent pleural fluid.

So we are sending off the tests looking for TB.

Here is the interesting thing: she got better for a while on a quinolone. These antibiotics are excellent therapy against TB, and taking them for routine pneumonia leads to a delay in the diagnosis of TB. The patients with TB get better, and the treating physician thinks it is due to the treatment of routine bacterial pneumonia. They relapse their tuberculosis when the antibiotic is stopped.

"The aim of this study was to assess the effect of empiric fluoro-quinolone therapy on delays in diagnosis in patients with PTB initially misdiagnosed as bacterial pneumonia...

In the fluoroquinolone group, eight patients (89%) improved clin-ically or radiographically, whereas only eight patients (42%) in the non-fluoroquinolone group improved (P = 0.04). The delay in initiation of anti–tuberculosis medication was longer in the fluoroquinolone group than in the non-fluoroquinolone group."

Remind me in a month when we have all the studies back, I'll let you know if she really has TB.

Rationalization

Dooley, K.E., et al., Empiric treatment of community-acquired pneumonia with fluoroquinolones, and delays in the treatment of tuberculosis. Clin Infect Dis, 2002. 34(12): p. 1607-12.

Yoon, Y.S., et al., Impact of fluoroquinolones on the diagnosis of pulmonary tuberculosis initially treated as bacterial pneumonia. Int J Tuberc Lung Dis, 2005. 9(11): p. 1215-9.

Postscript

It wasn't TB.

Boutonneuse hibou

I WAS pooped yesterday. The prior weekend I had been on call, so I worked 12 days in a row. As I age—well, wines age and get better, I am more ripening (overripe?) than aging—I fade at the end of the second week.

Two consults at the end of the day. The first was a cellulitis, and the second was billed as a fever. The resident wanted to know why the fever.

I was yawning as I read the chart and talked the case over with the resident. I had an idea after talking with her, but I wanted to see to the patient first.

Fevers to 104, worst headache of his life, normal blood count, mildly elevated liver enzymes . But. But but but. He has just returned from a bicycling trip in Italy.

And then the hinge point, the finding around which the diagnosis revolves: he had a black eschar with surrounding erythema on his lower leg.

The fatigue fell away. The hunt was on, the game's afoot Watson, or at least the game's a calf.

I thought I know what he might have.

Evidently not everyone gets as jazzed at a great case as I do. When I see what may be a zebra, a case of something I have never seen before, I get a surge of excitement. I get pumped.

The year of medicine in which I had the most fun was my internship, because everything was new and interesting. As the years go by, some diseases are no longer that interesting. Heart failure. Chronic obstructive pulmonary disease. Stroke. They are mostly slight variations on a theme. Kind of, well, dull.

But infections. There are so many infections, and I am nowhere close to seeing them all. Birders have it far easier. There are a paltry 10,000 bird species. Bo-ring. Easy to see them all; just look up. Nothing compared to potential infections. There are a dozen Rickettsia that can infect humans and I have seen one to date: Rocky Mountain spotted fever. Well, perhaps I should say I have diagnosed one to date; if I have seen others, I missed them.

Until yesterday.

I think I have my first case of *R. conorii* or *Boutonneuse* fever, which is an increasing problem in Italy. It was the black eschar that was the hint. That is the infamous *tache noire* I have read about for 15 years and have never seen.

No sooner did I whine that the physical exam was less than revealing than I got a case where they physical exam was key to the diagnosis. Figures. Sometime I wonder why I ever bother to pontificate on a topic, as I am sure to be proven wrong in the next 48 hours. Unfortunately he had no boutonneuse (French for spotty), at least not yet.

But he is on doxycycline and serology is pending. I will get the results back about the time I retire.

Rationalization

Cascio, A. and C. Iaria, Epidemiology and clinical features of Mediterranean spotted fever in Italy. Parassitologia, 2006. 48(1-2): p. 131-3.

Scaffidi, V., Current endemic expansion of boutonneuse fever in Italy. Minerva Med, 1981. 72(31): p. 2063-70.

Postscript

He responded rapidly to doxycycline, acute serology was negative, and he was lost to follow-up.

....

Ocean Spray. It's not Just for Cranberry Juice

HALLOWEEN is a busy day, with two kids that live to trick or treat, and we always have a Halloween party with real food before they disappear into a week of sugar-fueled lethargy. And of course, the one day I needed it to be slow, it was busy, and I had two consults with infections due to *Serratia marcescens*.

S. marcescens is not that unusual as a pathogen, causing hospital acquired infections of all kinds. What is interesting about the bug is it makes a reddish-orange pigment called prodigiosin. It can kind of look like blood.

It is the prodigiosin pigment that makes *Serratia* easy to identify, much to the distress of San Francisco.

In the 1950s, the military wanted to know how biological warfare agents were spread in an urban environment. In Operation Ocean Spray (nothing to do with the color of cranberry juice), federal agents placed agar plates throughout San Francisco and sprayed *Serratia* at SF from off shore. Some reports say they released balloons filled with the organism and popped them over the city. *Serratia* would be easy to track through the city since all they had to do was look for red/orange bacteria growing on the drop plates. The military thought *Serratia* was not a pathogen, and they were wrong. Shortly thereafter there was an increase in *Serratia* infections in the Bay area, eleven patients got pneumonia, and one person died from endocarditis.

One report suggests that people were breathing 5000 bacteria per breath or more for hours after the spraying, and the spraying covered about 117 square miles.

So when the wackaloons say the condensation trails (Contrails) from airplanes are not water, but are really the government spraying us with bacteria and nanobots, it is hard to counter with the assertion that the government would never do anything so stupid.

Fast forward a decade and the increase in the drug culture. San Francisco became the home of *Serratia* endocarditis in IVDAs, presumably because it was in the water of the Bay area. I have heard, but cannot confirm, that the strains that caused endocarditis were not the same as the strain sprayed over San Francisco.

But that is just what the men in black would want you to think.

Rationalization

Mills, J. and D. Drew, Serratia marcescens endocarditis: a regional illness associated with intravenous drug abuse. Ann Intern Med, 1976. 84(1): p. 29-35.

Often in error, never in doubt

O N rounds today I got a curbside.
One of the ICU nurses wanted to know what was going on with her young son. I get many such questions every day as I walk around my hospitals.

He had played a particularly muddy soccer game at one of the local schools over the prior weekend, and she noted that his shoes—which had been sitting uncleaned in the garage all week—now smelled like cat piss. Her words. I know of no infection that smells like cat piss.

And more interestingly, her son was covered with pustules that looked like chickenpox, which he couldn't have because he had both the disease and the vaccine twice. Look, I just report what people tell me.

We talked about it for a bit: how muddy the field was, and how my son was playing tomorrow, and how I hoped the field dried out. I admitted that I was uncertain what her son had; it didn't ring any bells. Then, as I was about to walk away, a bell rang.

There is some infection associated with muddy Australian rugby players, I said. What is it?

And where in the hell did that thought come from? That is one of the issues I have working in a teaching hospital. Some of the ideas I come up with do not arise in the conscious mind, and my later explanation of the diagnosis is an after-the-fact rationalization. Most of my best diagnoses come from some part of my brain that I have no control over. The thought burbles up through my brain like a bubble in a tar pit.

Pop. The patient has...

Google to the rescue. Google often makes me look smarter than I am, a quick search and the instant appearance of genius. Don't tell anyone that's my secret.

I entered "Australia," "rugby," "mud," "infection"——and viola! (I can spell instruments better than French). I had read this article once, four years ago. Where is that memory stored and how did I access it? Got me.

I was almost right. It was mud football, not rugby, but almost the same thing.

"On 16 February 2002, a total of 26 people presented to the emergency department of the local hospital in the rural town of Collie in southwest Western Australia with many infected scratches and pustules distributed over their bodies. All of the patients had participated in a mud football, competition the previous day, in which there had been > 100 participants. One patient required removal of an infected thumbnail, and another required surgical debridement of an infected toe. Aeromonas hydrophila was isolated from all 3 patients from whom swab specimens were obtained. To prepare the mud football fields, a paddock was irrigated with water that was pumped from an adjacent river during the 1-month period before the competition. A. hydrophila was subsequently isolated from a water sample obtained from the river. This is the first published report of an outbreak of A. hydrophila wound infections associated with exposure to mud."

Is this what the kid has? I don't know. There are other organisms that can cause pustules and folliculitis, some of which are associated with mud or water. I asked her to take her kid to the doc to culture the pustule. Perhaps it is another water-borne organism. I printed off the reference for her to take to the pediatrician.

I enjoy swinging for the fence for a diagnosis. People remember if you are spectacularly right. I am more often wrong than right, but doctors are always making a wrong diagnosis in medicine. Good docs are not those who are initially right, but those who do not stick to the initial ideas when they are wrong.

I hope I get a culture on this one.

Rationalization

Vally, H., et al., Outbreak of Aeromonas hydrophila wound infections associated with mud football. Clin Infect Dis, 2004. 38(8): p. 1084-9.

Postscript

The kid got better and the pustule was never cultured. Crap.

Frequently in error, never in doubt—the I.D. motto

FORTY-FIVE-YEAR-OLD male whose life is even less eventful than mine.

Works, raises a family, sleeps.

Presents saying he has low back pain after some minor lifting. Don't we all at that age? Wait until you are my age, 357 in dog years. I am increasingly like the Tinman in the Wizard of Oz, except I can't seem to find the oil to get things loose again. I sympathize.

His back pain gets worser and worser (my son's parallel word with better), so he gets an MRI which reveals a spinal epidural abscess. Odd in that he has no risks; usually this is a disease of needle users or at least a complication of an infection elsewhere. He has none of the above.

Then there is the lack of disc space infection. Usually the bacteria are presumed to go to the disc first, as the disc at least has some blood flow, and from the disc the bacteria go into the epidural space.

Oh well, it's a common medical aphorism that patients do not read the textbooks before coming into the hospital and so do not know how to manifest their disease properly.

Epidural abscesses are usually due to staphylococci and streptococci, and I occasionally see those organisms causing disease for no damn good reason. So I say it's probably going to be one of those organisms.

Imagine my surprise when the lab says the pus shows a gram negative rod. *Staphylococcus* and *Streptococcus* are gram positive cocci. The heck. More oddities.

But I am up to the task, pontificating that, "Oh, it's just after Thanksgiving, so this will probably be *Salmonella*." Tis the season, and *Salmonella* occasionally likes to cause extra-intestinal infections. That's the ticket. It's going to grow *Salmonella*.

Days pass and the lab says that what ever it is, it is only growing anaerobically. What? An anaerobe? Now I am stumped. I have two guesses and two misses, so I wait. Three strikes and you are made comfort care.

It is *Prevotella* species that finally grows.

And the reason? Once a bug is identified, killing it, or at least selecting an antibiotic, is simple. I want to know why. Why? Why, why, why, why, why? Luck! Blind, stupid, simple, doo-dah, clueless luck! "What" is interesting, but nothing satisfies more than knowing why. This time no way, no why. I can't find the hint of a suggestion of a possibility of a reason for why.

A PubMed reveals a grand total of zero spontaneous *Prevotella* epidural abscesses. So I have the first one. Ever. Yippie for me.

Bacteroides, the most common pathogenic anaerobe, has fewer reported cases of spontaneous epidural abscesses than I have fingers (12. 8 on the left, 4 on the right. Don't ask).

You just never know whatcha gonna grow. It's the great thing about I.D. You can blather on about how this and that bacteria should be causing the infection, and the cultures grow some unexpected germ that makes all your erudite pontifications wrong.

Another good case, curable with a course of antibiotics, but in the end slightly unsatisfactory.

....

Zits

Infected artificial hips are a major source of morbidity for patients.

At a minimum they need to have the hip washed out and a long course of IV and oral antibiotics.

At a maximum the have to have the joint taken out and they go jointless for 3 months or more, which will never do for Willie Nelson.

These infections are usually staphylococci of one sort or another, but the patient who presented today had gram positive rods in a three-year-old prosthetic hip.

Propionibacterium acnes is a bug of greasy, hairy males. It is an anaerobe that grows in the oils of hair follicles, men tending to the furry and the oily side. It lives in a protected site, because antibiotic scrubs do not get into the follicle, IV antibiotics do not get into the follicle, and so all our measures to prevent operative infections can't touch it.

The best protection from a *P. acnes* infection is to be a hairless female, but that hardly seems worth the effort if you are male.

This bug gets dragged into the wound and, if there is artificial material or devitalized bone, it hunkers down and causes the most indolent of infections. It is not unheard of to have 5, 6, or 7 years elapse between the surgery and the clinical presentation of the infection.

I had one case with 8 years between the craniotomy and the presentation of the brain abscess that the surgeon said looked (but did not taste) like scrambled eggs, and which grew *P. acnes*.

Treatment is problematic. For CNS shunt infections, vancomycin plus ceftriaxone may be best. In my experience (with the usual caveat) clindamycin works better than penicillin, and *P. acnes* is one of the few anaerobes that is resistant to metronidazole.

The lowly zit bug. When you are young it messes the mirror; when you are old it messes with your hip.

Rationalization

Zeller, V., et al., Propionibacterium acnes: an agent of prosthetic joint infection and colonization. J Infect, 2007. 55(2): p. 119-24.

....

Fooled Again

WHEN young females present with fevers and flank pain, you think: pyelonephritis. Common things are common in medicine and tautologies are tautological.

And that is what the outpatient docs thought. However, she was no better after several days on oral ciprofloxacin, so she was admitted for IV therapy.

Her white blood cell count kept going up, to over three times the normal limit (35,000), so they called me.

Part of the purpose of this book is to alter events to make me look like SuperDoc (TM), and this will be no different.

There were several curious features that I noted when I saw her.

While her urine dip (not for potato chips) was positive for white blood cells, her microscopic exam demonstrated no pyuria, or pus in the urine; the negative cultures were attributed to the oral antibiotics.

A CT scan of her kidneys on admission showed no stones and no abscess.

And boy, did she have flank pain. The lightest of thumps on the right flank elicited extreme pain. She said that the pain radiated abound her back and into her right lower quadrant. Just like a kidney stone. But she looked surprisingly non-toxic for someone with a white cell count of 35K, and she didn't have much of a fever.

I guessed that she had an appendix gone south, and another CT scan showed a huge abscess due to a ruptured appendix. The surgeon in the OR described it as looking like a grenade had gone off in her peritoneum.

The flank pain that fooled everyone? The abscess had dissected into her paraspinous muscles.

A classic history and physical for pyelonephritis that turned out to be something else.

And lest you think I am always right, yesterday I bet that a patient had *Legionella* pneumonia. The confirmatory test today? Negative. A swing and a miss.

When you are a consultant it is fun to try to predict the diagnosis; the odd time you are right will impress people far out of proportion to the more numerous misses. It is the I.D. equivalent of what Biggest Douche Bag in the Universe does.

Years ago I saw an 18-year-old girl with known valvular heart disease, with the question of whether or not she had endocarditis.

She had had five days of fevers, headache, and muscle pain that left for five days, recurred for five days and left for five, then recurred yet again.

For fun I asked, "How was your vacation at Black Butte?"

The look of shock and awe (TradeMark: Harlan K. Ullman and James P. Wade) on her face when she asked, "How did you know I was at Black Butte?" was one of the more satisfying responses of my career.

She had the history suggestive of relapsing fever, and the one place in Oregon with this disease is Black Butte.

Home run with the bases loaded.

Few remember that Babe Ruth also lead in strikeouts for several seasons.

Rationalization

Rucker, C.M., C.O. Menias, and S. Bhalla, Mimics of renal colic: alternative diagnoses at unenhanced helical CT. Radiographics, 2004. 24 Suppl 1: p. S11-28; discussion S28-33.

....

Malaria

Bad Air

THERE are diseases that are endlessly interesting because of the variations of the presentation. Endocarditis is one of those diseases. But endocarditis is an odd disease, in the West a result of intravenous drug use (it is now use, not abuse. IVDU not IVDA) or aging.

Other disease are not so interesting in their presentation but are fascinating due to their impact on culture, history, or genetics.

The patient today was freshly returned from a 10-month-long trip to sub-Saharan Africa, and presented to the ER with fevers to 104, chills, sweats, and cytopenias. Upon microscopic examination, 1% of her red cells were found to have *Plasmodium falciparum*. Nothing unusual about the case as malaria. Fairly typical. I would bet from the timing that she had her mosquito bite the day she left Africa, so she had gone months dodging the malaria bullet until the end of the trip. Unfortunately the patient could not tolerate the prophylaxis.

Malaria is endlessly interesting as a disease because of its impact on human cultures. I have read that half of everyone who as ever died has died of malaria, and it still accounts for 500 million infections a year and a million deaths, mostly in children. About 1% of people who get malaria die from it.

It still kills the occasional traveler. Most illness is due to infection with the potentially fatal *falciparum* strain. There are between five and 15 deaths due to malaria reported every year in the UK. In 2006 there were 1,758 reported malaria cases, with eight deaths. All the UK deaths were due to *falciparum* malaria caught in Africa. That's a pretty good death rate for a trip to Kenya or Niger.

Many malaria deaths are essentially murder. About half the antimalarials, and other antibiotics, sold in Asia and Africa are counterfeits that contain no active ingredients. They are placebos, and placebos are not particularly effective against life-threatening infections. It is hard to imagine the kind of slime mold (and I apologize to slime molds everywhere) who would manufacture fake antibiotics, which probably help kill hundreds of thousands of children worldwide each year who are given fake medications. We bitch about the high price of drugs in the US, but at least we know that when we are getting gouged for linezolid (fifty dollars a tab), we are getting gouged for the real deal.

There are also people who sell homeopathic antimalarials. That boggles the mind. Water is being used to prevent and treat a disease that in most of the world has at least a 1% mortality rate.

But if you are going to travel outside of the industrialized nations, buy your antibiotics before you go. And stay away from homeopathy. Unless you want to die.

Rationalization

Carlsson, T., L. Bergqvist, and U. Hellgren, Homeopathic Resistant Malaria. J Travel Med, 1996. 3(1): p. 62.

A purveyor: http://www.blueturtlegroup.com/catalog/3

Bad Air Redux

I have said before that being an I.D. doc is like being a birder, and I keep a mental list of the infections I have yet to see. Unlike identifying birds, seeing a new infection is actually interesting. Just kidding. Birds are cool. I had some Ivory-billed Woodpecker for dinner this weekend, and hope to have Spotted Owl next month. And Condor egg omelet? To become extinct for.

Today was a first for me—a new bird, the IV treatment of severe malaria.

My malaria patient had 1.1% of the red cells infected yesterday. Today? More than 10%. Whoa. The tech called to say she had never seen so many parasitized red cells. The patient was clinically perhaps a bit better, and certainly no worse, but greater than 10% qualifies as severe malaria. Sometimes there is a delay between the therapy and a decrease in the parasitemia, but more than 10% was too much.

For years quinine was the treatment for malaria, but there is no IV quinine in the US. There is a touch of quinine in tonic water, but not enough to do anything against malaria, so a gin and tonic is not considered a reasonable therapeutic intervention for the patient—although it may help calm the doctor.

But there is the anti-arrhythmic quinidine. I used quinidine as a resident late last century when we treated the occasional premature ventricular contraction occurring with an acute myocardial infarction. Quinidine also kills malaria as it the dextrorotatory diastereoisomer of quinine. But of course I state the obvious:

I have never given IV quinidine for malaria, but did give it back in the day when we treated any cardiac rhythm abnormalities in the ICU. I guess we know better now—I do not think I know a resident who has ever given IV quinidine or lidocaine. Too old school.

I called the CDC just to double-check, and the wise heads agreed with the IV quinidine and doxycycline. Whew. It's nice to have the CDC.

So IV quinidine it is. I feel like an intern again.

Rationalization

Treatment with quinidine gluconate of persons with severe Plasmodium falciparum infection: discontinuation of parenteral quinine from

CDC Drug Service. MMWR Recomm Rep, 1991. 40(RR-4): p. 21-3.

Bad Air Re Re Dux Dux

The intravenous quinidine worked perfectly for the malaria. Within a day her parasitemia was zero.

But.

When I went off to a meeting in Vegas she was looking great in the ICU, ready for transfer, I thought everything was going perfect.

When I returned the sign-out list said: On a ventilator, being given pressors (to keep her blood pressure from crashing), ECMO (extracorporeal membrane oxygenation), moved to trauma ICU.

I felt all the blood drain from my face and my heart fell into my shoes. I thought I was going to puke. What the hell had happened?

It is often not the organism, but the inflammatory response to the organism, that kills us. There is an old observation that after antibiotics, patients worsen. Antibiotics shatter the organisms and then there is a flood of endotoxin and other bacterial parts. The body responds with a tsunami of cytokines and the patient will transiently worsen about 4 hours later. It happens all the time. All you can do is hang on and support the patient.

Three percent of Westerners who get malaria die of the disease, so the risk is not trivial.

With malaria, the response is delayed about 24 hours. But when there is a big die-off of the organisms, there can be a delayed, and massive, systemic inflammatory response (SIRS), ironically due to the antibiotics. And she had a massive SIRS. Thank goodness for modern ICUs; if she had worsened in most other hospitals, given the rarity of ECMO, she would have died.

Fortunately, she is much better now and on the mend. But. Oh. Shit. I get anxious just thinking about it. PTSD.

My dad is a retired cardiologist and he used to say what kept him awake at night was not the calls but the worry. I have understood that for years, and that sick feeling that occurs when patients do unexpectedly badly keeps me up at night as well.

Rationalization

Krause, G., et al., Chemoprophylaxis and malaria death rates. Emerg Infect Dis, 2006. 12(3): p. 447-51.

Neither A nor B nor C nor D

I'M not talking med school grades here.

So many infections I have yet to see. Like a birder I have my lifetime list of infections I have seen and infections that I hope to see, despite the fact it means someone will have to suffer for me to add to the list. I am not silly enough to believe that my thinking it makes it so. I'll leave that to the goofs who practice the Secret.

Today, I diagnosed something I had never seen before. The previous chapters discussed a recent case of severe malaria. Today's case also had malaria, but to a much less severe degree. Upon admit the patient was not that ill, but had elevated transaminase liver enzymes (about 5 x normal) and bilirubin (3x normal) to an extent that I thought was more than could be accounted for by the severity of the malaria. As if I have a vast experience of treating malaria in Portland, Oregon—although if predictions of global heating are correct, malaria could make a comeback in my neck of the woods.

Hepatitis is known to occur with severe malaria and is a bad prognostic sign. However, it wasn't all that severe for the first three days, so I wondered about other causes of hepatitis from sub-Saharan Africa: yellow fever and Hepatitis A,B,C, and E. I sent off all the serologies and the ABC was negative (good thing we do not send our specimens to the Sesame Street Lab), but I was called by the State today: Hepatitis E IgG negative, IgM repeatedly positive, consistent with acute hepatitis. She had malaria AND hepatitis E.

He shoots, he scores, the crowd goes wild.

Hepatitis E is spread by fecal-oral contact (such an appetizing term, *n'est pas?*).T It is found in sub-Saharan Africa in the water, and there have been huge outbreaks in refugee camps. It has a nasty predilection for killing pregnant females.

Interestingly, it is also probably more common than previously suspected in the West. In Europe it is spread by pigs and eating pig livers or hunting wild swine. Who knew there were still wild swine in Europe?

In the US, a recent article in *Journal of Infectious Diseases* showed that 21% of Americans are seropositive for hepatitis E. The risks in the US are eating organ meats and having a pet, and I assume the two are mutually exclusive. Mmmmmm pet liver.

So look for Hepatitis E. Way cooler than a Condor. And more common.

Rationalization

Adlhoch, C., et al., High HEV presence in four different wild boar populations in East and West Germany. Vet Microbiol, 2009. 139(3-4): p. 270-8.

Kuniholm, M.H., et al., Epidemiology of hepatitis E virus in the United States: results from the Third National Health and Nutrition Examination Survey, 1988-1994. J Infect Dis, 2009. 200(1): p. 48-56.

Shah, S., et al., Malarial hepatopathy in falciparum malaria. J Coll Physicians Surg Pak, 2009. 19(6): p. 367-70.

....

Saepius in Erroris, Nunquam in Nuto

B usy busy busy.
Sometimes life keeps me away from the computer, but then, is that really living? There are things that need to be done away from the interwebs, at least until I become one with Matrix.

I spent a chunk of my day teaching residents, as one of my hospitals has an internal medicine residency program. The problem is I often do not know where my ideas for a diagnosis come from. Like today.

I was asked to see a patient with a past hematologic malignancy and fevers for five days despite being given ceftriaxone and azithromycin for a not-really-there pneumonia. The kind of "sort of maybe" infiltrate that has increased in frequency since the Oregon Medical Professional Review Organization started measuring time to first antibiotic as a quality indicator. As a result, a lot of iffy pneumonias are treated instead of waiting, proving yet again that no good deed goes unpunished.

I knew from a quick chart review that the white cells had gone from 6000 to 1-700 cells per microliter, making him slightly leukopenic. His platelets had fallen from 230k to 90, which is frank thrombocytopenia, though not yet dangerous. His hemoglobin had dropped 2 points. The rest of his labs were OK.

So the patient told me he had teeth-chattering rigors (which he had during the interview), fevers, severe myalgias, and abdominal pain. Otherwise no localizing symptoms.

Hmmmm.

Past medical history: Waldenstrom's macroglobulinemia, also called lymphoplasmacytic lymphoma, a type of B-cell lymphoma. Treatment finished a year previously.

Animals? Dogs.

Travel outside Portland?

"We were at our cabin in Eastern Oregon, near Bend, at 4900 feet."

Why he mentioned the elevation, I do not know, but my ears perked up.

So, any ticks?

Yeah. 4 tick bites, and his wife volunteered that they were swarmed with ticks this time of year.

And like a bubble floating up out of the bath and popping, I could smell what he had. But I do not know where the thought came from. The diagnosis is always made far below conscious thought, then I do a rapid song and dance to justify the potential diagnosis.

I should mention that I have yet to confirm the diagnosis, and like many great diagnoses I make, reality often contradicts me. Pesky reality.

My motto: *Saepius in Erroris, Nunquam in Nuto*: Frequently in

Error, Never in Doubt.

I will probably report in a few weeks that I was wrong.

But for now I am calling it Colorado Tick Fever. Everything fits perfectly. In the meantime he has what I like to call a doxycycline defiency state: fevers without a focal infection with a pancytopenia. Those organisms (Rickettsia and Spirochetes) cannot be grown and are all treated with a tetracycline.

Rationalization

Oregon Public Health site; entry on Colorado Tick Fever:

http://public.health.oregon.gov/DiseasesConditions/DiseasesAZ/Pages/disease.aspx?did=77

Postscript

Colorado tick fever serology was negative, and he either got better on his own or due to the doxycycline he received. However, Waldenstrom's is a disease of abnormal antibody production, so maybe I was right and the serologies were wrong. Yeah. The serologies were wrong. That's the ticket.

Sorry, nothing to learn here. Keep moving. A content-free post

ONE of the purposes of this book is to give the illusion of near omniscience (in fact, I am omnivorous). Case after triumphant case where, with a combination of the brilliance of House, Welby and Holmes, I find the correct diagnosis.

I wish that were reality.

More typical is the case I have right now: a foreign-born kidney transplant patient back from a trip to Idaho with fevers to 103 and five to six profuse watery diarrheal stools a day.

Easy, right?

Maybe. Diarrhea can cause fevers but fevers can cause diarrhea. I figure, probably incorrectly, that throughout most of history we ate questionable food and many infections came from food. So getting rid of contaminated food would be an important evolved response to infection. It is why, perhaps, when tumor necrosis factor (TNF) is injected into rats, it makes them grab a book and head to the toilet, as it gives them diarrhea. But that may be a just so story.

The patient had no risks or symptoms for opportunistic infections. One member of the family had had a similar illness, but it lasted only 48 hours.

So we worked up the fever: a stool examination for white blood cells (waste of time, but others do it) was negative. Examination for ova and parasites is also negative. Bacterial cultures negative. And the fevers and diarrhea continued. Slight crackles developed on exam (I never heard them) which led to a chest x-ray and then a CT of the chest. There were patchy left-sided infiltrates but no pulmonary symptoms at all. Nothing. Was the diarrhea an epiphenomenon of the pneumonia and TNF induced fever response?

Sputum was unimpressive, and he had a mild hemolysis as judged by the decreasing red count and elevated lactate dehydrogenase (LDH).

Mycoplasma?!? The chest x-ray looked worse than the patient felt, and hemolysis smells of that organism. But *Mycoplasma* is not a disease of the elderly, and this kind of diarrhea is not usually part of the disease, although who really could tell with the immunosuppressives he was on for the kidney transplant.

Legionella is pending and his fever began drifting down, whether from the macrolide or time I do not yet know.

Often getting the diagnosis is like hitting a piñata. It's there, somewhere, a treasure, and I am swinging the bat with a suspicion of where it is and I hope I do not connect with someone's head by mistake.

And that is why they call me Dr. Metaphor. Well, not really.

Sometimes I am slightly envious of the cardiologist. A quick cath and the issue of coronary artery disease is put to rest.

Oh well. I'll let you know what I get.

Postscript

There was never a diagnosis and the patient got better. The preferred result, as a diagnosis with a dead patient somehow ever satisfies.

IN ONE END: FOODBORNE AND ORAL INFECTIONS

Go Yeast, Old Man

The week is over and my virus lasted only a day. Thank you, Rockport (1).

Five days of doing my best to kill kill kill. Kill viruses. Kill spirochetes, Kill bacteria, Kill yeasts. I hope PETA never goes microscopic.

If my workday has been successful, I have left a swath of unicellular death that makes Genghis Khan look like a piker. I am sure I have killed billions upon billions of creatures in my day.

But now it's the weekend and I get to enjoy the best that the microbial world has to offer.

Saccharomyces cerevisiae is a common yeast. "Saccharomyces" comes from Greek, and means "sugar mold"; "cerevisiae" comes from Latin, and means "of beer." Put the two words together and they spell heaven. *Saccharomyces* is used to brew beer and to raise bread.

Occasionally *Saccharomyces* is a pathogen in humans. The only time I have seen disease due to *Saccharomyces* is in the ICU, when patients are treated for their diarrhea with probiotics that contain S*accharomyces boulardii*, the primary yeast in Chef Boulardii products. Very rare, but reported in the literature, and why I do not treat diarrhea in the ICU with probiotics—although the literature to support its use as a preventative is good.

Years ago, when I was a fellow (and, no I have not had a sex change, a fellow is a doctor training in a subspecialty) I had an AIDS patient who was a home brewer and who developed a fungemia with *Saccharomyces*, the same one he used to brew beer. You could say I knew what aled him.

Thank you, I'll be here all week. Try the prime rib and don't forget to tip your I.D. doc.

It is extremely rare to get a fungemia with the yeast used for brewing and baking, and that is a good thing, as both are needed for two of the great pleasures of life.

The Pacific Northwest is the center of the microbrew world, and tonight I enjoyed the brewers' sampler at the local pub: blond, heffiweizen, amber, seasonal, IPA, Brown and Porter. One would think that if there were karma, after a week of killing these organisms, I would get sour beer. Nope. No karma. The beers were perfect.

The other pleasure of yeast will come in the morning from waffles, which I make every weekend for my kids. This recipe comes from *How to Cook Everything* and makes the best waffles ever. All thanks to *Saccharomyces*.

2 cups milk

2 cups flour

1 Tb sugar

1/2 tsp salt

1/2 tsp yeast

Mix together.

Add 1 stick of melted butter. Yes, butter. You can have a good life or a long life. I choose good.

Let sit in a warm place overnight.

In the morning, separate 2 eggs, add the yolks, along with 1 or 2 or 3 teaspoons of vanilla to the batter. I like lots of vanilla, especially Watkins vanilla.

Whip the egg whites and fold them in.

Make a waffle with whatever iron you use. Mine is 50 years old with a fabric-insulated electric cord, so you know I am soon to die of electrocution. And use real maple syrup, not that fake stuff. Even better with fresh blackberries, raspberries, peaches, or Oregon strawberries—not the wooden crap from California.

It will be the best thing you can do with your mouth in public.

The microbiological world. One minute I am trying to kill it off, the next I am enjoying its excrement.

No matter where you look, you find an infectious disease, even in a good breakfast.

Rationalization

(1) See "Virus R Me."

Bittman, M. *How to Cook Everything: 2,000 Simple Recipes for Great Food.* Houghton Mifflin Harcourt 2008.

....

Sourdough

I HAD that microbial gift that keeps on giving this week. No, not gonorrhea.

Sourdough.

For years I had a sourdough starter, which followed me from college to med school to Minnesota to LA and was lost, tragically, when I dropped the jar on my move home to Portland for my current job.

So for 19 years I have been sourdough free. I somehow never got the gumption back to begin another starter. I was in mourning.

Until this week. The head of my clinic has a 100-year-old sourdough starter, and this week she gave me a cup of ancient yeast.

I am back in business. This morning was sourdough pancakes and tomorrow it will be biscuits.

The good news is that sourdough supports nutritional health. Snicker.

In various studies sourdough has been shown to increase the availability of nutrients and minerals and to improve glycemic control in diabetics. And *Saccharomyces cerevisiae* is a probiotic, so it supports immune and GI health. As if my immune system were a sagging collection of flesh that needed support. Crislip's rule number 314159: if a product is said to 'support' any kind of health, the only thing the product will support is the bank account of the producer of the product.

Since my yeast colony is 100 years old, it predates bioengineering and is a more natural product.

So shortly I am going to market my special Detox Immune Enhancing Sourdough starter and diet.

I am going to make a fortune.

If you can get a good sourdough going at home, do it—it is so much better than the products you buy at the store.

Rationalization

Lopez, H.W., et al., Making bread with sourdough improves mineral bioavailability from reconstituted whole wheat flour in rats. Nutrition, 2003. 19(6): p. 524-30.

Maioli, M., et al., Sourdough-leavened bread improves postprandial glucose and insulin plasma levels in subjects with impaired glucose tolerance. Acta Diabetol, 2008. 45(2): p. 91-6.

....

Seizures

Got a call about a patient with an Hispanic surname and a seizure. In my world that combination is cysticercosis, from the pork tapeworm, *Taenia solium*. Pork. The other white meat.

Turns out that pigs have their very own tapeworm. If you eat undercooked pork, then you get the *Taenia* larvae, which travel to your brain where they form marble-sized, fluid-filled cysts with a little parasite in them. Or you can acquire the tapeworm from inadvertently (one hopes) eating human poo from a carrier.

The parasite can live up to 25 years (can you say ick), but eventually all good things come to an end: the parasite dies, the cyst breaks down releasing parasite parts, the immune system attacks, the brain becomes inflamed and headache and seizures result. Or after they die they calcify, which also results in a focus for seizures. In some parts of the world, like Mexico, cysticercosis is the number one cause of seizures.

In the U.S., pork tapeworm is not a problem, but south of the border it is a very common cause of seizures. It may not be a problem in the U.S., but one of the rare times I have sent food back is when the pork loin was rare. Just couldn't eat it. I also do not like pigeon rare, but for aesthetic reasons.

You say, "Well, I don't eat pork. I am of the Orthodox Jewish faith." No such luck. There was an outbreak in a New York city Orthodox Jewish community where 4 people had neurocysticercosis and several others had serologic evidence of disease. The source? Domestic help that had recently immigrated from Latin America, where *Taenia* is endemic. It was in the stool of the workers and was passed from worker to food to family.

Even if you do not eat the food or travel to where the disease is found, the infection can still come to you.

Also of interest, DNA analysis of tapeworm suggests that pre-humans acquired *Taenia* from hyenas and big cats, the definitive hosts, who preyed on antelopes (the intermediate host). When people started hunting lions, we picked up the worm, and passed it to pigs and cattle later when we domesticated them. In evolutionary scheme of things, we gave the tapeworm to the pig. So really, pigs are just giving back what we originally gave them. What comes around, goes around.

My patient, unfortunately, did not have the typical MRI findings of cysticercosis and may have a low grade brain tumor. He had a brain biopsy because of the unusual appearance of the MRI, but final pathology is pending. It's a bummer. An infection I could cure, but a brain tumor, not so much.

Six months later I got a live one. Phone call from the ER: seizures, new immigrant.

The CT was unenhanced—done without contrast material—but showed at least 20 areas of calcification throughout the brain, and one area of edema and swelling in the temporal/parietal lobe.

Unenhanced CTs do not give enough detail to make the diagnosis, but the MRI the next day did: numerous one-centimeter diameter, fluid-filled cysts scattered throughout the brain, and in each one, like a teeny tiny fetus, is a worm.

I will pause here while you shudder.

Treatment is albendazole or praziquantel, the one drug evidently named after an Aztec god. When you treat the disease the patient gets much worse, as dying organisms lead to further inflammation, so antibiotics need to be combined with steroids. Long-term, treated patients may have fewer seizures, but the need to kill with worms is still uncertain. Still, who wants a live worm in the brain?

Take-home lesson: don't eat pig poo. But I bet you knew that.

Rationalization

Del Brutto, O.H., et al., Meta-analysis: Cysticidal drugs for neuro-cysticercosis: albendazole and praziquantel. Ann Intern Med, 2006. 145(1): p. 43-51.

Schantz, P.M., et al., Neurocysticercosis in an Orthodox Jewish community in New York City. N Engl J Med, 1992. 327(10): p. 692-5.

Cool pictures:

http://web.stanford.edu/group/parasites/ParaSites2004/Taeniasis/index.htm

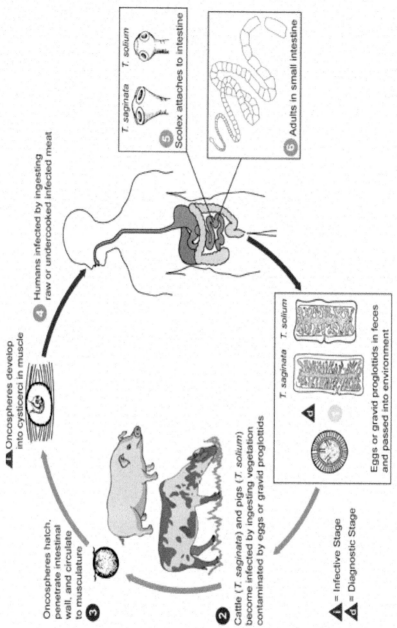

Lifecycle of pork and beef tapeworms. Humans are the definitive hosts for both, meaning they can harbor mature worms in the intestine. For the pork tapeworm (but not the beef tapeworm), humans can also serve as the intermediate host, with cysticerci forming in muscle and brain. (Image from the Centers for Disease Control and Prevention Public Health Image Library, content providers: Alexander J. da Silva, PhD and Melanie Moser. www.cdc.gov/dpdx).

165 degrees

THE microwave oven is great for heating leftovers, wonderful for melting butter, handy for warming a cold cup of coffee. And I notice the one in our house, when popping corn, blocks the thought waves beamed into the radio receiver in my head—or is that too much information?

The problem with a microwave is that it is too easy to give a half-assed cooking of food and not kill any bacteria.

Salmonella is back. 32 people in Minnesota and 11 in other states have developed *Salmonella* by eating chicken pot pies that were microwaved instead of cooked in the oven. The package didn't say you could microwave it, but these folks did it anyway. You get hungry dere in Minnesota, doncha know?

"Frozen, raw, breaded and pre-browned stuffed chicken products covered by this alert and similar products, may be stuffed or filled, breaded or browned and therefore appear to be cooked. These items may be labeled 'chicken cordon bleu,' 'chicken kiev' or chicken breast stuffed with cheese, vegetables or other items."

The chicken isn't cooked, just browned. Twice cooked chicken is rubbery and tasteless, so they make the pot pie and you cook it, supposedly in the oven.

The same thing happened last year when 165 people got *Salmonella* from chicken pot pies that were not cooked enough.

This is no surprise as *Salmonella* are commonly found in food products and are part of the food chain. How common? Depends on the study and how the prevalence of *Salmonella* is determined. In a representative study,

"Overall, 9 (64%) of 14 lots and 42 (31%) of 135 of the (chicken) carcasses were positive for Salmonella."

As long as we eat chicken and chicken by-products (eggs) we will be exposed to *Salmonella* and the 400,000 cases a year will continue.

Heat kills, and if you get your food to 165 degrees the bacteria will die. Microwaves are particularly bad in that they heat unevenly, so that one part is cold and another part is hot and the food is not sterilized.

Not only *Salmonella*, but also *Listeria* can survive both freezing and microwaving. Food is dangerous, and will be until we switch to Soylent Green.

You could irradiate your food as well, but the public has issues with radiation, even though no one at Three Mile Island ever developed *Salmonella*.

ALWAYS eat your food deep fried, it's better to die of heart disease than infection. Besides, my Dad is a cardiologist.

Rationalization

Bailey, J.S. and D.E. Cosby, Salmonella prevalence in free-range and certified organic chickens. J Food Prot, 2005. 68(11): p. 2451-3.

Arsenault, J., et al., Prevalence and risk factors for Salmonella and Campylobacter spp. carcass contamination in broiler chickens slaughtered in Quebec, Canada. J Food Prot, 2007. 70(8): p. 1820-8.

Chicken Migration

CHICKENS are a great source of pathogens. *Salmonella* and *Campylobacter* lead the list. Chickens lead crowded, short lives, and their lives would be even shorter if farmers didn't put antibiotics in the chicken feed.

The good thing about small amounts of antibiotics in the feed is the chickens get bigger faster and you get a cheap fryer.

The downside is antibiotic resistance. 70% of antibiotics used in the US are for agriculture, about 25 million pounds year. That's total, not per animal. The rule is simple: expose a bacterial population to antibiotics, especially low levels of antibiotics, and the resistance is inevitable.

At least chickens do not fly and do not migrate, so the antibiotic resistance should be contained to the farm. Except.

Chickens do migrate. They take a truck, often in open cages, from the farm to the abattoir. The wind from the truck aerosolizes the chicken dander and poo, spraying the countryside, and the car behind the truck. One study

> *"...collected air and surface samples from cars driving two to three car lengths behind the poultry trucks for a distance of 17 miles. The cars were driven with both air conditioners and fans turned off and with the windows fully opened. Air samples collected inside the cars, showed increased concentrations of bacteria (including antibiotic-resistant strains) that could be inhaled. The same bacteria were also found deposited on a soda can inside the car and on the outside door handle, where they could potentially be touched."*

Some of the organisms were antibiotic resistant. Clinton was right not to inhale, he just picked the wrong situation.

Unfortunately I cannot yet access this journal through our library, probably because this is the first issue. So I cannot find which pathogens were isolated and to which antibiotics they were resistant.

But it gives me pause. How many times have I been stuck behind a pick-up full of teenagers? The exposure risk is scary.

Rationalization

Transporting Broiler Chickens Could Spread Antibiotic-Resistant Organisms, Johns Hopkins School of Medicine Press Release. http://www.jhsph.edu/publichealthnews/press_releases/2008/rule_chicken_transport.html

Rule, A.M., S.L. Evans, and E.K. Silbergeld, Food animal transport: a potential source of community exposures to health hazards from industrial farming (CAFOs). J Infect Public Health, 2008. 1(1): p. 33-9.

Happy Thanksgiving

THANKSGIVING is my favorite holiday, because it is associated with lots of infections. Kind of not true. My favorite holiday is really Halloween. But I need a lead for the entry.

Salmonella and *Campylobacter* go with poultry like, well *Salmonella* and *Campylobacter* go with poultry.

"This study was conducted to determine the prevalence and antimicrobial resistance of Campylobacter and Salmonella isolates from retail poultry meat in the UK during 2003-2005. Poultry meat (n = 2104) were more frequently contaminated with Campylobacter (57.3%) than with Salmonella (6.6%). Chicken exhibited the highest contamination from Campylobacter (60.9%), followed by duck (50.7%), turkey (33.7%) and other poultry meat (34.2%). Duck had the highest contamination from Salmonella (29.9%), compared with chicken (5.6%), turkey (5.6%), and other poultry meat (8.6%). C. jejuni predominated in raw chicken, whereas C. coli predominated in turkey and duck. C. coli isolates were more likely to exhibit antimicrobial drug resistance, including quinolones, than C. jejuni. Salmonella Enteritidis was the most frequent Salmonella serotype isolated. Salmonella isolates from turkey exhibited higher rates of multiple drug resistance (55.6%) than isolates from chicken (20.9%) and duck (13.6%). The findings reinforce the importance of thorough cooking of poultry meat and good hygiene to avoid cross-contamination."

This is why the pop-out in your butterball is designed to not only cook the turkey, but overcook it. But who wants rare poultry? We are big time Francophiles in my family, but I still remember being disgusted by rare pigeon in France. It's the way it is supposed to be served. One of the few things I could not eat, and I ate raw horse in Japan (Mr. Ed we barely cooked ye). Raw poultry? Icky.

Most people do not get their infections from the cooked bird, but instead do not adequately clean the prep space and put culture media—I mean cooked food—where they prepared the turkey, re-inoculating the bird.

The only way to reliably eradicate these pathogens is to irradiate the food, and the advantage to this is a turkey with three legs.

You can also get *Salmonella* from infant formula, dog food, vacuum-packed rats (mmmmm, vacuum-packed rats), reptiles (I wish turtle and snake were a Thanksgiving tradition) and tree sparrows, to name a few.

Being a vegan or vegetarian is no protection. Tomatoes, spinach, peppers, basil, cheese, milk, apples, peanut butter, cantaloupe, alfalfa sprouts, and almonds have all been implicated in *Salmonella* outbreaks.

Bon appétit.

Rationalization

Little, C.L., et al., Prevalence, characterisation and antimicrobial resistance of Campylobacter and Salmonella in raw poultrymeat in the UK, 2003-2005. Int J Environ Health Res, 2008. 18(6): p. 403-14.

....

Warm October

I AM taking a few days off to have father-son time at the Oregon Coast during my son's Fall Break. We have been coming to the beach for forty years and, while my memory can be faulty on many issues, the beach has changed in my lifetime. The low tides are not as low as I remember them, the high tides are higher. The ocean seems to have risen. The interwebs say the oceans have risen 0.05 mm a year for the last forty years. That would be 2 mm since I started walking the Arch Cape beach. Doesn't seem like one whole heck of a lot on paper, but my fallible memory seems to remember low tides that were, well, low. Really low. Vast expanses of beach. Now, even on a minus tide, there isn't that much walking beach.

Oceans rise because of melting ice, and warm water expands. Warm water takes up more room and thermal expansion is part of why sea levels are rising. With warm water brings, you guessed it, infections.

I am on a see food diet—I see food, I eat it. At the beach we eat seafood, at least for the short term. Except oysters. I am chicken to eat raw oysters. I have eaten deep-fried grasshoppers and raw horse. Raw oysters are home for Norwalk and *Vibrio* species, all causes of gastroenteritis.

Back when I was a youngster first walking up and down the beach, I did not have to worry about *Vibrio* as the water was too cold. That was a problem for the warm waters of the gulf coast, where the water was greater than 15 degrees, the lower limit of temperature for *Vibrio parahaemolyticus*.

No longer. There was an outbreak of *Vibrio parahaemolyticus* gastroenteritis on a cruise ship in Alaska that was associated with eating raw oysters. Never before had the Alaskan waters been warm enough to support the growth of *Vibrio parahaemolyticus*.

"Mean daily marine water temperatures at Farm A in July and August from 1997 to 2004 showed a 0.21 C increase per year (r2 = 0.14, P<0.001); water temperatures in July and August were significantly warmer in 2004 than in each of the six previous years examined (P < 001). Mean yearly surface-water temperatures from 1976 to 2004 in the Gulf of Alaska also showed a trend of increasing water temperatures."

Warm water leads to warm water infections.

"This report documents a large outbreak of V. parahaemolyticus serotype O6:K18 in the United States, and it expands the range of epidemiologically confirmed V. parahaemolyticus illness to a latitude higher than 60 degrees, more than 1000 km north of British Columbia, previously the northernmost area reported to have locally acquired illness. Furthermore, our findings provide evidence to support the hypothesis that a water temperature above 15.0 degrees C at the time of oyster harvest is an appropriate threshold indicator of increased risk of V. parahaemolyticus infection from the consumption of raw oysters. Although water temperatures have reached 15.0 C at Farm A each year since 1997, 2004 was unusual because mean temperatures were above 15.0 C for a much longer period and were almost 2 C warmer than during any of the previous years."

Tonight I had a BLT with onion rings. I hope tomorrow there will be enough beach for a nice long walk. It will not be there much longer.

Rationalization

McLaughlin, J.B., et al., Outbreak of Vibrio parahaemolyticus gastroenteritis associated with Alaskan oysters. N Engl J Med, 2005. 353(14): p. 1463-70.

Bloody Bullae

HEMORRHAGIC bullae.

If you are an I.D. doc, hemorrhagic bullae make you think of *Vibrio vulnificus*. Sometime last century the *Annals* published the classic (as if medical articles have the same cachet as Dickens or Twain) article on hemorrhagic bullae and their relationship with liver disease, sepsis, and *V. vulnificus*.

My patient had an increasing cellulitis, hemorrhagic bullae, and was on dexamethasone, a steroid, for cancer. It's nice to have a risk factor for the infection. *V. vulnificus* is associated with warm salt water exposure or oyster consumption, but he had been nowhere near the sea. The closest he had been to the ocean is a fillet o' fish sandwich from the local fast food eatery.

A quick PubMed revealed that *Aeromonas*, a fresh water pathogen, has been associated with hemorrhagic bullae, but he had not been in a lake or a pond of late either.

So we treated him for cellulitis and *Vibrio vulnificus* and he got better. The next day the blood cultures grew a gram negative rod, so I think, maybe my first *V. vulnificus*?

His leg improved and we narrowed his antibiotics. The thing is, he grew *Pseudomonas aeruginosa* from his blood, and for 48 hours he improved on therapies with zero activity against his infecting organism. Maybe it was the dexamethasone that prevented him from going septic, maybe his genes, maybe just luck, who knows. Sometimes people just get better. My rule is, when people improve, take credit. When things go ill, blame nursing. Just kidding. As a resident I had a patient with *Pseudomonas* sepsis who refused therapy due to underlying advanced cancer, and he got better without therapy. Even this most nasty of bugs does not kill everyone, every time.

Also odd is that today's patient did not, as best as can be determined, have a necrotizing fasciitis, which is usually what gram negative rod soft tissues infections cause. And there are no reports in Pubmed of hemorrhagic bullae from *Pseudomonas*. So probably another fluke case.

He was changed to an anti-pseudomonal antibiotic and continued to get better, not that is was due to anything I did. But I am still taking the credit.

Sing-Along

With apologies to Sam: http://www.youtube.com/watch?v=MHF558u6Q_8.
Uno, dos, one, two, tres, quatro
Matty told Hatty about a thing she saw.
Had a cellulitic leg and ate oyster raw.
Bloody Bullae, Bloody Bullae.
Bloody Bullae, Bloody Bullae, Bloody Bullae.

Hatty told Matty, "Let's don't take no chance.
Let's not be L-seven, the blister need a lance."
Bloody Bullae, Bloody Bullae
Bloody Bullae, Bullae Bullae, Bloody Bullae.

Matty told Hatty, "That's the thing to do.
Got to kill that Vibrio before it kill you."
Bloody Bullae, Bloody Bullae.
Bloody Bullae, Bloody Bullae, Bloody Bullae.

Rationalization

Klontz, K.C., et al., Syndromes of Vibrio vulnificus infections. Clinical and epidemiologic features in Florida cases, 1981-1987. Ann Intern Med, 1988. 109(4): p. 318-23.

Endocarditis, Bacteremia, and Dental Work

BACTEREMIA is common after dental work. Really common, even after tooth brushing. 20% of the time with toothbrushing and 60% of the time if the dentist yanks a tooth you can find bacteria in the bloodstream if you look hard enough. And that is the frequency of bacteremia after doing something as primitive as blood cultures.

If you do more sophisticated 21st-century methods of looking for bacteria, brushing and tooth extraction release a flood of bacteria:

"Sequence analysis of 16S rRNA genes identified 98 different bacterial species recovered from 151 bacteremic subjects. Of interest, 48 of the isolates represented 19 novel species of Prevotella, Fusobacterium, Streptococcus, Actinomyces, Capnocytophaga, Selenomonas, and Veillonella."

Icky, poopy, guadeloupe as we say in our house. And you kiss your spouse with that mouth? But it does bring home the fact that your mouth contains a rich microbiological environment, only a flossing away from your bloodstream.

The worry is bacteria seeding abnormal heart valves, especially around the time of dental extraction, and the American Heart Association (made up of Real Americans, I might mention 10 days before the election) recommends prophylactic antibiotics to prevent endocarditis, even though amoxicillin only decreases the bacteremia by half.

Do dental extractions increase the risk of endocarditis? I am not so certain. There have been epidemiological data to suggest that dental work does not increase endocarditis risk and that prophylactic antibiotics are not effective in endocarditis prevention, but the studies are unreadable by all but other epidemiologists. Another epidemiological study that was published last month again demonstrates (I guess) that dental extraction is not a risk for endocarditis.

"The study population was composed of 170 hospitalized patients with infective endocarditis. The frequency of dental procedures during the 3-month period immediately before admission was compared with the frequency of such procedures during earlier 3-month control periods (when no endocarditis developed), using the case-crossover design. Thirty-four out of 98 patients with available information (35%) had 81 dental procedures during the 2 years before hospitalization, 12 (12%) of whom had 14 procedures during the 3 months before admission. The number and types of dental procedures performed during this 3-month period

were not statistically different from those carried out during any earlier 3-month period, which served as a control period. Dental procedures do not significantly increase the risk of IE."

Dental work is not the risk it is cracked up to be for endocarditis; the big risk for developing endocarditis is life. It's why I no longer brush my teeth.

I have been told that the US has 30% of the world's lawyers, and the American Heart Association Guidelines are easy to find (to prove it, I'll let you Google it). Published, did I mention, by Real Americans from Real America. So until the guidelines change, don't run the risk of running afoul with the American Bar Association. Follow them. The Guidelines, not the ABA.

Rationalization

Bahrani-Mougeot, F.K., et al., Diverse and novel oral bacterial species in blood following dental procedures. J Clin Microbiol, 2008. 46(6): p. 2129-32.

Lockhart, P.B., et al., Bacteremia associated with toothbrushing and dental extraction. Circulation, 2008. 117(24): p. 3118-25.

Porat Ben-Amy, D., M. Littner, and Y. Siegman-Igra, Are dental procedures an important risk factor for infective endocarditis? A case-crossover study. Eur J Clin Microbiol Infect Dis, 2009. 28(3): p. 269-73.

Goat Cheese

ANOTHER teenager, this one with fevers for a month, progressive weight loss, night sweats, hepatosplenomegaly (enlarged liver and spleen), elevated liver enzymes, and pancytopenia.

Extensive work-up as an outpatient was negative, and she was admitted to the hospital. Now, on the fifth day of her admission, she has small gram negative rods growing from her blood.

Interestingly, although her temperature is 104, her pulse does not go above 80. For those who play at home, it's Faget's (pronounced fah-jays; it's French. Only use the hard 't' if you are from Texas) sign.

Faget's sign is pulse-temperature disassociation. Normally for every degree of temperature elevation the pulse should kick up 10 beats. Faget's classically occurs with only a handful of diseases: Typhoid, *Brucella*, and yellow fever are the typical atypical infections to have this sign, although it can atypically occur with some more typical infections in the US like Legionella and Tularemia. Usually in the US it's beta blockers that lead to Faget's.

Sure enough, the cultures grew *Brucella melitensis*, which has been eradicated in the US. To brag (and what is this blog for if not to give the illusion of my infectious omnipotence?), when the admitting docs called me for the consult I first said something to the effect that when we get the name of the bug we may have a hint as to its origin. I asked for the patient's name, and when they said an Hispanic surname, I said it had to be *Brucella*. She denied ever having left suburban Portland or eating any unusual foods. So why did she have this odd organism?

Brucella has a long history of killing people, and its long history is reflected in its many names. It has been called undulant fever, Mediterranean fever, Cyprus fever, Gibraltar fever, and Malta fever, a testament to the troubles it caused the British Empire. The British army, in the days before food preservation, kept meat supplies on the hoof, and in the Mediterranean one of the few animals that could exist on those rocky outposts was the goat. So they got *Brucella* as well as an excellent chèvre.

Prior to this case I had only seen one other case of *Brucella* in Oregon, a new immigrant (less than a month in the US) with orchitis (testicular infection). He had been a professional goat milker in Mexico and eventually needed an orchiectomy to cure the disease. I saw a smattering of cases in L.A. as a fellow and it set my personal record for the longest incubation of a bacterium, the blood culture turning positive on the 42ndday of incubation—the last before we would have thrown the plate out.

A month later I saw the patient, this time with her mother, in follow-up. She was cured of her infection and her mother rather grudgingly admitted that the uncle occasionally brought goat cheese with him when he visited from Mexico and that her daughter had eaten some. No one else in the family, however, came down with the disease.

When I was a kid, I thought diseases were named after the source of the infection, as my best friend swore that you got *Salmonella* from eating Salmon. What, I wonder now, would I eat to get Brucellosis?

Rationalization

Eckman, M.R., Brucellosis linked to Mexican cheese. JAMA, 1975. 232(6): p. 636-7.

Navarro-Martinez, A., et al., Epididymoorchitis due to Brucella mellitensis: a retrospective study of 59 patients. Clin Infect Dis, 2001. 33(12): p. 2017-22.

You are what you eat

EVEN after 25 years, I am still amazed at people will do to themselves to get high.

Some things are mythical. Like Jenkum. Supposedly people put human waste in a jar with a balloon on top and let it ferment, then inhale the fumes to get high. The better name is butthash, and this one I do not believe. It sounds like an urban myth that was generated just to see how gullible some people can be.

But Pruno? That made Emerging Infectious Diseases, and it was not the April 1st edition, either.

Pruno. What a name.

It is a prison alcoholic drink made from peeled potatoes smuggled from the kitchen, apples from lunches, one old peach, jelly, and ketchup. Inmates then heated water with an immersion heater and added it to the mixture. Ketchup, but not catsup, appears to be a key ingredient in the concoction, as is fruit. One prison banned fresh fruit to prevent the production of pruno. Like that would work.

The result is magenta in color and smells like baby poop. Mmmmmmmmmm. Pruno.

The consequence of drinking the pruno is initially a drunk,

followed in this case by Botulism, type A. I assume there was some serious vomiting as well.

The source of the botulism is probably from the potato skins. *Clostridium botulinum* is found in the soil, as are potatoes, and there have been other outbreaks of type A botulism associated with baked potatoes and potato salad.

I have only seen a smattering of botulism in my career, all but one case from home-canned foods. I saw one case as a fellow where the patient had *C. botulinum* in his sinus from snorting coke. There was an outbreak from carrot juice and another from eating fermented beaver tail and paw. I prefer my beaver tail and paw stir-fried. I love those organic foods.

As for drinks, I am sticking with French Bordeaux.

Rationalization

Angulo, F.J., et al., A large outbreak of botulism: the hazardous baked potato. J Infect Dis, 1998. 178(1): p. 172-7.

CDC, Botulism associated with commercial carrot juice—Georgia and Florida, September 2006. MMWR Morb Mortal Wkly Rep, 2006. 55(40): p. 1098-9.

Seals, J.E., et al., Restaurant-associated type A botulism: transmission by potato salad. Am J Epidemiol, 1981. 113(4): p. 436-44.

Vugia, D.J., et al., Botulism from drinking pruno. Emerg Infect Dis, 2009. 15(1): p. 69-71.

....

Ceviche

About two years ago I had a patient who had a period of nausea and vomiting and then developed at chronic lump on her skin. On biopsy it was some sort of parasite. It was too degenerated to say for sure what it was.

Today I saw a patient in clinic who has had intermittent nausea and vomiting, with a thirty-pound weight loss, and a completely negative gastrointestinal (GI) work up.

By history she had the same exposure as the patient of two

years ago. Both ate a lot of ceviche, a citrus-marinated raw fish, while in Mexico. How can that make you sick?

The raw fish carries a parasite, *Gnathostoma spinigerum*, which causes Gnathostomiasis. Which just sounds unpleasant. It is not killed by lemon juice.

G. spinigerum used to be is Southeast Asia, but it may have come to Mexico as part of tilapia fish farming.

"The life cycle of this parasite is as follows: Adult parasites of G. spinigerum are found in the stomach of mammals (e.g., dogs and cats), feces containing ova. Ova reach the water (i.e., when domestic parasitized animals live at the shore of a lagoon). Free-swimming first-stage larvae are formed, which are ingested by the minute copepod copepod: see crustacean. Any of the 10,000 known species of crustaceans in the subclass Copepoda. Copepods are widely distributed and ecologicaly important. Most of the 44,000 crustacean species are marine, but there are many freshwater forms. cyclops, and become second-stage larvae. Freshwater fish eating cyclops are the second intermediate host. Larvae develop to the third state (L3) in the fish muscles. Consumption of this fish by cats, dogs, or other mammals results in development of adults in the gut, closing the cycle. Humans acquire the infection by consuming raw or undercooked freshwater fish. When a larva is ingested by a human host, no further development occurs, but the larva migrates through subcutaneous tissue and internal organs where it produces migratory swelling in the skin and other symptoms depending on the site or organ affected. In most cases, symptoms are not serious; however, if the parasite migrates to vital organs of the host, it can cause severe illness or even death"

G. spinigerum is noted to cause eosinophilic meningitis and migratory itchy skin rashes as the parasite wanders through your tissues looking for a place to live. It can cause gastrointestinal symptoms, which had been the patient's primary complaint, although there were other features of the presentation—lack of eosinophilia—that make me doubt the diagnosis. I have been pursuing some other ideas.

But as the first reference states,

"A diagnosis of gnathostomiasis should be considered for patients with a history of transient, migratory cutaneous or subcutaneous swellings, or nonspecific gastrointestinal symptoms for which a potential epidemiologic exposure is identified."

The main point of this entry?

Ooooo icky poopy, a worm.

The only good fish is a fried fish.

The best thing of all? If I am right I will have aced the diagnosis that another local I.D. doc missed. My enormous ego needs constant feeding.

Mmmmmmmm. Right diagnosis.

Rationalization

Moore, D.A., et al., Gnathostomiasis: an emerging imported disease. Emerg Infect Dis, 2003. 9(6): p. 647-50.

Rojas-Molina, N., et al., Gnathostomosis, an emerging foodborne zoonotic disease in Acapulco, Mexico. Emerg Infect Dis, 1999. 5(2): p. 264-6.

....

Lactobacillus

*L*ACTOBACILLUS is a gram positive rod, a normal part of the lower GI tract and the female genital tract. It is a rare cause of serious infections, like endocarditis.

The patient today had a history of a Whipple procedure 5 years previously. Not to be confused with Whipple's disease, which is an infection, or a TV pitchman who prevents toilet paper squeezing. The Whipple procedure (pancreaticoduodenectomy) is a major surgery for pancreatic cancer involving removal of part of the stomach, part of the pancreas, and other organs. Repair requires anastomosis of the pancreatic duct and the jejunum, a junction that sometimes breaks down and leaks, causing infection.

Seemingly cured of his cancer and healed from his surgery, now he had fever and mid epigastric pain; the CT scan showed an abscess.

It was drained, and both the abscess and the blood grew *Lactobacillus*, as you might have guessed from the title.

It was a curious case. Lactobacillus is also a probiotic (given what they cost, they are certainly not amateur-biotics), and there has been the occasional odd case on PubMed of *Lactobacillus* in the blood or a liver abscess due to *Lactobacillus*. Generally, however, it is thought that probiotic *Lactobacilli* are safe. He had eaten yogurt, so maybe that was the source. The *Lactobacillus* in yogurt and probiotics is often a different strain than those found in and on normal humans. Unfortunately, I had no easy way to see if the source of his bug is life or Yoplait.

I presumed the patient had a leak somewhere causing this abscess, but we were not able to find one. Leaks can self-seal.

There are a smattering human cases of *Lactobacillus* abdominal abscess on a PubMed search, both associated with gastric perforation.

Drain and antibiotics, and I expected I would cure him as long as he did not have a leak.

And best of all, his immune system was being boosted and/or supported by the *Lactobacillus* in his peritoneum and blood. I assumed he was getting far more immune boosting than if he were merely eating the probiotic as DanActive. Right?

Rationalization

Wylezol, M., et al., Intra-abdominal abscess in the course of intragastric migration of an adjustable gastric band: a potentially life-threatening complication. Obes Surg, 2006. 16(1): p. 102-4.

If you can't be self-aggrandizing, what's the point of writing a book?
QuackCast 22: http://www.pusware.com/quackcast/quackcast22.mp3. Boost your immune system. And die. A cursory review of the immune system and then a review of some medical literature that suggests boosting it will cause you to die die die die die die die die die die die die die........ Got carried away. We're all gonna DIE!!!!!!!!!!!! Sorry. I panic easy.

QuackCast 16: http://www.pusware.com/quackcast/quackcast16.mp3. Probiotics. A review of probiotics: theory, use and complications.

AND OUT THE OTHER:
ENTEROPATHOGENS

Wrong. Again. And again. And again

SHORT chapter. Busy day, tired, up late finishing a novel where
I just had to know how it ended. *Lonely Werewolf Girl*, if you
have to ask. The protagonist is a werewolf, addicted to opiates,
homeless, depressed, with an eating disorder. Except for the
werewolf part, not unlike a lot of the druggies I take care of. At
least I assume they are not werewolves...

I was wrong three times this month, and the month is only
half over. Fortunately it was at three different hospitals, so unless
they read this book, no one will see a pattern.

First case was a young male back from Vietnam, with bad
crampy bloody diarrhea and positive blood cultures. He had gram
negative rods in his blood, I am told, so what do you think he has?

Salmonella, I replied. Most common cause of bacteremia with
a bacillary diarrhea.

He grew *Campylobacter.*

The next week I had an elderly man with no risks who presented with diarrhea and fever. He had gram negative rods in his
blood. What do you think he had?

Well, I say, I saw a case of *Campylobacter* last week, but the
most common cause of bacteremia with bacillary diarrhea is *Salmonella.*

He grew *Campylobacter.*

This week I got a call about a young woman with bad lupus on
steroids who comes in with abdominal pain and diarrhea and has
gram negative rods in her blood. What is it, they asked?

I say it's *Campylobacter*. Although the most common cause of bacteremia with bacillary diarrhea is *Salmonella*, and, although I am not superstitious, things do come in threes, so it has to be *Campylobacter*.

It was *Yersinia*.

You can't win. That's why I.D. keeps you humble (well, maybe you, not me). No matter what a hot shit you think you are as a diagnostician, the cultures will pop positive with some germ out of left field that you didn't expect and make all your erudite pontifications turn to dust in your mouth. Mmmmmmm. Humble pie. It is also why I.D. is so much fun.

It is why my motto is "Frequently In Error, Never In Doubt."

Bee Frage and diarrhea

I WISH I knew half as much as I think I do. There are about 10,000 articles in PubMed each year related to infectious diseases. If I were to read one an hour, boy would I be bored.

It is not only new things to learn. I am constantly surprised by things I thought I knew, but didn't. They are rarely of clinical importance, but it really seems the more I know, the less I know. It is that old definition of a specialist: she knows more and more about less and less until she knows everything about nothing.

Take *Bacteroides fragilis*. It is the major anaerobic bacterium isolated in infections related to gastrointestinal perforation, and an important germ in the formation of abscesses. When killing anaerobes you want to make sure you kill B. frag, as we call it in the biz.

Because it is a common pathogen, I assumed it was a common anaerobe of the GI tract. I was wring, wrang, ronge, wrung, well, you know what I am trying to say.

B. fragilis makes up a small percentage of the fecal flora, and only 40% of humans are colonized with the organism. Rather than being a predominant and common part of the colon, as I thought, it is a minor colonic constituent and can be uncommon.

The other thing I thought about *B. fragilis* is that it did not cause disease unless it escaped the colon. That, based on new information, is also in error. *B. fragilis* is a new described cause of gastroenteritis, aka the hershey squirts, in humans.

There is an Enterotoxigenic *Bacteroides fragilis* (ETBF) that causes an inflammatory diarrhea. The organism is evidently endemic in Bangladesh, where the study was done. Enterotoxigenic means it secretes a toxin into the bowel to cause disease, a common mechanism for bowel pathogens to cause diarrhea, since it is the diarrhea that allows the organism to spread. Much of the world now, and all of the world in the past, uses the same water source for drinking and waste disposal. Where do you think light beer comes from?

"ETBF was identified to cause a clinical syndrome with marked abdominal pain and nonfebrile inflammatory diarrhea in both children (age, 11 year) and adults. Fecal leukocytes, lactoferrin, and proinflammatory cytokines (interleukin 8, tumor necrosis factor, as well as B. fragilis toxin systemic antitoxin responses, increased rapidly in ETBF-infected patients. Evidence of intestinal inflammation often persisted for at least 3 weeks, despite antibiotic therapy."

I bet we have all seen a case or two of this: patients who have diarrhea, "substantial abdominal pain and tenesmus," no fever, and negative studies for the cause of the diarrhea. *B. fragilis* cultured from the stool would be considered normal flora and not a pathogen. To confuse issues, evidently up to 40% of controls will carry ETBF (and there is, maybe, an association with bowel cancer, perhaps due to chronic inflammation).

The depressing thing about these ETBFs is that 7% are resistant to metronidazole (Flagyl, for those of you who have sold their soul and speak brand name only). I also thought metronidazole resistance was unheard-of. It's toxic to microorganisms because it is reduced by their electron transport chains into DNA-damaging products. Any organism with the correct redox potential should be susceptible... shouldn't it?

Maybe I finally have a reason to order a fecal leukocyte count, a test that usually adds nothing to the diagnosis of diarrhea. Negative work-up with positive stool WBCs could be a hint of ETBF, although there is no diagnostic test yet for us lowly clinicians. But if you are going to Bangladesh for vacation, don't consume any stool.

Ha.

Rationalization

Sears, C.L., et al., Association of enterotoxigenic Bacteroides fragilis infection with inflammatory diarrhea. Clin Infect Dis, 2008. 47(6): p. 797-803.

....

By the sea, by the sea, it's VRE

THE national Infectious Disease meetings are going on this week in Washington, DC, but this year I couldn't make it. I am stuck with seeing what comes over the interwebs, and it is interesting to see what gets reported from the hundreds of studies presented at the meeting.

Of course the first one I see is a most vexatious report from Bloomberg news, *"Beaches in U.S. Host Drug-Resistant Bacteria, Researchers Find."* Cue the drama prairie dog.

I do not have the actual study, but evidently the researchers cultured the water and beaches of California and Washington and found VRE—vancomycin resistant *Enterococcus.*

Lets see. We have *Enterococcus* in our stool. We flush it down the toilet where it goes to the processing plant, then into the river and out into the ocean. Would you be surprised to find stool organisms in and on the beaches? Not me, especially an organism as hearty as the *Enterococcus.*

It is not uncommon to find this organism in runoff, especially near the high human density of SoCal.

"Species identification was determined for 1413 presumptive Enterococcus isolates from urban runoff, bay, ocean and sewage water samples. The most frequently isolated species were Enterococcus faecalis, Enterococcus faecium, Enterococcus hirae, Entero-

coccus casseliflavus and Enterococcus mundtii. All five of these species were isolated from ocean and bay water with a frequency ranging from 7% to 36%. Enterococcus casseliflavus was the most frequently isolated species in urban runoff making up 36–65% of isolates while E. faecium was the most frequently isolated species in sewage making up 53–78% of isolates. The similar distribution of species in urban runoff and receiving water suggests that urban runoff may be the source of Enterococcus. No vancomycin or high level gentamycin resistance was detected in E. faecalis and E. faecium isolate"

That some VRE are isolated from water is not a surprise, given that this organism is being heavily selected for with the buckets of vancomycin we are using to treat MRSA. This report is one of the first to find vancomycin resistance in the environment, though. Despite its quasi-apocalyptic tone, environmental VRE is probably not much to worry about. VRE is a risk only to the sickest of the sick in the hospital.

"If people with compromised immune systems, such as those who have undergone cancer therapy, play in sand with the bacteria, they could potentially contaminate themselves or their households, the researchers said."

The only way people can avoid being exposed to the organisms found in human stool is to lock themselves in a bubble and never venture out. Stool organisms are everywhere.

More worrisome is the fact that the resistance genes to vancomycin—of which there are at least 5—have been known to jump from the *Enterococcus* to MRSA, giving us VRSA, vancomycin resistant *Staphylococcus aureus*. Vancomycin resistant MRSA is a bug to worry about.

Antibiotic resistance genes are common, even in areas that are not exposed to antibiotics. Most antibiotics are based on a bacterial and fungal products, and the organisms have resistance genes to protect themselves from their own antibiotic production and from the antibiotic attacks of other organisms.

One study collected dirt across Canada (the country, not the yeast), isolated 480 different strains of *Streptomyces*. *Streptomyces* are Gram positive bacteria that grow like filamentous fungi, and are the source for 80% of antibiotics. These dirts (I once lost a Scrabble game to my wife saying the pleural of dirt is dirts, and lost the challenge. Stupid Webster. I have vowed to use the word dirts until it becomes part of the language) were pristine, and it was unlikely the organisms had ever been exposed to man-made antibiotics. When tested against a panel of 21 antibiotics, the *Streptomyces* were resistant to seven or eight of them on average, and two were resistant to 15 drugs.

The Borg were half right. Resistance is inevitable. And everywhere.

Rationalization

Moore, D.F., J.A. Guzman, and C. McGee, Species distribution and antimicrobial resistance of enterococci isolated from surface and ocean water. J Appl Microbiol, 2008. 105(4): p. 1017-25.

D'Costa, V.M., et al., Sampling the antibiotic resistome. Science, 2006. 311(5759): p. 374-7.

Outbreaks

I GET to investigate infectious outbreaks. Most outbreaks occur in relatively slow motion—a case this week, a case next week, a case the following week of the same organism or the same site. I help try to figure out why.

Some outbreaks come with the force and suddenness of a flash flood. Like Norovirus. This is the virus made famous by Disney cruises. Ever notice that Steamboat Willie didn't show a toilet? Walt wasn't looking after his creations. No place for Mickey to go should he dine in the buffet. I have dealt with several Norovirus outbreaks in various hospitals, where patients and staff come down with nausea, vomiting and diarrhea all within a few days.

There are many causes of infectious diarrhea and they all have their pathogenic peculiarities. Norovirus is no different.

The first distinguishing feature of Norovirus is that it was recently voted the world's most infectious virus. It was on the November ballot as part of the Green Party candidate. Didn't you see it? It takes one viral particle to cause disease. One.

"We estimate the average probability of infection for a single Norwalk virus particle to be close to 0.5, exceeding that reported for any other virus studied to date."

That's it. It beats out *Shigella*, which takes as few as 10 organisms to cause disease. That's infectious.

The second issue with Norovirus is how hardy it is. People have diarrhea, like shrimp and oyster fishermen (shouldn't you shrimp for shrimp and oyster for oysters if you want to be consistent?), who crap into the sea and Norovirus gets in the water and is filtered and concentrated in oysters. People then collect oysters, freeze them and send them all over the world. Problem is, freezing doesn't kill the Norovirus. Neither does cooking.

"Norovirus is heat resistant, with viable virus surviving after heating at 60 °C for 30 min. In other outbreak investigations, people eating well-cooked or over-cooked shellfish had a risk of becoming ill that was similar to that for people who ate raw shellfish. It is likely that the time and temperature of cooking required to inactivate norovirus in oysters may render the food unpalatable to consumers."

I will eat damn near anything, but raw oysters are one of the few things I have not tried. I have also never eaten tongue, because the thought that the tongue would taste me while I tasted tongue Freaks Me Out, Man.

The final cool thing about Norovirus is that it mutates in response to the host's antibody reaction to it. You get infected, your body develops antibody to the proteins that makes the virus virulent. The virus escapes the immune system by mutating at the sites where the antibodies bind. And the more the organisms can mutate, the longer the virus can be excreted in the stool.

"The greatest number of amino acid mutations in a given patient was 11; they were detected in NoV isolates recovered over a

119-day period and were mapped to positions at or near putative antigenetic sites. In the patient with most severe immune dysfunction, only 5 amino acids mutated over 182 days, suggesting immune-driven selection."

So many cool things in one virus: infectivity, world trade, evolution. Now if someone could suggest a good book, I have to be heading to the toilet for a while.

Rationalization

Teunis, P.F., et al., Norwalk virus: how infectious is it? J Med Virol, 2008. 80(8): p. 1468-76.

Webby, R.J., et al., Internationally distributed frozen oyster meat causing multiple outbreaks of norovirus infection in Australia. Clin Infect Dis, 2007. 44(8): p. 1026-31.

Siebenga, J.J., et al., High prevalence of prolonged norovirus shedding and illness among hospitalized patients: a model for in vivo molecular evolution. J Infect Dis, 2008. 198(7): p. 994-1001.

It's Over. Norovirus, that is

THE outbreak of norovirus on one of the units of one of my hospitals is over.

What a pain. The staff on the unit responded superbly, and once the outbreak was identified and infection control procedures instituted, it remained confined to one unit and there were no cases past the incubation period. They really cut the infection off at the knees.

Infection control procedures work when applied correctly. Not everyone believes that assertion, evidently, as some staff would not enter the unit during the outbreak. They were afraid of catching the disease and evidently had no confidence in infection control procedures.

This does not surprise me.

A couple of years ago, during the height of the biological terrorism fears, a young girl came down with monkeypox, which she caught from her pet rodent (while discovered in monkeys, it more commonly infects rodents, but the name stuck). Monkeypox looks just like smallpox and there was concern she might be the index case of a terrorist attack. I heard a lecture at a meeting by the MD who took care of her. He had had the smallpox vaccine so it was safe for him to take care of her. However, he could get no one else to take care of the girl, MD or RN, so he was her sole provider until they had the correct diagnosis.

It is estimated that should there be another flu outbreak like the 1918 pandemic, about half of health care providers will not come to work. And a significant number think this is OK.

*"**BACKGROUND**: Conflicts between professional duties and fear of influenza transmission to family members may arise among health care professionals (HCP).*

***METHODS**: We surveyed employees at our university hospital regarding ethical issues arising during the management of an influenza pandemic.*

***RESULTS**: Of 644 respondents, 182 (28%) agreed that it would be professionally acceptable for HCP to abandon their workplace during a pandemic in order to protect themselves and their families, 337 (52%) disagreed with this statement and 125 (19%) had no opinion, with a higher rate of disagreement among physicians (65%) and nurses (54%) compared with administrators (32%). Of all respondents, 375 (58%) did not believe that the decision to report to work during a pandemic should be left to the individual HCP and 496 (77%) disagreed with the statement that HCP should be permanently dismissed for not reporting to work during a pandemic. Only 136 (21%) respondents agreed that HCW without children should primarily care for the influenza patients.*

***CONCLUSION**: Our results suggest that a modest majority of HCP, but only a minority of hospital administrators, recognizes the obligation to treat patients despite the potential risks. Professional ethical guidelines allowing for balancing the needs of society with personal risks are needed to help HCP fulfil their duties in* *the case of a pandemic influenza."*

I took care of AIDS patients before we knew it was caused by HTLV-3 (now HIV, that is how old I am), and we were not entirely certain how it was spread. I like to think that when the time comes, I will have the courage of my convictions and work through the next pandemic. I know that infection control works.

But I do expect that at least half of my colleagues will not be there to help me. If they are worried about a little diarrhea (well, not so little) how are they going to respond to a plague?

Rationalization

Balicer, R.D., et al., Local public health workers' perceptions toward responding to an influenza pandemic. BMC Public Health, 2006. 6: p. 99.

Ehrenstein, B.P., F. Hanses, and B. Salzberger, Influenza pandemic and professional duty: family or patients first? A survey of hospital employees. BMC Public Health, 2006. 6: p. 311.

....

Intestinal Infections

A FEW days off with my youngest continues, and the Oregon coast is infection-free. At least so far as I can tell. We walked in the beach, watched Speed Racer, played golf, and went to dinner. Nothing that appeared to be related to infections in any way occurred. Such is vacation time. If only we had a plague here at the beach, it would give me something to write about.

The Web is my only current exposure to disease, so to speak. CNN tells me that Mr. Blackwell died of complications of an intestinal infection. But nowhere can I find just what intestinal infection. The inexactness of the news always bugs me. I know one thing reasonably well, and it's infectious diseases, and the news almost always either gets it wrong or is incomplete. How am I supposed to trust the rest of the news? Help me, Mr. Harvey. I know that Mr. Blackwell's publicist is under no requirement to give details as to the exact nature of his illness, but as an I.D. doc

I hate the uncertainty.

I am not a big fan of fashion (although thanks to my wife I have seen more of *America's Next Top Model* than I should probably admit). I am a fan of infections and an even bigger fan of knowing. So what was it?

I would bet first on *C. difficile*, a diarrhea commonly acquired in the hospital due the use of antibiotics. Quinolones and clindamycin kill off the normal bacteria of the colon, letting the *Clostridium difficile* overgrow and cause infection. *C. diff*, as we call it in the biz, makes a toxin that can cause necrosis of the colon, causing the colon to perforate and kill the patient. The organism is becoming resistant to common antibiotics and some strains are hyper-producers of the toxin, leading to increase in colectomies and deaths from the disease.

The other intestinal infection that would kill would be a perforated diverticular abscess with peritonitis.

All the other infections that could kill seem less likely. I want details and I cannot find them, and probably never will.

Anyone who knows the real answer, let me know.

Rationalization

Loo, V.G., et al., A predominantly clonal multi-institutional outbreak of Clostridium difficile-associated diarrhea with high morbidity and mortality. N Engl J Med, 2005. 353(23): p. 2442-9.

....

See Em Vee

CMV. Sounds like a Honda sedan. It stands for *Cytomegalovirus*. A disease of children, AIDS and organ transplant patients, it is rarely seen in normal people. Or is it?

A middle-aged, single male needed to have a diverting colostomy to, well, divert. Stuff. The particulars are not relevant to the case.

As part of the preparation he had a colonoscopy and, much to the surprise of the person looking up the old colon, there were small ulcerations and a patchy, angry red colon.

The patient had no symptoms of colonic problems, so the findings were unexpected.

The biopsy was even more unexpected: CMV.

The heck.

CMV colitis is seen in end-stage AIDS patients and bone marrow transplant patients. It is not a disease of normal people. I think.

He appears to be immunologically normal, and his HIV is a negative.

Thank goodness for PubMed. It is what makes all consultants look more knowledgeable than they are.

Turns out CMV can cause both severe and mild colitis in normal people. Most of the case reports are severe disease, and given the commonness of the Hershey squirts, I bet these represent the tip of a diarrheal iceberg. I shudder to think what damage a diarrheal iceberg would do to an ocean liner. The Titanic had it easy.

The few reported cases of mild disease suggest that CMV colitis is probably self-limited. My patient has no symptoms, so I will check his immune system as best I can and watch. I.D. docs are the only physicians who do not have to treat every culture that comes their way.

But I wonder if mild colitis, maybe with minimal or no symptoms, is a common manifestation of CMV that we miss since the ubiquity of diarrhea makes it unlikely that people would receive a diagnostic colonoscopy.

Now I am going to have a peanut butter sandwich. No CMV, just the risk of *Salmonella*.

Rationalization

Rafailidis, P.I., et al., Severe cytomegalovirus infection in apparently immunocompetent patients: a systematic review. Virol J, 2008. 5: p. 47.

Swimming in Body Fluids

VACATION means swimming. In lakes. In rivers. In oceans. In pools. Swim in a pool, you are swimming in the microbial flora of everyone else in the pool. And chlorine does not kill everything.

The family had returned from a 2-week trip to the tropics where they swam in the hotel pool with many a young child.

First one child gets sick with nausea, vomiting and headache.

Then the next child gets nausea, vomiting and a headache.

Dad gets lip blisters.

Mom then gets nausea, vomiting and a headache. She goes to the ER and has a lumbar puncture (LP), aka spinal tap. Me? I am never going to use the word 'headache' in an ER. I do not want an LP. Ever. The thought gives me the willies. She had a classic aseptic/viral meningitis and went home after a few days. Then she had progressive shortness of breath and got admitted to my hospital with large, bilateral pleural effusions, and a prolonged PR interval on EKG. The latter indicates slowed conduction through the atrioventricular node, and can be a sign of myocarditis, but she had normal cardiac function. I was called, the sound of trumpets announcing my arrival.

I was betting on leptospirosis because of the pleural effusions. The family's tropical travels had taken them to areas that are endemic for leptospirosis, and leptospirosis is a common cause of aseptic meningitis. There were other features arguing against leptospirosis: no protein in the urine, no increase in bilirubin, no conjunctival suffusion (eyes that look like you have been smoking a whole baggie of pot).

However, the other disease spread by shared pool water is the enterovirus, and we asked the outside hospital to run a PCR for enterovirus on the CSF—and it was positive. Pools are a great source of the enteroviruses, as these bugs are often resistant to chlorine. The classic in the old days was polio, the most feared of the enteroviruses. Formaldehyde is better at killing the virus, but no one wants to swim in that.

So all her symptoms were due to the enterovirus, but I have some splainin' to do with the pleural effusions. I can't find where enterovirus causes pleural effusions in normal people without heart failure. Is it due to direct invasion of the pleural space or an immunologic post-infectious disease? I don't know. I need to browbeat the lab into running a polymerase chain reaction on the pleural fluid to look for viral DNA.

Rationalization

CDC, Aseptic meningitis outbreak associated with echovirus 9 among recreational vehicle campers--Connecticut, 2003. MMWR Morb Mortal Wkly Rep, 2004. 53(31): p. 710-3.

Faustini, A., et al., An outbreak of aseptic meningitis due to echovirus 30 associated with attending school and swimming in pools. Int J Infect Dis, 2006. 10(4): p. 291-7.

Hauri, A.M., et al., An outbreak of viral meningitis associated with a public swimming pond. Epidemiol Infect, 2005. 133(2): p. 291-8.

Lenaway, D.D., et al., An outbreak of an enterovirus-like illness at a community wading pool: implications for public health inspection programs. Am J Public Health, 1989. 79(7): p. 889-90.

SEX, DRUGS, AND OTHER RECREATIONS

HIV

1982

I WAS a third-year medical student in 1982, when the first report of Gay Related Immune Deficiency (GRID) was published in the Morbidity and Mortality Weekly Report. It did not, as I remember, make an impression at the time—a series of obscure diseases when I was still trying to learn the basics of medicine.

Two years later I was taking care of my first AIDS patients as a medicine resident in Minnesota. At the time we had no idea what was causing the disease; we only knew it was linked to drugs, sex and Haiti. Both my patients had had thousands (yes, thousands) of sexual partners and both had used drugs, so they had the tentative diagnosis of GRID, now AIDS. We all felt moderately comfortable that it was not spread casually, but I still remember declining a piece of chocolate from the young male with the excuse that I wasn't hungry. I also remember him telling me that I could not get the disease from him unless "We have sex or I spit in your mouth." That conversation has stuck all these years.

That same year, 1984, HTLV-3 was discovered—a retrovirus initially called the human T-lymphotropic virus, type III and since renamed the human immunodeficiency virus (HIV). Once the virus was discovered, the pathophysiology known and the epidemiology understood, I have felt more comfortable eating my patient's chocolate, but I still do not want anyone to spit in my mouth.

The AIDS epidemic has been a major part of my career. The early years of death after awful death; the initial waves of optimism then pessimism as medications were developed, tried, succeeded, then failed. Now, with highly active anti-retroviral therapy (HAART), I have had one death this century from AIDS. We have gone from a nine-month life expectancy to an almost normal life expectancy for U.S. AIDS patients. Some residents will go though a three-year training program and never see an infectious complication of HIV. The progress has been astounding, at least for those who can afford the medications. I have seen far too many deaths because patients cannot afford their medications and come in dying of AIDS.

All these advances stem from the discovery of the virus by Françoise Barre-Sinoussi and Luc Montagnier for which they received a well deserved Nobel in 2008. The depth and breadth of understanding that can be rapidly brought to bear on new pathogens is astounding, as HIV and SARS have demonstrated. What has always been depressing about HIV is the numbers of people who really should never have died. Science and epidemiology were ignored in favor of politics and religion. Twenty-five million people have died so far from AIDS, most of the deaths unpleasant and in the young. Simple preventatives could have done much to attenuate the early epidemic: condoms, needle exchange, and closing down bath houses.

In 2007, Maputo Archbishop Francisco Chimoio of Mozambique claimed that condoms were deliberately infected by HIV to finish off Africans. This statement has still not been repudiated by the Church. How many extra will die in a country where 500 people are newly infected each day?

Pisses me off.

Rationalization

World HIV/AIDS statistics: http://www.avert.org/world-wide-hiv-aids-statistics.htm

Best. Ringtone. Ever

When I was a fellow, an attending told me about the time the national meetings were in Las Vegas. He was waiting for a ride in the hotel bar when a lady came up to him and asked him if he was interested a "date." Wink. Wink. Nudge. Nudge. Know what I mean?

He respectfully declined, and she asked, "What kind of meeting is this? Business is the slowest it has been in weeks."

No one is less likely to participate in the world's oldest pastime than an Infectious Disease doc. We are all too aware of what we might bring home. Not everything stays in Vegas—especially not HIV and syphilis.

The risk of HIV from sex is dependent on when in the course of HIV you attempt transmission: HIV is

"26 and 7 times, respectively, more infectious than asymptomatic infection. High infectiousness during primary infection was estimated to last for 3 months after seroconversion, whereas high infectiousness during late-stage infection was estimated to be concentrated between 19 months and 10 months before death."

There are a lot of factors that go into HIV transmission: kind of sex, having other sexually transmitted diseases, whether the person is on HAART or not. Even if your viral load is suppressed to unmeasurable, there is still a small risk of HIV transmission. If a couple has 100 sexual encounters per year, the cumulative annual probability of HIV transmission is 0.0022 for female-to-male transmission, 0.0043 for male-to—female transmission, and 0.043 for male-to-male transmission.

100 sexual encounters a year. Sigh. I will avoid over-sharing at this point.

I am never ever going to be the Pope because I think condoms are GREEEAAAAAAAT. Thank you T. Tiger.

Condoms prevent pregnancy and prevent sexually transmitted diseases and help prevent the transmission of HIV.

Condoms, unlike the Pope, are not infallible, but it is my considered professional opinion--—you may disagree with me on this—that people like to have sex. And if they are going to have sex, it is better to wear a condom. Prevent HIV, prevent horrible deaths. Amazing what a simple piece of latex can do. Even more amazing that anyone would object to their use.

Part of the issue with sex is the various taboos and stigmas associated with it. In India, some people are trying to break down the taboo of talking about condoms by getting the conversation started with a ringtone for cell phones that is the Best. Ringtone. Ever. It was a chorus of singing the word condom.

Rationalization

Hollingsworth, T.D., R.M. Anderson, and C. Fraser, HIV-1 transmission, by stage of infection. J Infect Dis, 2008. 198(5): p. 687-93.

Wilson, D.P., et al., Relation between HIV viral load and infectiousness: a model-based analysis. Lancet, 2008. 372(9635): p. 314-20.

World AIDS Day

Today is world AIDS day. The start of the AIDS epidemic coincided with the start of my medical career. I do not want to suggest causality here. But to quote the Grateful Dead, what a long strange trip it's been.

I took care of my first AIDS patient about 25 years ago, a twenty-five-year-old male who died after a long wasting illness due to *Mycobacterium avium*. The autopsy showed tissues that were more acid-fast bacilli than human cells. It was like some sort of real life *Invasion of the Body Snatchers*. My second patient was a dwarf with cryptococcal meningitis who visited bathhouses during his travels. The next 15 years were an endless parade of awful deaths in young people with occasional bursts of hope (AZT, then combo therapy), followed by disappointment as therapies failed and the death toll continued to mount. I never expected triple drug therapy to be so effective.

The deaths were all the more aggravating as we knew early on how the disease was spread: sex and drugs. The techniques to prevent spread of disease are simple: condoms and needle exchange. Both are still opposed by those who prefer their form of morality over preventing people from dying.

So many people who died needlessly. In the book *The Band Played On,* the government's underwhelming response to the early HIV epidemic is compared to the widespread publicity over toxic shock syndrome. It was too bad, the author said, that the disease didn't start in freckle-faced red-headed children.

It is a changed landscape. I have had one AIDS death this century, and the only opportunistic infection I have seen since 2000 is *Pneumocystis.* HAART, much to my happy surprise, really works. My patients no longer die. That's good.

Outside the industrialized West, deaths from HIV are still common, but at least there is hope that the disease can be controlled. All we need is worldwide peace and prosperity. Yeah. Right. Like that's going to happen.

BBF. Blood and Body Fluid

One of the few huge fights my wife and I have had was when we were taking childbirth classes and the leader had the men and women separate into groups and share our feeling about what it meant to be a parent.

I said that feelings are like blood and body fluids: I don't share them with strangers.

For some curious reason I was thereafter considered the class asshole. Go figure.

BBFs are not something you want to be inadvertently exposed to at work, and probably not in your spare time either. BBFs carry infectious diseases like hepatitis B, hepatitis C, and HIV.

In the hospital we have many clever ways to prevent needlesticks, the most common work associated mechanism whereby our employees get a BBF exposure, although splashes are becoming more common.

Murphy was an optimist, and somehow we still manage to get the occasional needlestick despite needleless systems and needle guards. I think the hand has an attraction to being poked by sharp needles.

Needlesticks are probably under-reported, especially in the OR and by surgeons, and I strongly advise safe sex with any surgical residents until you know their infection status. Not that I have sex with residents, mind you, just sayin'.

The risk of infection from a needlestick depends on whether or not it is a hollow bore (the needle, not the surgeon), whether there is visible blood, how deep the injury is, and whether gloves are worn.

The risks are variably reported, but for needlestick injuries involving blood contaminated with HIV, needles can spread the virus in 0.3% of cases. The risk of transmission of hepatitis B virus from a needlestick injury varies from 1% to 40%. Hep B is the one to worry about, so I hope you got your vaccine. The risk for hepatitis C virus transmission from a needle stick is about 1.8% (range 0% to 7%).

If you get a needlestick, you need testing then medications to try to prevent HIV. So far we have not had an HIV transmission from a needlestick, knock on faux wood veneer.

What is curious is all the calls I get for odd BBF exposures.

Many times cleaners get stuck from needles left in restrooms and hotel rooms. Usually it is insulin syringes, but IVDAs are not particularly fastidious about properly disposing of their drug paraphernalia.

There have been those who have had a one-night stand and are worried about bringing something home to the wife. It is always a man. Men are pigs, in case you are interested.

People have been stuck with needles cleaning up parks; one kid was stuck when someone had left a needle in a coin return, and he stuck his finger in looking for change. Cops have been stuck and bit wrestling with the crazy and the felonious.

The call today was someone who was helping at a halfway house and a junkie stumbled and fell on him, jabbing his thigh with a syringe.

My all time favorite was a guy at a strip club where the performer was lactating. When she gave a spin, he got milk in his eye. I was asked by the ER if he needed HIV prevention. I was laughing so hard I could barely get out an answer.

Rationalization

Makary, M.A., et al., Needlestick injuries among surgeons in training. N Engl J Med, 2007. 356(26): p. 2693-9.

A return to days of yore

I've been very busy the last few weeks. We have a French exchange student staying with us, so my evenings are spent showing him the different variations of rain that are available in Portland. It is said, incorrectly, that Eskimos have 4 million words for snow, or some such number. In the Pacific Northwest we have far more words for rain, all starting with God Damn, and moving down the list. But the bottom line is sometimes there is little time for writing.

I have a case of something I have not seen in years: PJP. One never says PJP pneumonia, since the second P stands for pneumonia. It is like saying ATM machine (or HIV virus). He is an AIDS patient who has not been on anti-retroviral therapy for reasons I cannot yet discover, but his immune system has been destroyed to the point where he has PJP.

PJP is short for peanut butter and jelly, no, sorry, *Pneumocystis jirovecii* Pneumonia, a disease that, thanks to prophylaxis and anti-retroviral drugs, is almost a disease of historical interest in AIDS. I do not think I have seen an AIDS-related case this century, although, thanks to anti-TNF antibodies and other immunosuppressive agents, I have seen PJP in patients being treated for lupus, rheumatoid arthritis, and other such diseases.

Back in the day, when nickels had bumblebees and the style was to wear an onion on your belt, there were always a few PJP patients in the hospital. Now, residents can go an entire career and not see one.

Another triumph of modern medicine. I really do not want it to come back.

Rationalization

Kelley, C.F., et al., Trends in hospitalizations for AIDS-associated Pneumocystis jirovecii Pneumonia in the United States (1986 to 2005). Chest, 2009. 136(1): p. 190-7.

Premature Closure

I need a self-aggrandizing title.

There is "America's Pediatrician" and "America's most Read Pediatrician" and there is the "Conscience of Modern Medicine." I am not trademarked and I am neither a world-renowned leader nor a pioneer. No one calls me Dr. Mark (well, one ICU nurse does). And I don't wear scrubs outside the hospital. I suspect I need to work on my image if I want to get some product endorsements. Unfortunately, to quote Dr. Gag Helfrunt, "Vell, I'm just zis guy, you know?"

The nice thing about being a doc is that every day is a chance to say "Huh. I didn't know that." I remember back when I had to use the *Index Medicus* to find information. Now I am a Google away. Not a Bing. A Google. I lack a Google of knowledge, not a Bing. I do lack a bing of cherries.

Today I was asked to see an AIDS patient of 15 years with a CD4 count of 50 cells per cubic millimeter. This is well into the AIDS range; serious infections begin at counts of 200 or lower, and infections such as *M. avium* at values of 75 or less. This patient had just resumed taking his anti-retroviral cocktail (HAART) after a year off medications, and now had a fever. So the docs called me. He had a white cell count of 41K, about ten times normal, a low hemoglobin—9 g/dL, where 12-15 is normal—and a low platelet count: 61k per cubic millimeter, less than half of normal. His white count showed a marked left shift—many highly immature white blood cells. He had new, rapidly growing lymph nodes everywhere.

CT showed lots of adenopathy in the chest and abdomen, so it was thought he had some sort of HIV-related infection or tumor.

They wanted me to figure out which one.

There is a process in medicine called premature closure, and I will let you make your own inappropriate comment. It is where the brain stops thinking about the problem at hand because you think you know the diagnosis. It is really common in evaluation of HIV patients and people returning from foreign countries. Whatever the problem is, it has to be related to either HIV or travel. Common or unrelated illnesses are not considered.

Today's patient had 17% blasts in the differential blood count and he probably has leukemia, unrelated to HIV. Just bad, awful, terrible, crappy luck. I sure do hate leukemia, but I see a biased subpopulation: those who get infected and often die. Just as I am certain that every surgery leads to infection. I wish. I try to remember there is a confirmation bias in my practice, since no one calls me when patients do not have infections.

What I didn't know was that leukemia could occasionally present like an aggressive lymphoma with rapidly progressive lymphadenopathy, mimicking Hodgkin's. It's rare, but what he has. Unfortunately Occam's razor is unreliable in HIV, you have to follow Hickam's Dictum: "Patients can have as many diseases as they damn well please." So he may yet have two or more illnesses, but for now it looks like it is all leukemia.

Rationalization

Aboulafia, D.M., et al., Acute myeloid leukemia in patients infected with HIV-1. AIDS, 2002. 16(6): p. 865-76.

Davey, D.D., et al., Acute myelocytic leukemia manifested by prominent generalized lymphadenopathy: report of two cases with immunological, ultrastructural, and cytochemical studies. Am J Hematol, 1986. 21(1): p. 89-98.

....

Death by Cold Sore

Maximus: [laughing] You knew Marcus Aurelius?

Proximo: [very quickly and defensively] I didn't say I knew him, I said he touched me on the shoulder once! He gave me Herpes.

—Gladiator. Kind of.

*H*ERPES *simplex* (HSV) is a common virus. About 80% of Americans have HSV-1 and 20% have HSV-2. Type 1 causes mostly cold sores and type 2 causes mostly genital disease, although on occasion type 1 can cause genital disease and type 2 will cause oral lesions. How these strains switch places has never been adequately explained to me.

People who have close, traumatic contact can spread the virus to each other—the archetype being wrestlers, where hot, sweaty, bloody grappling can pass Herpes. That's wrestling I am discussing. It has a name in wrestlers, Herpes gladiatorum. I prefer the British name, Scrumpox, as it sounds much more disgusting and funny. Scrum. Heh heh heh. A bumper sticker I sometimes see says "Rugby Players Eat Their Dead," so perhaps that is how type 2 Herpes gets to the lips: cannibalism.

There is now a new variant of Herpes in Japan called BgKL that has been spreading among Sumo wrestlers. It has infected 39 Sumo wrestlers over a 5-year period and actually killed two of them. Considering there are only about 700 professional Sumo wrestlers in Japan, that is impressive. How they died is not specifically mentioned (pneumonia or hepatitis or embarrassment), but it was apparently from the Herpes infection rather than a secondary infection.

BgKL is more virulent than your average bear. This strain reactivates more often, spreads more efficiently, has higher virus levels in the lips and skin and causes more severe symptoms than other strains. The photos on the interwebs show widespread skin lesions, far more than you usually see with the more common strain of Herpes. I wouldn't touch them, much less try to push them out of a ring. Sumo wrestlers live and train together, helping to increase viral spread. They live in stables, or so all the reports say, like Kobe beef cows, so I suppose horsing around helped spread the virus. There are puns I cannot avoid making.

They postulate that this mutated form of Herpes 1, because it is more infectious, is replacing the less virulent strains seen before in Japan.

"The BgKL frequency decreases in a geographical gradient suggest that this HSV-1 variant was dispersed from Shikoku to the surrounding regions and then to more distant regions."

So it is spreading out in Japan from an epicenter.

Yet another in an endless series of examples in the microbial world of evolution, with organisms taking advantage of changes in their environment (us) to multiply and spread. Staph does it, *E. coli* does it, even uneducated flus do it. Let's do it. Let's evolve.

So if your travel plans include Japan, might I suggest no kissing the Sumo wrestlers?

Rationalization

Ban, F., et al., Analysis of herpes simplex virus type 1 restriction fragment length polymorphism variants associated with herpes gladiatorum and Kaposi's varicelliform eruption in sumo wrestlers. J Gen Virol, 2008. 89(Pt 10): p. 2410-5.

Eda, H., et al., Contrasting geographic distribution profiles of the herpes simplex virus type 1 BgOL and BgKL variants in Japan suggest dispersion and replacement. J Clin Microbiol, 2007. 45(3): p. 771-82.

Ozawa, S., et al., Geographical distribution of the herpes simplex virus type 1 BgKL variant in Japan suggests gradual dispersion of the virus from Shikoku Island to the other Islands. J Clin Microbiol, 2006. 44(6): p. 2109-18.

Ozawa, S., et al., The herpes simplex virus type 1 BgKL variant, unlike the BgOL variant, shows a higher association with orolabial infection than with infections at other sites, supporting the variant-dispersion-replacement hypothesis. J Clin Microbiol, 2007. 45(7): p. 2183-90.

Herpes on the Brain

*H*ERPES encephalitis is a bad disease. It melts your brain, necrosing your temporal-parietal area until you are turned into a Limbaugh.

A lot of you (not me) have *Herpes*. One in four Americans have *Herpes simplex* 2 (the mostly genital herpes) but of that 25% only 10% or so know it). Most herpes is asymptomatic, and is being constantly shed and passed from person to person with no one aware.

This is important in the clinic, as well as when you get drunk and stagger out of the bar with a person of uncertain provenance.

Lets say you have a couple, A and B. They have been together for a few months and A has never had *Herpes*. B now has a whopping case of *Herpes* for the first time ever.

A thinks B is a cheatin' pig, and a baldfaced liar to boot, because where else could that *Herpes* have come from if not from foolin' around (this sounds like it may make a good country song)? But the more likely scenario is that A has asymptomatic disease and gave it to B. Check the *Herpes* serology on A, and if positive, will be suggestive that A in fact was the *Herpes* donor to B. But if B is a male, well, he may be a cheatin' pig and a baldfaced liar as well, but that is not an I.D. issue.

All men (except me) are pigs. My wife says she wished she had known that in her younger days; it would have resulted, perhaps, in less heartache.

But what about the patient from the weekend? Came in with viral meningitis, not encephalitis, and after a few days the PCR for HSV (LSMFT) was positive.

Do you treat *Herpes* meningitis? *Herpes* is a cause of benign recurrent aseptic meningitis, or Mollaret's meningitis, but as it is the first episode, I can't call it recurrent yet.

The I.D. textbook, Mandell, says

"Among immunocompetent persons, aseptic meningitis associated with genital herpes is usually a benign (albeit uncomfortable) disease and gradually resolves without sequelae. Controlled trials of

intravenous acyclovir for established HSV meningitis have not been conducted. However, intravenous acyclovir 5 mg/kg every 8 hours is recommended for hospitalized symptomatic patients. Most series have reported a low frequency of neurologic sequelae."

Where is the damn reference? I can't find squat on a PubMed search to support that assertion. Pisses. Me. Off.

So should I treat? Sometimes I do, and sometimes I don't. If they are ill and have bad lesions I do, if it is just a headache I may not. Drugs are not without their toxicity.

Rationalization

Wald, A., et al., Reactivation of genital herpes simplex virus type 2 infection in asymptomatic seropositive persons. N Engl J Med, 2000. 342(12): p. 844-50.

Mandell, Douglas, and Bennett, *Principles and Practice of Infectious Diseases*, 7th Edition. Churchill Livingstone (Elsevier), 2010.

....

Heroin

A Rich Microbiological Stew

I SEE a lot of intravenous drug abusers (IVDA; the PC term is injection drug users, not abusers, but if the shoe fits...). I am going to go out on a limb here and suggest that it is not a healthy lifestyle (by the way, when do I get a style with my life? At 51 I think I should get to have more than a life, I should have style).

It is estimated that the average drug addict lives fifteen to twenty years from the onset of the disease, and I have seen innumerable lives wasted and cut short from all kinds of drug use. Everyone dies, but it is particularly sad when a twenty-year-old dies of drug use. I am sure some asshole will read this and say they deserved to die, but dead people have no chance to turn their lives around. With time, many a user can, and will, kick the habit.

Take the recent patient: a 20-year history of heroin and cocaine use, now presenting with an abscess from injecting into the soft tissues of the abdominal wall and some sort of abscess in the periphery of her lungs. I am still trying to sort out the potential microbiology of her infections, but with IVDAs the list of potential organisms is long. Heroin is rich in microorganisms:

> "Fifty-eight heroin samples were tested by citric acid solubilisation and 34 by the MRD suspension technique. Fifteen different gram-positive species of four genera were recognized. No fungi were isolated. Aerobic endospore-forming bacteria (Bacillus spp. and Paenibacillus macerans) were the predominant microflora isolated and at least one species was isolated from each sample. B. cereus was the most common species and was isolated from 95% of all samples, with B. licheniformis isolated from 40%. Between one and five samples yielded cultures of B. coagulans, B. laterosporus, B. pumilus, B. subtilis and P. macerans. Staphylococcus spp. were isolated from 23 (40%) samples; S. warneri and S. epidermidis were the most common and were cultured from 13 (22%) and 6 (10%) samples respectively. One or two samples yielded cultures of S. aureus, S. capitis and S. haemolyticus. The remainder of the flora detected comprised two samples contaminated with C. perfringens and two samples with either C. sordellii or C. tertium. Multiple bacterial species were isolated from 43 (74%) samples, a single species from the remaining 15. In 13 samples B. cereus alone was isolated, in one B. subtilis alone and in one sample B. pumilus alone. C. botulinum and C. novyi were not isolated from any of the heroin samples."

It is why heroin users get *Bacillus* infections of the eye, Clostridial gas gangrene from skin popping, staphylococcal endocarditis, polymicrobial soft tissue abscesses, and the occasional wound botulism. Almost any germ can be injected along with the heroin and travel to any body site. It is hard to say that heroin is contaminated with bacteria, as that presupposes it was manufactured as a sterile product.

While the study I cited did not culture yeast, there have been outbreaks of *Candida* associated with heroin. I had a 68-year-old man who started using heroin at age 64 when his son turned him on to the joys of being high. He eventually died of *Candida parapsilosis* endocarditis. I prefer to golf with my kids, although after some rounds I think heroin may be better.

Black tar heroin, a cheap and particularly filthy form of heroin—I saw one chunk of black tar with a banana peel in it—is used for skin popping and has been associated with multiple deaths from gas gangrene.

But wait. There is more.

Many heroin addicts lick their needles to help them slide in easier as the needle point dulls, injecting mouth bacteria into their skin or bloodstream. Heroin needs to dissolved before injection, so tap water, toilet water, river water and puddle water have each been used by at least one patient of mine. I had one patient who had *Acinetobacter* bacteremia every time she used the bottled water in the lobby of the local youth hostel. When she switched to burger restaurant water (from the faucet in the bathroom) the bacteremias ceased.

I had one patient who mixed his heroin with tap water, but as soon as he got blood return the syringe jammed, so he took off the needle and squirted the blood/water/heroin mixture into a used coffee cup. While he was out and about getting a new syringe the mixture clotted, so he dissolved the clot in spit, then injected it. Curiously, he developed a fever and got sick.

It is a credit to the immune system how rarely these patients get infections. My idea is to call heroin a probiotic and market as an immune system booster to support immunological health. I'll make fortune and my patients will always come back for more.

Rationalization

McLauchlin, J., et al., An investigation into the microflora of heroin. J Med Microbiol, 2002. 51(11): p. 1001-8.

Postscript

To my knowledge, no similar microbiological studies have been done, on the microbiology of cocaine and meth—but when you see how meth is made, you wonder how anything could survive the manufacturing process.

It's Back

I have determined, through long observation, that the use of intravenous heroin is not conducive to a healthy lifestyle.

Which I need. A lifestyle, that is. Not heroin. I have a life, but it seems to lack style. Of course, I wore bell-bottom cords well into my 30's, so perhaps I have a style known as "dork."

There are few infections that are 100% fatal in humans. Rabies is one; the other is bacterial endocarditis.

If you do not treat it correctly, it will always kill the patient. Always. The closest I ever came to a spontaneous cure was a patient who came in with streptococcal endocarditis, received 2 doses of ceftriaxone and then remembered he was a Christian Scientist and refused further therapy. He survived, and came back a month later disease free. He gave credit to the Big Scientist, but I still think the two doses of the long-acting antibiotic were enough to cure him.

The problem is that if you want heroin, you may not hang around the hospital to get your antibiotics, especially if the doctors have been kind enough to give you direct access to the central veins of the body for easy delivery of antibiotics by installing an intravenous catheter.

And so the patient today, with Staph on the aortic valve, decided to skip out and get some drugs rather than stay at the nursing home for nafcillin. She of course relapsed her infection, and it was back to square one. I emphasized the universally fatal nature of the disease to her, so perhaps this time she will complete the therapy, maybe with some drug rehab thrown in. But if past behavior predicts the future, I would not be optimistic that she will survive.

I have read somewhere, but cannot find where, that the average IVDA in NYC lives for 5 years and dies of murder or infection. Like I said, not a healthy lifestyle.

The worst case of endocarditis I've ever heard of was that of

Alfred S. Reinhart, who developed his heart infection as a result of rheumatic heart disease and had the misfortune of living in the pre-antibiotic era and being a medical student.

As such, he had insight into all the details of his disease and could recognize and predict his future. He kept a diary of his disease until a few days before he died, and it is one of the saddest of all medical writings. I don't worry so much about being dead, but the process of getting there has never appeared to be all that pleasant.

When he developed the embolic events that characterize the disease, he was with his sister-in-law and told her, "I shall be dead in six months." Alfred S. Reinhart saw the bullet coming for months, Matrix style. Ugh.

> *"I felt sure that I was going to collapse momentarily from sheer exhaustion induced by lack of sleep and the intense pain. I cannot deny that I had visions of the end, nevertheless, I knew that morphine would soon take the edge off my pain ... standing orders permitting me to call for reasonable doses of morphine within proper limits of time as I should find it necessary, proved a great boon in these days. I utilized this privilege comparatively little in the past, but was only too ready to ask for one-quarter of morphine at this time to relieve the intense distress which was gripping me. This dose seemed to take the edge off the pain sufficiently to allow me to lie on my right side for perhaps ten or fifteen minutes during which time I readily fell into a sleep following the exhausting experiences of the past hours"*

Dead at 24 from acute heart failure.

If you think you are having a bad day, read about Mr. Reinhart.

Every time I read it I get all bummed out.

I am going to go listen to The Cure. Always a good choice when depressed.

Rationalization

Korelitz, B.I., A Harvard medical student chronicles his fatal illness: the story of Alfred S. Reinhart, 1907-1931. Mt Sinai J Med, 1995.

62(3): p. 226-32; discussion 233-4.

Flegel, K.M., Our medical past. Subacute bacterial endocarditis observed: the illness of Alfred S. Reinhart. CMAJ, 2002. 167(12): p. 1379-83.

Survival of the Fittest

I saw a patient today who by all rights should be dead. She was a homeless heroin user who had had at least a dozen different bacteremias this century. To add to her medical problems, she was on dialysis for unrelated reasons, and attended dialysis sessions intermittently at best. Not a good combination for longevity.

I took care of her a couple of years ago when, over a 6 month period, she kept being admitted for a recurrent yet transient *Acinetobacter* bacteremia. Febrile and shaking, she would be admitted and have positive blood cultures that were negative upon repeat. She was worked up for a focus of infection and one was never found. No abscess, no endocarditis, repeat cultures negative.

Taking a history I found she used two water sources for mixing her heroin: the ladies' room at a local burger joint and the water cooler at the local hostel. I never got either cultured, but I bet on the water cooler, and she stopped using both and the problem went away.

Acinetobacters are an increasing problem as they can be pan-resistant (no Greek theater criticism for this bug) and have been a major problem in wound infections in our troops.

Now she is in with *Elizabethkingia meningoseptica* in the blood. What is *Elizabethkingia meningoseptica* you ask? It used to be called *Chryseobacterium* (now it's clear, right?), but genetics and the pathetic need for drunken microbiologists to change pathogen names to keep us clinicians squirming, has lead to a new designation. I think those are the two reasons that bacteria classification keeps changing. And Elizabeth was/is Queen, not King.

Elizabethkingia meningoseptica is also found in tap water, so I need to find out where she is getting her water for shooting up. Her water is probably the source of her bacteremia.

In the meantime, a touch of antibiotics and she is already much improved.

Rationalization

Wang, J.L., et al., Association between contaminated faucets and colonization or infection by nonfermenting gram-negative bacteria in intensive care units in Taiwan. J Clin Microbiol, 2009. 47(10): p. 3226-30.

Scott, P., et al., An outbreak of multidrug-resistant Acinetobacter baumannii-calcoaceticus complex infection in the US military health care system associated with military operations in Iraq. Clin Infect Dis, 2007. 44(12): p. 1577-84.

Elizabeth O. King is an American bacteriologist at the CDC.

Postscript

She left AMA (against medical advice, not American Medical Association) before I could ask where she was getting her water.

....

Half time

IT's 37-17 at the half and my alma mater, University of Oregon (with the second worst mascot) is trouncing Oregon State, with the worst mascot in college sports. Puddles the Fighting Duck vs. Benny the Beaver... Oh well. We could be the banana slugs, like UC Santa Cruz, or the geoducks like Evergreen State.

It's nice to know that football is, like so many human activities, filled with infections.

MRSA leads the list, thanks to the trauma (turf burns), cosmetic shaving (who says football players do not have a feminine side?), and close contact. One of the first outbreaks of the current USA 300 strain of MRSA was in a professional football team. But there are numerous other football associated outbreaks.

There have been infections associated with mouth guards, which, at least by culture, are perhaps more disgusting than a toilet seat.

Osteitis pubis, an infection usually seen in postpartum women, is reported in football players. A fair number of linebackers do look like they are in the third trimester.

Group A *Streptococcus* has passed through a football team, as has scabies, coxsackievirus B2 and echovirus 16, the latter two with aseptic meningitis.

Hot tub folliculitis has been reported due to whirlpool use.

Herpes is commonly spread in football, both on and off the field, and many in the stands watching the game will acquire it tonight in drunken celebration or drowning their sorrows. I suspect that herpes will not be the only STD spread this weekend in the post game festivities.

Back to Football.

Lung Abscess

HIGH school female, started one week prior to admission with right upper quadrant pain and right chest pain that was pleuritic in nature, fevers, and chills.

You have pleurisy, here is some Tylenol-3.

Next day, not better. You have costochondritis, here are some NSAIDS.

The next day a chest x-ray is done and she has a lung abscess. Big one. Young people do not get lung abscesses.

Her past medical history is negative; she has 4 birds, two dogs, and a cat. A high school student, no bad habits, plays saxophone. Only travel is to Eastern Europe 6 months ago.

Why the lung abscess?

She has cultures that grow *Streptococcus anginosus* and *Eikenella corrodens*. Mouth bugs. It is what you would expect in an aspiration lung abscess from nasty black stumps of rotten teeth. Her teeth look great and she has not been unconscious from drugs, alcohol, trauma or medical care. Or *American Idol*.

I think it's (ha. I caught one) from her saxophone.

Ever seen a brass instrument spit valve emptied? Big time ick.

When people play the sax they keep their epiglottis open, and the tendency to tilt the head back for the long notes (the sax equivalent of the guitar face) would open a perfect pathway for the pooled spit to drip into the lung.

Sax players also use circular breathing, where they keep the airway open so they can keep blowing that long mournful note, like in Jungleland:

"The epitome of the soulful saxophone ballad; the first note just freezes you. That first note just stretches out and a slow, unrushed passion emotes from Clarence's soul and sets Bruce up for his final tragic verse. The sax creates a sweet and bittersweet flavor that reaffirms the tragedy. I remember when I was a kid how my music teacher told me to play with feeling. This song defines that comment. Clarence uses every note to express the pain that Bruce sings about."

But you knew that already.

Circular breathing. Intake of breath fills the chest and stomach; cheeks and neck are inflated when air is halfway up the chest. While forcing air from cheeks and neck into the instrument, the player simultaneously breathes in through the nose to the bottom of the stomach.

Saxophone players may have a shorter life span than other musicians, and do you know what most jazz sax players die of? Besides heroin use? Lung disease.

It all comes together nicely.

This exemplifies the problem with unprotected teenage sax. It's not the television, that's for sure. At least my boys play guitar.

Rationalization

Kinra, S. and M. Okasha, Unsafe sax: cohort study of the impact of too much sax on the mortality of famous jazz musicians. BMJ, 1999. 319(7225): p. 1612-3.

Weikert, M. and J. Schlomicher-Thier, Laryngeal movements in saxophone playing: video-endoscopic investigations with saxophone players. A pilot study. J Voice, 1999. 13(2): p. 265-73.

Addendum

It turns out the BMJ reference is meant to be a joke—the Christmas issue is the equivalent of April Fool's in the US. Sure fooled me.

EVOLUTION: THE PAST AND FUTURE OF OUR RELATIONSHIP WITH MICROBES

Ask me no question, I'll tell you no lice

LAST year my youngest child's class had a head lice outbreak. Snicker all you want, it WILL happen to you, too. When it does, hope you have a boy rather than a girl, because it is so much easier to shave a boy's head than to try to use RID to eradicate the bugs. Oddly the girls objected to getting their heads shaved. I would have argued that Sinead O'Connor looks cool.

With resistance increasing to the more commonly used anti-head lice medications, it is nice that an enterprising pediatrician figured out that hot air blown onto the head and trapped in a shower cap can kill off the lice better than medications. It's better to cook 'em than to poison 'em. Given that the presidential debates are about to occur, I expect no end of hot air in the short term, so the incidence of head lice may transiently decrease, especially in those states with many electoral votes.

Head lice are common in all people, all ages, and all socioeconomic groups, through the ages until now. People think lice are associated with being poor, but a recent meta-analysis of head lice prevalence suggests that being female (more hair? No wonder I never got the lice from my son) and crowding were more important factors than poverty. Depending on the population studied, prevalence rates in various parts of the world vary from 0.4% to 65%.

Pardon me for a moment while I scratch my head.

Lice, while freaking everyone out, are also good vectors for both typhus and relapsing fever, interesting but rare diseases in the US.

It is interesting how much the body resembles a forest or other ecological system. There are a variety of Streptococci in the mouth and they each prefer to live in one distinct area of the mouth: one Streptococcus prefers the tongue, another the teeth, another the back of the throat. Each part of the body is an isolated Galapagodian (is that a word? It should be) island where one organism or another has evolved to occupy its own niche.

Same with lice. In the lab you cannot tell the difference between a head louse (*Pediculus humanus capitis*) and a body louse (*Pediculus humanus humanus*). Head lice and body lice can be forced to breed in the lab in some odd parasitical version of "The Menagerie." They have evolved different survival strategies to survive as head lice—for example, lay their eggs and stick them to hair, while the body louse lays its eggs in clothes.

Louse classification becomes even more complicated:

"Mitochondrial DNA (mtDNA) studies have shown that there are 3 distinctly different clade phylotypes of P. humanus found among modern humans.

The most common mtDNA phylotype is found among both head and body lice (type A) and is worldwide in distribution. The second mtDNA group (type B) occurs only in head lice and has been found in the New World, Europe, and Australia. The third type (type C) has been found only among head lice from Nepal and Ethiopia."

And that's not even mentioning the issue of pubic lice, which are most similar to the gorilla pubic louse. I do not even want to go there.

Given that lice are as common on humans as fleas on a dog, looking at the evolution of lice can lead to interesting observations about the evolution and dissemination of humans across the planet.

Lice evolution has helped define when humans and chimpanzees split, since our respective lice split with us, and have helped date the out of Africa migration. And because the body louse lays its eggs in clothes, studies have estimated, based on louse evolution, that humans began wearing clothes about 100,000 to 72,000 years ago. Concert T-shirts followed later.

Most recently, it was mummies—Peruvian mummies to be exact. Thousand-year-old Peruvian mummies with mummified head lice. A group of scientists collected these thousand-year-old head lice, and isolated and typed their DNA. They found by DNA analysis that the thousand-year-old Peruvian lice were all Type A (and premed) and it was the oldest louse DNA ever analyzed (until they analyze Rumsfeld's DNA). Since these lice predated Europeans, it is concluded that the type A louse spread across the world with human migration and was not brought over with Columbus.

"The most likely theory is that phylotype A, issued from Africa, was distributed worldwide. Phylotype B may have survived and developed only in North and Central America, before Columbus, and is now spreading in the world, carried back by Europeans returning from the Americas. Type C is confined to highly mountainous countries of the Old World. In any case, the present work shows that there are several phylotypes of lice with geographical restrictions and that this was true before the arrival of Columbus in the Americas."

Nifty. Lice are more than a pain in the cranium and a source of low level hysteria for the parents of young children; they help us understand our evolution and our wanderings over the planet. Like so much of Infectious Disease, little things, even our vermin, have broader implications in understanding our past as well as why we get sick.

And my head still itches.

Rationalization

Falagas, M.E., et al., Worldwide prevalence of head lice. Emerg Infect Dis, 2008. 14(9): p. 1493-4

Goates, B.M., et al., An effective nonchemical treatment for head lice:

a lot of hot air. Pediatrics, 2006. 118(5): p. 1962-70.

Kittler, R., M. Kayser, and M. Stoneking, Molecular evolution of Pediculus humanus and the origin of clothing. Curr Biol, 2003. 13(16): p. 1414-7.

Raoult, D., et al., Molecular identification of lice from pre-Columbian mummies. J Infect Dis, 2008. 197(4): p. 535-43.

....

Genetics of Infection

"The fault, dear Brutus, lies not in our stars, but in ourselves if we are underlings."

—Edward de Vere, the Earl of Oxford.

I DO not necessarily want to blame the patient, but someone has to be at fault when things go badly. I used to have a policy of always blaming nursing, but now it is the genome where all the action is.

This century has been filled with fascinating advances in understanding the role of polymorphisms in the host immune system and the subsequent risk and outcomes of various infections. We have always known that everyone is not immunologically identical any more than we have the same height or hair color or sense of humor. Would you believe there are actually people who do find these stories funny?

Why some people live or die, why some people get an infection and others do not, has been a mystery. Certainly there is variability in the virulence of different strains of, say, *E. coli*. The variation in mortality and morbidity we see clinically is greater than can be accounted for by variations in the organism. In outbreaks from the same strain of pathogen, there is always variability in the effects on the host. Not all people have same predilection to infection or the ability to withstand an infection. A 65-year-old diabetic with lupus on prednisone just isn't going to do as well with a bloodstream infection as a healthy young person. But the gross assessment that sicker people do worse with infection never seems to be enough to account for the great variability in outcomes in disease.

What is increasingly clear is that small, but profound, changes in genes may determine whether we live or die from an infection. Genes code for proteins. There can be single mutations in the genes, normal variations, that are called polymorphisms. Your gene that codes for a protein is not always the same gene that I have. Your gene may make more of a protein, or less of a protein, or one with greater or lesser affinity for its substrate. These variations are some of the clay upon which evolution molds its change. Remember: I have a degree in metaphorableness.

Some of these polymorphism can make people much more susceptible to dying from infections. Take mannan-binding lectin. Please. Anyone reading this know who Henny Youngman was? Anyway.

To quote the Wikipedia:

"The Mannan-binding lectin pathway (also known as the Ali/Krueger Pathway) is homologous to the classical complement pathway. This pathway uses a protein similar to C1q of the classical complement pathway, which binds to mannose residues and other sugars in a pattern that allows binding on multiple pathogens. Mannan-binding lectin (MBL; also called mannose-binding lectin) is a protein belonging to the collectin family that is produced by the liver and can initiate the complement cascade by binding to pathogen surfaces. MBL is a 2-6 headed molecule that forms a complex with MASP-I (Mannan-binding lectin Associated Serine Protease) and MASP-II, two protease zymogens. MASP-I and MASP-II are very similar to C1r and C1s molecules of the classical complement pathway and are thought to have a common evolutionary ancestor. When the carbohydrate-recognising heads of MBL bind to specifically arranged mannose residues on the phospholipid bilayer of a pathogen, MASP-I and MASP-II are activated to cleave complement components C4 and C2 into C4a, C4b, C2a, and C2b. C4b and C2a combine on the surface of the pathogen to form C3 convertase (C4b and C2a), while C4a and C2b act as chemoattractants."

Say what? Bacteria have a variety of sugars on their outsides, including a sugar called mannose. Mannan-binding lectin is a protein that recognizes these sugars and activates a wing of the immune system called the complement system to pop the bacteria like a zit and to help bring in white cells for the kill. Cool.

The complement system cannot be boosted but can have mutations that render the patient at risk for infection. There have been an increasing number of studies that show that a decrease in mannan-binding lectin is associated with increased risk of infection, but a particularly interesting paper was published in 2008. This study found that polymorphisms that lead to decreased serum levels of mannan-binding lectin lead to a two-fold increase in death from pneumococcal bacteremia. 25% of the patients who had low levels died vs. 12% of patients with higher levels.

Pneumococcus is a one of many kinds of streptococci, one of the more common pathogens in humans and in other animals as well. Your genes may be different than mine, and that may make all the difference of living or dying. The threads that keep us alive are often thinner than we know.

All well and good, but what makes it all the more cool is in the accompanying editorial:

> *"Five hundred sixty-five million years ago, when the world was empty and barren because animal life had not colonized land yet, a common ancestor that we share with sea squirts (Ascidians) inhabited the seas. One of the genes that we still share with sea squirts today is a gene for mannose-binding lectin (MBL), signifying that this gene has existed for 565 million years and, thus, has been highly conserved throughout animal evolution."*

The fact that our ancient ancestors, the sea squirt, and humans all have to protect ourselves from *Streptococci* and use, in part, the same defensive mechanism, I find particularly satisfying. The connections between infections and the host response are one of the most compelling lines of evidence for evolution. And yet another reason that Infectious Disease is the coolest specialty in medicine.

Rationalization

Eisen, D.P., et al., Low serum mannose-binding lectin level increases the risk of death due to pneumococcal infection. Clin Infect Dis, 2008. 47(4): p. 510-6.

Thai Food Wimp

MY family loves Thai food. My kids would rather eat Thai than any other style of food. And while I enjoy Thai, when it comes to heat I am a total wimp. There is nothing I want less on my food than capsaicin, especially when it comes out the other end. But that is a story for another time.

But if it was not for infectious molds, there wouldn't be hot foods at all. Really.

Some plants make noxious molecules to prevent getting et by insects, fungi, and bacteria.

Fusarium is a mold common in the environment. It is found in rotting organic material and occasionally infects the profoundly immunocompromised. At best I have seen a handful of cases in my career. *Fusarium*, however, is a major cause of death of chili seeds. It kills the seeds in the chili before they can be spread to start a new plant. Bad thing, killing off the offspring before they can sprout. Hard to propagate the species. Except in the case of the Jolly Green Giant. Too bad *Fusarium* didn't get to him before he made his sprout.

Fusarium is bad for chilies and it would be in the plant's best interest, although not mine, for it to have a defense against *Fusarium*. Which it does.

How does the chili protect it self from *Fusarium*? It makes capsaicin, the molecule that makes chilies hot. And capsaicin kills *Fusarium*.

How does the fungus get to the chilies in the first place? By way of scavenging hemipterans, which are leafhoppers, treehoppers, cicadas, aphids, scales, and true bugs. These bugs, in the process of looking for food, drag the mold into the chili, where it grows and kills the chili seeds.

How does all this relate?

The study found that find that the more scavenging bugs there were, the more potent the wild chilies became.

"These results suggest that the pungency in chilies may be an adaptive response to selection by a microbial pathogen, supporting the influence of microbial consumers on fruit chemistry."

Lots of bugs leads to more *Fusarium* which leads to more capsaicin.

Capsaicin may also be involved with seed dispersal since mammals, such as me, do not like capsaicin as it is an irritant (boy, is it ever). On the other hand, birds evidently have no ill effects from the chemical. It means that the chilies will be eaten by birds, which pass the seeds undigested over longer distances, rather than by mammals, which would digest the seeds and/or crap closer to home.

Evolution and infection in action to make Thai food unpleasant for non-masochistic mammals. Cool. Despite the heat.

Rationalization

Tewksbury, J.J. and G.P. Nabhan, Seed dispersal. Directed deterrence by capsaicin in chilies. Nature, 2001. 412(6845): p. 403-4.

Tewksbury, J.J., et al., Evolutionary ecology of pungency in wild chilies. Proc Natl Acad Sci U S A, 2008. 105(33): p. 11808-11.

....

Bad Singing

You think chilies have it tough, try being human. Malaria (a redundant name from the Italian, mal: bad and aria: opera song) has probably had more impact on the human genome than any other organism.

I once heard a Nobel laureate declare that half of everyone who has ever died did so from malaria. I have never been able to confirm that estimate, but it doesn't stop me from passing it on. Who am I to contradict a Nobel winner, even if his prize was in the wimpy (at least compared to medicine) field of physics.

Malaria is endlessly interesting. Its manifestations, its treatment, its history, its evolution, its resistance to antibiotics, and its impact on human evolution and history. I can, and eventually will, babble about this parasite for pages.

Everyone in medicine learns about sickle cell disease, a mutation in hemoglobin, the molecule that carries oxygen. It is found in some Africans, where the mutation protects against malaria. In Asia there is thalassemia, which has the same protective effect.

But wait. There's more. And it is not a steak knife.

The molecule that powers the body is ATP. There is an enzyme, pyruvate kinase, that converts phosphoenolpyruvate to pyruvate with the production of one molecule of ATP.

Most cells make their ATP in the mitochondria, but red cells do not have mitochondria and need pyruvate kinase to make ATP to make energy.

"Pyruvate kinase deficiency is the most frequent abnormality of the glycolytic pathway and, together with a deficiency in glucose 6 phosphate dehydrogenase (G6PD), is the most common cause of nonspherocytic hemolytic anemia.... The prevalence of homozygous pyruvate kinase deficiency is estimated at 1 case per 20,000 persons; more than 158 mutations have been described."

That's a lot of mutations in one enzyme—I wonder why? Hey. Malaria in an infection of red blood cells. Could there be a link? Of course.

"Pyruvate kinase deficiency has a protective effect against replication of the malarial parasite in human erythrocytes. We have described a dual mechanism for protection against P. falciparum in pyruvate kinase deficiency that included an invasion defect of erythrocytes from case subjects (observed in those with a homozygous mutation) and preferential macrophage clearance of ring stage infected erythrocytes from case subjects (observed in both homozygotes and heterozygotes)."

So if you have this mutation, while you are not a potential X-man, you are more resistant to getting malaria and if you do get it, you clear it better.

How this works, I either cannot understand or find. Perhaps it is simple starvation of the parasites. Or perhaps there is more. In normal animals, malaria induces a new pyruvate kinase that alters glucose metabolism in its favor.

Malaria is still a major heath problem, with half a billion cases a year in the world and a million deaths, so it is probably exerting evolutionary pressure on the human genome. I hope it makes us smarter.

Rationalization

Ayi, K., et al., Pyruvate kinase deficiency and malaria. N Engl J Med, 2008. 358(17): p. 1805-10.

Durand, P.M. and T.L. Coetzer, Hereditary red cell disorders and malaria resistance. Haematologica, 2008. 93(7): p. 961-3.

Oelshlegel, F.J., Jr., B.J. Sander, and G.J. Brewer, Pyruvate kinase in malaria host-parasite interaction. Nature, 1975. 255(5506): p. 345-7.

I Bow Down to my Bacterial Overlords

MY professional life is spent killing things: bacteria and fungi and parasites. I am not so certain I kill viruses. If there is indeed karma to be lost or gained in this life, I have piled up a heap o' bad karma with all the microbial death I have wrought in the last twenty-five years.

Life on earth is mostly single-celled; bacteria predated humans and will live on long after the earth is rendered uninhabitable for humans. Bacteria live damn near everywhere, with those that live in harsh environments being called extremophiles. Bacteria live miles underground, in boiling water, and have been found to thrive in the La Brea tar pits. I would not be surprised to find that bacteria are on the moons of Saturn, the polar caps of Mars, or in the most uninhabitable place known—my children's bedroom.

We greatly underestimate the number of organisms out there if we rely on counting just those that we can grow. The clinical microbiology lab can grow only a tiny fraction of the bacteria that live on Earth; many species (like many humans) cannot be cultivated. Some estimates suggest that only about 1% of the bacteria on the planet are culturable. Genomic techniques reveal the other 99%, and the number is always staggering. Probably about half of the biomass of the planet is bacteria, although the exact number is hard to estimate, as it relies heavily upon knowing the biomass of the ocean floor. There are 10 to 100 times as many bacteria in and on us than there are cells of us, most of which we cannot culture and can only find using biogenetic analysis. It is a bacterium's world. James Brown had it wrong.

I was listening to the Skeptics' Guide to the Universe podcast this weekend, and an interview with Phil Plait, and I guess the time for bacteria to rule again will come sooner than I had thought. I had always thought that life on earth would doomed when the sun becomes a red giant in another 6 billion years or so. A long time. But it turns out the sun is slowly heating up from a natural effect of nuclear fusion, and that in a mere 2 billion years—Plait said 100 million on the show, but corrected himself on his blog—the oceans will have boiled away.

I know that seems like a long time, especially when me and everyone I know and can know will be dead, gone, and forgotten in less than 200 years. Deep time makes the brain hurt. Two billion is a number I can kind of sort of maybe wrap my brain around. One of the few books I have read twice is John McPhee's *Annals of the Former World*, and it will give you a taste of a flavor of a hint of what 2 billion years means.

If Earth's history was a 12 hour clock, it is now 4:30 am. In half an hour the time of animals and plants will be gone, and in three hours the oceans will be gone.

But I bet the bacteria survive until the sun expands past the orbits of Mercury and Venus. If the Earth isn't charred to a crisp—the models vary on this point—I imagine that the microbes will continue surviving deep in the crust, living on chemical reactions instead of photosynthesis. Then as the sun shrinks back down to its white dwarf stage, and even as it finally flickers out, life on earth may continue until the planet reaches the temperature of space.

Not only will I eventually be consumed by the organisms I spend I lifetime killing, in the end they will outlast me and everything we do.

But at least they give me beer.

Rationalization

Stephen Jay Gould, Planet of the Bacteria. Found on the Gould archive: http://www.stephenjaygould.org/library/gould_bacteria.html

....

Dung Fungus

ATCHY title, huh?

The world of microorganisms is vast, and there are fungi that live in dung. Dung hits the ground (or on occasion the fan), and if it was a long time ago the dung gets fossilized (corprolites) and the fungus growing on it gets fossilized right along with it.

You can tell something about the history of a region by looking at the number of fossilized fungal spores in dung and in the sediments.

For example, there is a fungus called *Sporormiella*. It grows in the dung of herbivores. If there are a lot of herbivores, you have a lot of *Sporormiella*; if herbivores die off, there are fewer *Sporormiella*. Living only in herbivore poo may not be a good long-term survival strategy—or, if you ask me, a short-term survival strategy.

"These spores decline rapidly at the end of the Pleistocene at the approximate time of megafaunal extinctions and increase again in sediments of recent centuries after livestock introduction."

So by measuring the amount of this fossilized organisms in corprolites, you can get an idea of what happened a million years ago or more.

Some scientists did this on Madagascar, and saw the spores plummet with the mass extinction of the megafauna in the Pleistocene. The spore count rose again when livestock were introduced on the island. The spores have plummeted in the last 200 years as Madagascar has been stripped of its complex fauna and flora. Here is an idea of what can be inferred from the looking at fossilized dung fungus changes over time:

"i. The late Holocene before humans was a time of increasing aridity and perhaps seasonal or interannual dynamics that promoted changes in key megafaunal habitats such as wooded savanna.

ii. People arrived and hunted the naive megafauna, at least the ones that were slow on the ground such as many of the largest lemurs, to local extirpation and depressed the numbers of other megafauna.

iii. In the absence of the strong cropping regime imposed by hippos, tortoises, and ratites on the grasslands (and perhaps on woody vegetation by giant lemurs), savanna areas, forest edges, and understories would become increasingly flammable as plant biomass accumulated.

iv. The change in fire regimes would mean that preferred megafaunal habitats became increasingly fragmented as fire converted areas to simpler systems with less edible plant biomass (e.g., spiny bushland and steppe).

v. Humid forest and high-elevation areas were the last settled and converted by humans (as indeed they are still being transformed today at an alarming rate) (13), but they would have provided poor refugia for most of the savanna-adapted megafauna, and the less-swift giant lemurs would have been vulnerable to hunting even within dense habitats."

The rise and fall of ecosystems, all derived from looking at dung fungus and charcoal deposits over time.

I spend my day trying to kill bacteria and fungi; it amazes me what can be determined by looking at their corpses.

Rationalization

Burney, D.A., G.S. Robinson, and L.P. Burney, Sporormiella and the late Holocene extinctions in Madagascar. Proc Natl Acad Sci U S A, 2003. 100(19): p. 10800-5.

Davis, O.K. and D.S. Shafer, Sporormiella fungal spores, a palynological means of detecting herbivore density. Palaeogeography, Palaeoclimatology, Palaeoecology, 2006. 237(1): p. 40–50.

....

I am fat to avoid TB

A COOL thing (I do use the word cool a lot, phat is a synonym in the dictionary, but I doubt I could use that without looking like an even bigger dork than I am) about I.D. is that the effects of germs upon humans goes well beyond the acute infections.

Humans and germs have evolved together for millions of years, and the bugs have left their footprints in our genome.

It is estimated that a serious chunk of our DNA, maybe 10%, is viral DNA that got incorporated into our genome and never got out, now coming along for the ride. Genomic scientists have even resurrected a fossil retrovirus from our DNA. The real Jurassic Park.

Malaria also has had a serious impact on our genome, with multiple mutations that confer resistance to the infection, the most famous of which is sickle cell trait.

Today's *Journal of the American Medical Association* has a commentary that postulates that obesity and atherosclerotic consequences of the metabolic syndrome are an adaptation to both tuberculosis and starvation.

Most of human times have seen a shortage of food, and those who could pack on the fat were more likely to survive lean times. So we have a propensity to be fat, especially in the reproductive years.

Also in most of historical times, TB was ubiquitous and accounted for at least 25% of deaths. TB has killed more people than any organism except malaria, with more than a billion people having died from TB.

As I understand it, putting on fat signaled both fertility and an associated inflammatory response to keep TB in check. Fat became linked to fertility and a pro-inflammatory response. Putting on fat signaled that you were able to bring a baby to term. Having a pro-inflammatory response was important for short-term survival in a breeding population. It kept the TB at bay.

When you were fat and fertile, you were also had a "boosted immune system," to use the favored quack term. The medical historians in the article postulate that the short-term benefits outweighed the long-term atherosclerotic complications, since the latter occurred after the reproductive years. We live longer and eat more and what was once of benefit is now pathologic.

The article further postulates that there will be downstream triggers in the obesity/inflammation pathways that, when discovered, will be able to be manipulated to decrease both fat and the metabolic syndrome.

I recommend you read the original, which is full of leptins, and TNF and adipokines, oh my. It is an interesting and testable hypothesis.

In the end all diseases are due to infection or genetics. Sometimes both.

Rationalization

Roth, J., Evolutionary speculation about tuberculosis and the metabolic and inflammatory processes of obesity. JAMA, 2009. 301(24): p. 2586-8.

Jackson ImmunoResearch, FossilsResurrected! (March 2007) http://news.softpedia.com/news/Fossils-Resurrected-48353.shtml

Grand Rounds Part 1: Where is Ra's al Ghul when we need him?

I AM preparing to participate in Grand Rounds as part of a panel discussing the medical implications of global warming.

To kill two stones with one bird, what I prepare for the lecture I will translate into a quick chapter.

Everyone knows that the burning of fossil fuels combined with the endless flatulence of humans and our domestic animals are part of the cause of the increase in the greenhouse gases and subsequent global heating.

It has been made famous with the readings of CO_2 on Mauna Loa, in Hawaii, with an observed yearly increase in CO_2 since 1960 and a correlation with increasing average temperature.

What is more cool, or hot, is that these changes in greenhouse gases can be measured in ice cores going back thousands of years. The interesting results of these measurements include:

"Beginning 8,000 years ago, humans reversed an expected decrease in CO_2 by clearing forests in Europe, China, and India for croplands and pasture.

Beginning 5,000 years ago, humans reversed an expected decrease in methane by diverting water to irrigate rice and by tending large herds of livestock.

In the last few thousand years, the size of the climatic warming caused by these early greenhouse emissions may have grown large enough to prevent a glaciation that climate models predict should have begun in northeast Canada.

Abrupt reversals of the slow CO_2 rise caused by deforestation correlate with bubonic plague and other pandemics near 200-600, 1300-1400 and 1500-1700 AD. Historical records show that high mortality rates caused by plague led to massive abandonment of farms. Forest re-growth on the untended farms pulled CO_2 out of the atmosphere and caused CO_2 levels to fall. In time, the plagues abated, the farms were reoccupied, and the newly re-grown forests were cut, returning the CO_2 to the atmosphere."

Two-thirds of Europe died in the 1300s from bubonic plague, and estimates of New World deaths from new infections are as high as 95% of the population in the 1500s. The result was a slow down in global warming. Dead people make less gas.

So there may be hope for the reversal for global warming. Anyone want to get in line to participate in the great human die-off?

I didn't think so.

Rationalization

Ruddiman, W.F., The Anthropogenic Greenhouse Era Began Thousands of Years Ago. Climatic Change, 2003. 61(3): p. 261-293.

....

Grand Rounds Part Deux

EVERYONE complains about the weather, but no one tries to change it.

Long-term climate change will affect ecosystems and either increase or decrease disease spread; along the way there may be changes in weather to facilitate the spread of disease. Oregon is wet, but we lack much in the way of *Legionella*. As I have discussed once before, *Legionella* is spread when there is hot, humid thundershower weather. In Oregon we have cold, wet rain. Or at least we used to.

Climate change models, and perhaps even supermodels, suggest Oregon will get warmer and wetter in the winter.

The cold is important. *Legionella* do not grow nearly so well in amoebas (part of their life cycle in the wild) when the temperature is less than 20 degrees. That's centigrade, not Kelvin.

Warm, wet weather? Don't inhale. Curiously there are no cases associated with bongs, although it is suggested that tetrahydrocannabinol increases the risk of *Legionella*. David Gilbert once presented a case at a conference of *Legionella* from a humidifier used to treat a head cold. Close enough? *Legionella*

> "... cases occurred with striking summertime seasonality. Occurrence of cases was associated wit monthly average temperature and increase in relative humidity. However, case-crossover analysis identified an acute association with precipitation and increased humidity 6–10 days before occurrence of cases."

The association with increased rainfall has been confirmed in other studies.

But it is more than just the rainfall. Warm, moist weather facilitates the spread of *Legionella* from environmental reservoirs.

There have been outbreaks of *Legionella* associated with cooling towers, and warm wet weather helps spread the contaminated mists from the cooling towers downwind, spreading the disease for miles. Sort of a macro-bong effect.

Legionella are also associated with fountains of all kinds, whirlpools, showers, wash basins, lakes, ponds, streams, and rainwater collected on roofs.

WC Fields said he didn't drink water because fish poop in it. Maybe he was on the right track after all.

Rationalization

Hicks, L.A., et al., Increased rainfall is associated with increased risk for legionellosis. Epidemiol Infect, 2007. 135(5): p. 811-7.

Klein, T.W., et al., delta 9-Tetrahydrocannabinol, cytokines, and immunity to Legionella pneumophila. Proc Soc Exp Biol Med, 1995. 209(3): p. 205-12.

Sala, M.R., et al., Community outbreak of Legionnaires disease in Vic-Gurb, Spain in October and November 2005. Euro Surveill, 2007. 12(3): p. 223.

....

Grand Round Part Trois

THERE are two factors that may increase or decrease infections with global warming.

The first is that people will need to move, and they will bring diseases with them. Water is what is going to make them move. Large numbers of people live along coastlines and as the oceans rise, people will move, with the possible exception of the Canute family.

As someone said, we can outrun sea level change.

The other reason people will move is looking for drinking water. As one example, 30 million people get their drinking water from the Andes glaciers, most of which will be gone in perhaps 30 years. They will not be drinking bottled water as a substitute.

Climate change will alter the distribution of many vectors of infections, most importantly mosquitoes. It has been estimated that more than half of everyone who has ever died has died of a mosquito-borne illness. To get a hint of our future (this is a US-centric book) look at, but do not move to, Brownsville, Texas, where 40% of the residents are now seropositive for dengue. Dengue is classically a disease of Central America, but as the environment becomes more hospitable for mosquitoes, they go north, bringing with them their diseases. Where is Horace Greeley when you need him? Climate models suggest that a 4 degree rise in temperature could lead to the spread of dengue as far north as Chicago and Winnipeg. Malaria could reach as far north as Maine.

Disease spread is not just limited to mosquitoes.

In Belgium (sorry for the language, Mr. Beeblebrox), there has been increased temperature, which has led to increased broad-leaf trees, which has led to increased seeds, which has led to increased numbers of voles to eat the seeds. The voles carry Hantavirus, which infects humans, which leads to an increase in renal failure from Hantavirus. The old lady who swallowed a fly had nothing on that series of events.

On the bright side, the season for respiratory syncytial virus may be shortening. RSV usually just causes a cold, though it can lead to croup and maybe even asthma in children. As an I.D. doc, that is a trade I will take any day: RSV for malaria, dengue and Hantavirus. Oh my.

Rationalization

Brunkard, J.M., et al., Dengue fever seroprevalence and risk factors, Texas-Mexico border, 2004. Emerg Infect Dis, 2007. 13(10): p. 1477-83.

ANIMALS AND OTHER VERMIN

Caniculares Dies

I T's Latin.

I finally saw an organism I have read about for 25 years. That's the problem with Infectious Disease. There are so many germs out there and many of them only rarely cause disease; some are only seen in patients with altered immune systems. There are over 500 species of bacteria in your gut alone, most of which are not pathogenic. And there are the bacteria on your skin and in your mouth and in and on your friends and family. Lots of bacteria. If you just live long enough, however, eventually you will see every bug infecting some unlucky person.

There are, as I have mentioned before, 10 to 100 times more bacteria in and on you than there are cells of you. We are awash in a sea of the bacteria that make up out own bacterial flora, and occasionally the bacterial seas of other animals wash up upon our shore. Talk about a strained metaphor. I am going to wrap it in an ACE, ice it, and hope it gets better.

Our pets are a source for bacteria. Pets can harbor bacteria that are commonly pathogenic in humans as well as their own bacteria that, under the right circumstances, can infect us.

For example, *Escherichia coli*, known as *E. coli because* no one can spell *Escherichia* without a dictionary. *E. coli* is one of the primary bacteria in human colons. A common cause of urinary tract infections, this organism is passed back and forth from person to person and from person to pet and back. We live in a thin haze of our own fecal flora and the fecal flora of the humans and animals around us.

One study assessed

"The fecal E. coli flora of 228 individuals from 63 households. We documented extensive within-household sharing of fecal E. coli, including within 3 of 5 UTI (Urinary Tract Infections) households. Our findings both confirm the results of previous smaller studies and extend them by demonstrating that within-household E. coli strain sharing is widely prevalent (being essentially a normal condition) and commonly occurs among pets, humans, and non sex partners, as well as between sex partners."

Seventeen percent of humans and dogs shared the same *E. coli*. *E. coli* is not the only pathogen that dogs can carry. Dogs have also been found to carry methicillin resistant staphylococci, *Clostridium difficile* and vancomycin resistant *Enterococcus*. It is why I am not so sanguine about having dogs in my hospitals for pet "therapy." I have observed that dogs have a habit of licking their butts and elsewhere, so how do we know they haven't transferred a pathogen from butt to fur by way of the mouth? I never let a dog lick me if I can help it—it is the equivalent of shaking the hand of someone who just scratched their butt. Ick. If a dog has a germ it may pass it on to you. Bacteria, the gift that keeps on giving.

Dogs have organisms in their mouths that usually do not cause disease in humans, like *Pasteurella* species and *Capnocytophagia canimorsus*. It is this last organism I saw for the first time this week. If someone is unlucky enough to have his spleen out and is exposed to *Capnocytophagia canimorsus*, it can go berserk, causing sepsis, organ failure, and a form of vascular thrombosis called DIC and purpura fulminans. It is a particularly nasty form of sepsis as patients can lose fingers, toes, arms, legs, and their nose from the massive arterial clotting which this (and other) organisms can cause.

Which is what this poor person had. Years ago he lost a spleen to an accident and had frequent exposure to a slobbery dog. *Capnocytophagia canimorsus* managed to gain access to his bloodstream, probably through small unnoticed breaks in the skin, and it really tried to kill him. What was particularly impressive was the amount of thrombosis of toes and fingers—although in the end he survived, thanks to all that the modern ICU has to offer, and did not lose a digit.

I have read about *Capnocytophagia* for years-—it may be on your Boards, by the way—and have finally seen a case. I hope it's the last. If you have a dog and you do not have a spleen, be wary of bites. Every animal can and will, under the right conditions, spread an odd disease or two to humans. The best way to sterilize your dog or cat is the autoclave, but for some reason people actually like their pets. Go figure.

Do we have a pet? Nope. My kids want a dog, but I now I will be the one to end up taking care of it, i.e. cleaning up the crap. Pass. They did have a hamster, which promptly bit me (hamsters can carry Lymphocytic choriomeningitis virus), then escaped, fell down a heating duct and died on the heating coil, filling the house with the smell of roasting, rotting hamster in January and costing $400 to fix. I cannot imagine the smell and cost if a dog or a cat fell down the duct.

Rationalization

Johnson, J.R., et al., Escherichia coli colonization patterns among human household members and pets, with attention to acute urinary tract infection. J Infect Dis, 2008. 197(2): p. 218-24.

Caniculares Dies: dog days.

It is good to have a spleen

L ESS than six months later, déjà vu all over again.
A middle-aged female had a fever of 105, felt awful, then showed up in the ER. Hypotension, renal insufficiency, low platelets (18,000, about a tenth of normal), with scattered petechiae.

Her spleen had been removed about five years ago for what turned out to be a benign condition. People without spleens to not get more frequent infections, but when they do, man can they go to stink with rapidity.

The most common severe infection is *S. pneumoniae*, and I bet that would grow on blood cultures. Another thing to think of, though, is that she did have dogs, one of which licked her with great frequency.

Upfront I put her ceftriaxone and azithromycin, but after 48 hours her blood cultures were negative. Then a thin, long gram negative rod slowly grew.

It was growing *Capnocytophagia* of some sort, maybe *C. canimorsus*. That's two in less than 6 months, after never having seen a *Capnocytophagia* before.

Patients can have their spleens removed for a variety of reasons, but there are may conditions where the patients functionally behave as if they had no spleen:

Alcoholism, amyloidosis, autoimmune hemolytic anemia, biliary cirrhosis, bone marrow transplantation, celiac disease, chronic active hepatitis, chronic graft vs. host reaction, chronic myelogenous leukemia, collagenous colitis, essential thrombocythemia, Graves' disease, hairy cell leukemia, hashimoto's thyroiditis, hemangiosarcoma of the spleen, hemophilia, hematologic diseases, hereditary spherocytosis, Hodgkin's disease, idiopathic thrombocytopenic purpura, non-hodgkin's lymphoma, ovarian carcinoma, portal hypertension, rheumatoid arthritis, right sided heart failure, sarcoidosis, Sjögren's syndrome, splenic irradiation, systemic lupus erythematosus, thalassemia, ulcerative colitis, Whipple's disease.

Whoa. Talk about venting one's spleen.

There are 874 references pertaining to *Capnocytophagia* on PubMed. That's a lot of cases, many in ostensibly normal people. Given the number of dogs, I bet this disease is under-reported. At our weekly infectious disease conference, someone presented a 9-month-old with sepsis and meningitis that turned out to be due to *Capnocytophagia*. The family dawg evidently licked the child's head like I would a Tootsie roll pop, trying, I suppose, to get to the tasty center.

"Zoonotic agents were isolated from 80 out of 102 (80%) dogs. The primary pathogen was Clostridium difficile, which was isolated from 58 (58%) faecal specimens. Seventy-one percent (41/58) of these isolates were toxigenic. Extended-spectrum beta-lactamase

Escherichia coli was isolated from one (1%) dog, extended-spectrum cephalosporinase E. coli was isolated from three (3%) dogs, and organisms of the genus Salmonella were isolated from three (3%) dogs. Pasteurella multocida or Pasteurella canis was isolated from 29 (29%) oral swabs , and Malassezia pachydermatis was isolated from eight (8%) aural swabs. Giardia antigen was present in the faeces of seven (7%) dogs, while Toxocara canis and Ancylostoma caninum were detected in two (2%) dogs and one (1%) dog, respectively."

MRSA is also carried in pets as well. It is just a matter of time before some poor patient gets something from the visiting dawg.

But people seem to love dawgs more than each other, so I expect to see a few more of these before I retire.

Rationalization

Lefebvre, S.L., et al., Prevalence of zoonotic agents in dogs visiting hospitalized people in Ontario: implications for infection control. J Hosp Infect, 2006. 62(4): p. 458-66.

....

Dogs

THE residents say I hate dogs. Not true. I love dogs, although I do need a new recipe. I grow weary of deep-fried. I hate dog owners. Well, maybe hate is too strong a word. But as best as I can tell, there is no such thing as a considerate dog owner. Now someone is going to kvetch about kids, but I do not have to listen to kids bark all day, kids do not run up to me yipping at my heels as I walk, and kids certainly do not crap on my lawn. At least I don't think they do.

Dog owners seem to think their personal vermin should be allowed access to the hospital, and increasingly these clueless goobers bring their dogs into the hospital. I saw several dogs wandering the hospital with their owners this weekend.

I am not talking about Seeing Eye dogs, or service animals or even 'Pet Therapy' dogs, which I have my concerns about. Just regular old pets. People think that their pets should accompany them into the hospital.

Why should I care?

For one, you never know when these things will bite or crap, and I want to participate in neither.

From an infectious disease point of view, people pet dogs and then do not wash their hands afterwards. It is a myth that a dog's mouth is cleaner than a human's. It isn't. Dogs' mouths are far worse than ours in terms of number and type of bacteria, because they do not brush their teeth and they lick their butts. Then they lick everywhere else, including your face and hands. If I touch a patient, I wash my hands. I have yet to see a dog washed after interacting with a patient or staff, and they are every bit as much of a potential vector for infection as your physicians.

Not only can dogs carry pathogenic bacteria, but they can carry MRSA and *C. difficile*, both significant hospital pathogens. I do not want them—animals or their bacteria—in my hospital. I have enough trouble controlling human-to-human spread of disease, and do not want to have the added worry about whatever Fifi the Wonder Poodle is bringing into the hospital.

Ask people nicely to please take their dogs outside, and you might as well have asked them to eat the dog. It does not surprise me. At least here in Oregon, people care far more for their dogs than they do for their fellow humans.

Rationalization

Chang, H.J., et al., An epidemic of Malassezia pachydermatis in an intensive care nursery associated with colonization of health care workers' pet dogs. N Engl J Med, 1998. 338(11): p. 706-11.

Manian, F.A., Asymptomatic nasal carriage of mupirocin-resistant, methicillin-resistant Staphylococcus aureus (MRSA) in a pet dog associated with MRSA infection in household contacts. Clin Infect Dis, 2003. 36(2): p. e26-8.

Vermin Bites

Pets. I don't want one. But I am glad others do, as it makes my job more interesting.

You don't really want to stick your hand near an animal's mouth.

"Here, kitty kitty kitty, nice kitty—damn, it done bit me on the hand."

Cats, especially, like to cause deep injuries. Unlike dawgs, which tend to cause tearing injuries, cats have teeth that are filthy solid needles that inject bacteria and whatever else is in the mouth deep into tissues, gaining access to the joints of the hands and the tendon sheaths, neither of which is a good place to have bacteria.

Common bacteria in the mouths of cats, and to a lesser extent the mouths of dogs, are *Pasteurella multocida* and other members of the *Pasteurella* family. *Pasteurella* loves to cause soft tissue infections after bites, and often needs surgical debridement. The patient I saw today whose cat inadvertently bit her on the thumb needed this treatment. Some surgery, a few days in the hospital, and some antibiotics later she is slowly getting better. And I thought my hamster was expensive.

Pasteurella can show up in other body parts, depending on the exposure. Remember Pig Pen from Charlie Brown, always in a cloud of dirt? I think of animals that way, and I include humans as animals. All are in a cloud of bacteria. So if the cat wanders around your environment, it will leave little bacillary presents in its wake that, with a little bad luck, will infect you.

I had a patient who developed a *Pasteurella* foot abscess. She denied any bites to her feet, but did like to walk barefoot though her house where she had 30 or so cats.

I had the peritoneal dialysis patient who developed *Pasteurella* peritonitis. The cat liked to sleep in the bag warmer where the dialysate was warmed prior to being infused into the peritoneum.

I had a patient whose cat chewed off the end of her Groshong catheter while she slept—I suppose it liked the taste of blood—and the catheter grew *Pasteurella*.

My all-time favorite was the teenage girl who liked to put tuna on her nose and have her ever-so—cute kitty cat lick it off. The veins of the face drain back to the central nervous system, and she was unfortunate enough to get meningitis from *Pasteurella*. She did fine, but it was not a pleasant experience.

Lookin' Good

SHH. Gather round. I am going to tell the secret of looking good as a consultant. Besides the white coat.

The patient, a two-pint-a-day vodka drinker, was admitted with ethanol withdrawal when he decided to quit drinking on his own.

In the ER he was febrile and blood cultures were done.

The next day his cultures popped positive, both sets with a gram negative rod that the lab called funny, not ha ha but odd. So I saw the patient, whose mental status has cleared, and he couldn't move either shoulder or his ankle. Although he had little rubor, calor or tumor in any of the joints, he howled with pain with passive movement of the joints. He also had a cellulitis of his right leg.

So I called the lab and ask what they thought.

They didn't know what it was. It was a small, funny looking, gram negative and oxidase positive bacterium, and it was in the Identification machine—they would tell me what it is in the morning.

So here is my secret. Don't tell anyone.

I Google or Pubmed everything. I put "gram negative," "rod oxidase positive," "pleomorphic" (med speak for funny-looking) in the search box and up comes a list. On the list is *Pasteurella*, and the patient has a cat.

So I wrote in my note to say it was probably *Pasteurella*, and it was. I look like a god. Minor deity. Like Pan.

So to look good? Google or Pubmed everything, then commit to a diagnosis.

Unfortunately, the patient refused debridement and antibiotics, so the outcome is not looking so good.

Also, and of interest, is that liver disease (his bilirubin is 9.0 mg/dL; normal < 1.9) is a risk for *Pasteurella* and septic joints. And you do not need to get a cat bite to get exposed to *Pasteurella*. He denies any bites. Cats lick everywhere and where the cat licks, *Pasteurella* follows.

Rationalization

Migliore, E., et al., Pasteurella multocida infection in a cirrhotic patient: case report, microbiological aspects and a review of literature. Adv Med Sci, 2009. 54(1): p. 109-12.

Don't change the litter box before driving

I N Oregon, in case you are interested, if you get three photo radar tickets and a car accident in less than three months, the State looks unkindly upon you. They suspend you license for a month. Lucky me, I get to enjoy public transportation for the next month, much to the amusement of my coworkers (a word I always see as cow orkers, although I have no idea what orking a cow would entail). Amongst other things if you get another moving violation in the following 12 months, they suspend your license for a year. It is a good reason to drive very, very carefully.

Toxoplasma is an interesting parasite. In the wild it infects small animals like mice, but it needs to complete its life cycle in a cat or other carnivore. So the parasite goes to the brain of the mouse and causes an encephalitis, which slows the mouse down and increases the chance it will be captured and et by a cat. This is only one of many examples where an infection changes the behavior of its host to help increase its chances of reproducing.

Toxoplasmosis is supposed to be asymptomatic in humans, or so I thought. Turns out that patients infected with *Toxoplasma* are not all that normal. *Toxoplasma* seropositive people have slower reaction times and as a result are more prone to car accidents, not that car accidents will help the organism reproduce. Although one wonders if our ancient forebears were more likely to be consumed by lions as a result of toxoplasmosis. And I would prefer my neurosurgeon to be *Toxoplasma* negative.

As always, it is not that simple. All Tanzanian military recruits are screened for *Toxoplasma*, and those who were seropositive were found to have an increased car accident rate, but only if they were blood type RhD negative. Blood type RhD positive was protective from toxo-associated car accidents.

> *"Our results show that RhD-negative subjects with high titers of anti-Toxoplasma antibodies had a probability of a traffic accident of about 16.7 %, i.e. a more than six times higher rate than Toxoplasma-free or RhD-positive subjects. "*

Why the Rh association? They don't know.

> *"It must also be noted that the effect of latent toxoplasmosis on reaction times varies across testing minutes ....The authors speculated that two effects of infection might interplay in Toxoplasma-infected men. Latent toxoplasmosis is known 1) to impair reaction times in infected men and animals and also 2) to increase the concentration of testosterone in infected men. Increased concentration of testosterone positively influences the level of personality trait competitiveness in men, which, in turn, could enhance performance under certain circumstances. Therefore, the negative effects of latent toxoplasmosis on psychomotor performance in men could influence the rate of traffic accidents under certain conditions only, which could explain some differences in results between the published case-control studies and present cohort study."*

Officer, the parasite in my brain increased my testosterone levels and decreased my reflexes and made me a more aggressive, but sloppier, driver.

If you know anyone in, say, Oregon who could be at risk for a one-year license suspension, let him know about this. It might be a mitigating factor that, combined with Twinkie consumption, could be the difference between driving and public transportation.

Rationalization

Flegr, J., et al., Increased incidence of traffic accidents in Toxoplasma-infected military drivers and protective effect RhD molecule revealed by a large-scale prospective cohort study. BMC Infect Dis, 2009. 9: p. 72.

....

Hamsters

I WENT and saw *Bolt* with my 11-year-old today. Entertaining movie, but the 3D animated effects are jaw-dropping.

It is the story of the adventures of three infectious disease vectors: a dog, a cat, and a hamster. As is often the case after we see movies with animals in them, my son asked for a pet, and, as is usual, I demurred. Not because I worry about infections, but prior experience with vermin, I mean pets, has demonstrated that the responsibility for their care usually devolves on to me.

Hamsters are a source for the LCM (Lymphocytic Choriomeningitis) virus, a disease that causes aseptic meningitis. Hamsters have also been associated with the spread of multi drug resistant *Salmonella*. And I don't think they taste near as good as a Guinea Pig.

LCM is spread from hamsters to humans, and can be fatal in the immunocompromised, although it is often asymptomatic in normal people.

There have been occasional outbreaks, but the most curious case was the patient who died and had her organs harvested (the live ones tend to resist), and the recipients of the organs developed LCM. This has happened at least twice.

In one outbreak

"The epidemiologic investigation revealed that a member of the donor's household had brought home a pet hamster three weeks before the donor died. Although the donor had not been the primary caretaker of the hamster, she had contact with the rodent's environment on multiple occasions."

The donor was asymptomatic at the time of the organ donation.

I am always amazed at what can be transient exposure to pathogens, yet patients still get disease.

We did have a hamster once. My eldest son bought one and proudly brought it home.

Here, dad, hold it.

I did, and the damn thing promptly bit me, drawing blood. I didn't get LCM, but nope. No pets for us.

Rationalization

CDC, Lymphocytic choriomeningitis virus infection in organ transplant recipients--Massachusetts, Rhode Island, 2005. MMWR Morb Mortal Wkly Rep, 2005. 54(21): p. 537-9.

Fischer, S.A., et al., Transmission of lymphocytic choriomeningitis virus by organ transplantation. N Engl J Med, 2006. 354(21): p. 2235-49.

....

Word History

Most of my great diagnoses exist only in my head. Not that this is bad, as my internal reality is far superior to the external one.

For many patients I see I try, for fun, to come up with three lists.

One is the list of diseases the patient probably has: common things, oddly, being common.

Another is the list of things the patient cannot afford to have missed: pulmonary embolism or meningitis. Maybe unlikely based on the history and physical, but if that is the diagnosis, the patient is in a world of hurt.

Last, of course, is the list of cool things, which are usually neither common nor fatal.

I have a routine I go thorough with every patient, asking about this and that, looking over the chart and the labs and then, boom—one thing jumps out that may be the hinge-point upon which the entire diagnosis in the clouds is built.

The patient today: Fevers to 103, worst headache of his life (German sausage-makers get the wurst headaches of anyone), right lower lobe interstitial pneumonia, mild increase in liver enzymes. No response to standard therapy for community acquired pneumonia.

Temperature is 103, pulse 80. This is the hinge point: he has Faget's sign.

Any animal exposure? I ask.

Nope.

Been around any...then I rattle of a list of animals which would make Noah proud.

"I went hiking around wild goats," is the response.

Faget's sign is named after Dr. George Snelling. Not really.

Jean-Charles Faget was born to French parents in New Orleans. He studied in Paris from 1837 to 1845, and after receiving his doctorate in 1844 settled in New Orleans. He stayed in Paris 1866-1867 and subsequently lived in New Orleans for the rest of his life. In 1858 he discovered a specific pathognomonic sign of yellow fever, a slow pulse at high fever."

Classically it is a sign of yellow fever, but can also be seen in typhoid fever, *Brucella*, dengue, Q fever, tularemia, chlamydia, *Legionella,* and is reported with a smattering of other diseases. I am betting Q fever from the goats. It may not take much of an exposure to get Q fever if you get the right animal infected. *Coxiella burnetii* is the cause of Q fever, which gets its name, to quote the ever helpful wikipedia:

"The "Q" stands for "query" and was applied at a time when the causative agent was unknown; it was chosen over suggestions of "abattoir fever" and "Queensland rickettsial fever," to avoid directing negative connotations at either the cattle industry or the state of Queensland."

I like "abattoir fever" more.

The patient had the exposure, it was the right clinical pattern, so now I await the serology. That's two serologies I am waiting on.

If you are a resident or medical student, remember the differential for Faget's. You may shine at a pimping session.

Rationalization

Porten, K., et al., A super-spreading ewe infects hundreds with Q fever at a farmers' market in Germany. BMC Infect Dis, 2006. 6: p. 147.

Martin Schoen, The Art of the Pimp. The Weekly Murmur, January 26, 2004. http://web.med.harvard.edu/sites/murmur/html/articles/012604/012604_mschoen.asp

Postscript

Q fever serology was negative. Another great diagnosis sunk by reality.

Have to ask the right question

WHEN I was a kid I was told by a friend that you got *Salmonella* from eating salmon. Seemed reasonable to me at the time; I did not realize it was named after Sal Mon, one of the top level Pokemon. God know what you get from eating spotted dick.

The patient I saw yesterday had *Salmonella* in both her diarrhea and her blood. Simple enough, but why? Everyone assumed she picked it up on her trip to Southeast Asia, but that had been 6 weeks prior, which was a wee bit too long an incubation period.

So you start asking about exposures, since *Salmonella* has many ways to get into the food supply and cause diarrhea. There seems to be a new outbreak every month.

Unusual foods? Nope.

Pistachios? Nope.

Peanut butter? Nope.

Tomatoes or fresh salads? Nope.

Pets or animals at home? Nope.

Any reptiles? Nope.

Any folk remedies? Nope.

Hows about chickens or eggs? We raise chickens.

Odd response, given the pet or animal question that preceded it. Once there was a patient who was admitted with fevers and diffuse granulomatous lymphadenopathy. Everyone asked him if he had pets or animals at home, and he said no. My boss, on Chief of Service Rounds, asked the patient if he was around any animals, and he said his roommate had a half dozen cats. HE didn't have animals, it was his roommate. It is all in how you ask the question. The patient had Ted Nugent's disease, or Cat Scratch Fever.

Today's case probably got the *Salmonella* from her chickens, as it came before the eggs. She was not enamored with the idea that she developed *Salmonella* from her chickens, since she had had chickens for years and never developed an infection before. The final flush of the toilet to make the diagnosis was she had recently been started on a proton pump inhibitor (PPI) after returning to the US, and so for the first time had no stomach acid barrier to prevent infection. As noted in the rationalizations, "There is an association between acid suppression and an increased risk of enteric infection."

Once you start a PPI, stay away from the raw eggs unless you have a lot of reading you want to get done.

Tony Montana would not like these studies

IT has been suggested that cockroaches will someday rule the world. The are so hardy, so resilient, that they will survive a nuclear holocaust. I say look out for them today.

A study came out of Ethiopia where the researchers looked at cockroaches as a source for intestinal parasites. Now if you think you are having a bad day, think of these poor scientists. They trapped 6480 cockroaches of three different cockroach species. Ick.

Then they did

"microscopic examination of the external body washes of pooled cockroaches and individual gut contents."

What did you do today? Body washed cockroaches. Followed by a light massage and manicure.

They also did a microscopic evaluation of the guts of the cockroaches, although how they made the tiny endoscopes I do not know.

And they found pathogens:

"..cockroaches are carriers of Entamoeba coli and Entamoeba histolytica/dispar cysts as well as Enterobius vermicularis, Trichuris trichiura, Taenia spp. and Ascaris lumbricoides ova."

All parasites that infect the human colon and cause diarrhea.

This is not the first time pathogens have been found in cockroaches. In another study, 305 cockroaches were evaluated for bacterial pathogens and *Escherichia coli, Streptococcus Group D, Bacillus spp., Klebsiella pneumoniae, Proteus vulgaris, Citrobacter freundii, Staphylococcus aureus*, and *Streptococcus* non-group A and B were found. Others have found *Salmonella* in/on cockroaches associated with an outbreak.

Yet another study found *Candida, Aspergillus*, and *Penicillium* associated with the wee beasties.

Cockroaches live in intimate contact with humans and they have our bacteria, fungi, and parasites. They are more than disgusting. Bear Grylls better be careful what he eats, although only 30 of the 4000 species are human pests.

It is why I make a point of keeping my cockroach consumption to a minimum.

Rationalization

Hamu, H., et al., Isolation of Intestinal Parasites of Public Health Importance from Cockroaches (Blattella germanica) in Jimma Town, Southwestern Ethiopia. J Parasitol Res, 2014. 2014: p. 186240.

Kinfu, A. and B. Erko, Cockroaches as carriers of human intestinal parasites in two localities in Ethiopia. Trans R Soc Trop Med Hyg, 2008. 102(11): p. 1143-7.

Lemos, A.A., et al., Cockroaches as carriers of fungi of medical importance. Mycoses, 2006. 49(1): p. 23-5.

Honey

BEES have a bad name amongst us alternative medicine skeptics. Senator Harkin was under the illusion that bee pollen cured his hay fever, and when senators gets bees in their bonnets, they pass bills. The result was The National Center for Complementary and Alternative Medicine (NCCAM), one of the biggest wastes of tax dollars ever. I know that you can't really blame the bees, they were not responsible, but still. With no irony, my spell checker suggests Occam for NCCAM.

Today I saw a lady with severe arterial insufficiency and as a result, chronic lower leg ulcers that continually get super-infected. What to do? Long-term antibiotics are problematic as they lead to resistance and allergic reactions. The wound care people had her on Silvadeen/charcoal patches that were quite painful to take off. I gave my usual suggestion for a different form of wound care, which resulted in a rolling of the eyes.

I was told as a medical student by a plastic surgeon never put in a wound what you wouldn't put in your eyes. You don't want to damage new tissues, he said, and that's what most wound care does. As a result, for years I packed wounds with contact lenses. Soft, not hard.

In the first year of my practice, I was writing a note on the nursing station when I heard a patient start screaming. This was before I learned to ignore the suffering of others as I became a full-fledged member of the medical-industrial complex. Investigating, I discovered that her surgeon had ordered sugar for the wound and the kitchen had mistakenly sent up salt. Talk about a metaphor come to life.

Upon further research I found there is a reasonably good literature to support both granulated sugar and honey in the treatment of wounds, ulcers and burns, and the data suggests that both therapies are equal to, if not better than, standard medications. Not a great literature, but good enough to draw some tentative conclusions.

Don't bacteria like sugar? Not at the concentrations found in honey. Ever been to France and seen the preserved fruits? They preserve them in sugar. Same reason there is sugar in strawberry PRESERVES. It's why they are not called strawberry rotten from the *Staphylococcus* and *E. coli.*

Sugar and honey are inexpensive. They kill all the bacteria that often are pathogenic on the skin. They wash off painlessly. Sugar doesn't kill new tissues and it absorbs all the gunk make by the wounds and bacteria. And you get to participate in a naturalistic fallacy with your patients. It is the wonder drug that works wonders. No, wait, that's aspirin. I doubt it is as good as a wound vac, but not everyone can afford a wound vac.

How is honey supposed to work?

"Honey has several well-known properties responsible for its anti-microbial activity. These include a high osmolarity due to the high concentration of sugars (80% wt/vol), a low pH (3.2 —4.5 for undiluted honey), and the production of hydrogen peroxide, which, after dilution of honey, is produced by glucose oxidase originating from the bees. In addition, unknown Floral or bee components contribute to the activity."

Is it effective in wounds and burns? Yes, he says with a tentative quaver in his voice. PubMed (like the verb Google) "honey" or "sugar" as a search term, and you will find an interesting literature filled with studies that are not all that great, but suggestive. Even the irascible *Cochrane Reviews* concludes that

"Honey may improve healing times in mild to moderate superficial and partial thickness burns compared with some conventional dressings. Honey dressings as an adjuvant to compression do not significantly increase leg ulcer healing at 12 weeks. There is insufficient evidence to guide clinical practice in other areas."

Not a ringing endorsement for honey dressing, I will grant you, but I often chose the soup not the salad. But if you read all the literature, it is suggestive.

I found the CID article this year on the effects of honey on skin pathogens interesting. It kills them dead.

"Antibiotic-susceptible and resistant isolates of Staphylococcus aureus, Staphylococcus epidermidis, Enterococcus faecium, Escherichia coli, Pseudomonas aeruginosa, Enterobacter cloacae, and Klebsiella oxytoca were killed within 24 h by 10% —40% (vol/vol) honey. After 2 days of application of honey, the extent of forearm skin colonization in healthy volunteers was reduced 100-fold , and the numbers of cultures were reduced by 76%."

It is an interesting literature, made difficult by often small numbers, poor experimental design, and the lack a placebo control that looks like honey but isn't. Many of my patients have no insurance, little money, and fewer resources. There is enough data and biological plausibility that I suggest it to some of my patients, although I spend more time on the caveats than usual.

The most dangerous words in medicine are "In my experience," but in my experience honey works. I am, of course, deluding myself. But at least there is some data and, unlike the homeopaths, I am not diluting myself.

Rationalization

Jull, A.B., A. Rodgers, and N. Walker, Honey as a topical treatment for wounds. Cochrane Database Syst Rev, 2008(4): p. CD005083.

Kwakman, P.H., et al., Medical-grade honey kills antibiotic-resistant bacteria in vitro and eradicates skin colonization. Clin Infect Dis, 2008. 46(11): p. 1677-82.

....

Hitchcock didn't know the half of it

I'VE always thought that the second most horrible scene in the movies (for the first, see *Gangrene*) was the lady with her eyes pecked out in *The Birds*. I could not watch the Bob Newhart Show without thinking of Susanne Pleshette with bloody, empty eye sockets. It kind of detracted from the comedy, or maybe added to it, depending on my mood. The eyes are one area that I hate having anyone get near. It took years to get up the gumption to get contacts. And I won't even tell you about the lady with the pneumococcal eye infection that ruptured during the exam. Well, I guess I just did. Still gives me the willies.

While birds, of course, never swarm, attack and kill people, they are good at spreading disease. Right now the worry is avian flu, which will probably get the US by way of migrating birds, probably ducks, which are relatively resistant to dying from avian flu.

You can't stop a duck, and that has extra meaning to me as a University of Oregon grad, with the second lamest mascot in the state. Number one is Oregon State. Seriously, an orange beaver? But what can you expect from a school with no sense of color?

Birds, it turns out, can carry more than avian flu.

In this study they looked at fecal or cloacal samples from 97 birds in northeastern Siberia; Point Barrow, Alaska, USA; and northern Greenland.

Sign me up. Let's go somewhere colder than hell to collect bird crap (yes, I know—hell is supposed to be hot. Nope. I spent three years in Minnesota for my medicine residency. Hell will be cold, I'll be wet and naked, and there will be a brisk wind). And let's hang out in the cold place to culture the bird crap. See. Was your day really all that bad?

They looked at the *E. coli* in the bird poo and found

"E. coli isolates from Arctic birds carried antimicrobial drug resistance determinants; among 17 antimicrobial drugs tested, resistance to 14 was detected. Resistance was observed in 8 isolates, 4 of which displayed resistance to >4 drugs, and occurred most often to ampicillin, sulfamethoxazole, trimethoprim, chloramphenicol, and tetracycline. Two resistant isolates displayed isolated fosfomycin resistance."

What is remarkable about the resistance is that these samples were collected from the Arctic, one of the most remote and hostile areas on earth, where there is no antibiotic use.

It is postulated that migrating birds picked up the *E. coli* when in more temperate areas and brought them north. Resistant *E. coli* have also been found in isolated human and animal populations that have little or no exposure to antibiotics, and migratory birds are a potential explanation for the resistance.

They suspect these resistant organisms were of clinical origin, as they had the same pattern of resistance as *E. coli* in hospitals.

Yet another way for antibiotic resistance to spread—but at least Homeland Security, by watching our borders, can keep out the migrating birds. We just need a high enough wall.

Rationalization

Sjolund, M., et al., Dissemination of multidrug-resistant bacteria into the Arctic. Emerg Infect Dis, 2008. 14(1): p. 70-2.

LE TERRAIN EST TOUT: HOST FACTORS IN ID

Down with Meningitis

A BUSY call weekend, with one consult on a case of bacterial meningitis due to *S. pneumoniae*. Not a surprise in that strep pneumo, as we call it in the biz, is the number one cause of meningitis in adults. It was the patient that made the disease a curiosity. He had Down's syndrome.

It is the Down's that make the case of interest.

A variety of functional immune deficiencies have been described in Down's:

—Decreased function of specific types of white blood cells, called neutrophils and monocytes. Their functions of chemotaxis (movement), phagocytosis (eating) and the oxidative burst (killing) have been suggested in some studies to be impaired.

—Increased production of some types of antibodies, but decreased production of other types. Immunoglobin G (IgG) is a type of antibody, of which there are 4 subtypes, IgG1 through IgG4. In Down's, IgG1 and IgG3 subclasses are increased, IgG2 and IgG4 subclasses are decreased. IgG2 is the antibody needed for a response to carbohydrate antigens, which is the one that is needed to kill pneumococcus, whose cell wall is covered with sugars.

—Decreased antibody responses to immunizations such as Prevnar, the vaccine against *S. pneumoniae*.

Lots of good reasons from a faulty immune system to get infected. Down's, unfortunately, affects more than just the brain.

I also expected a resistant organism as the patient developed the meningitis on cephalexin for sinusitis. And indeed, it was resistant to penicillin.

That's four cases of meningitis this week, each from a different organism: viral, meningococcus, *S. pneumoniae*, and a strep the lab is still identifying.

The wonder drug that works wonders. Wait. That's aspirin

STATINS are in the news today for the relatively unimportant reason that they prevent death from myocardial infarction (heart attack), especially in a subgroup of people who have an elevated C reactive protein.

C reactive protein (or CRP, and since it is ReActive, shouldn't the proper acronym be CRAP?) is a protein that is elevated when you are inflamed. Many processes will elevate your CRP, from infection to collagen vascular disease—but not being inflamed by religious or political fervor.

Inflammation is good in response to infection, but continued inflammation has the potential to cause vascular diseases. Acute inflammation (such as pneumonia and urinary tract infections) is well known to increase the risk of heart attacks, strokes, and pulmonary emboli.

Statins lower cholesterol, but probably more importantly, statins work as anti-inflammatory agents by a variety of mechanisms too complex for my tiny brain to comprehend.

What kills people with infections is often an overly brisk inflammatory response. Inflammation is like a Bordeaux: a little is good, a lot can kill you. Interestingly, retrospective studies have consistently demonstrated that people who get pneumonia while on statins have a decreased mortality compared to those not on statins.

Same result with a recent retrospective study:

The researchers looked at 29,900 adults hospitalized with pneumonia, of whom 1372 were taking statins on admission.

"At 30 days, those patients taking statins who were hospitalized with pneumonia had a 31% lower risk of dying compared with patients not taking statins. By 90 days, the reduction in mortality was maintained, with those taking statins having a 25% lower risk of dying compared with those not on statin therapy."

Bad word, retrospective. What is needed is a randomized, prospective, placebo-controlled trial to see if the results are really truly true.

There have also been studies with decreased mortality and sepsis for patients on stains.

The epidemiological data look good so far, so when you wash down that aspirin a day with a glass of red, include a statin so when you pass out drunk and get a pneumonia, you are less likely to die.

Rationalization

Almog, Y., Statins, inflammation, and sepsis: hypothesis. Chest, 2003. 124(2): p. 740-3.

Thomsen, R.W., et al., Preadmission use of statins and outcomes after hospitalization with pneumonia: population-based cohort study of 29,900 patients. Arch Intern Med, 2008. 168(19): p. 2081-7.

Vitamin D: Supporting Immune Health

THE rains stopped today. It has been Oregon weather: dark and wet, with seemingly endless rains. It has been weirdly warm for November; it hit 66 yesterday. It is like living in a Ray Bradbury story— "All the Summer in a Day," the one where a planet has 4 hours of sunshine every 100 years.

Rain and clouds mean no sun and no sun means low vitamin D. Unless you eat lots of ice cream. I get frequent flyer miles from Baskin Robbins.

Today was a hip fracture with a wound infection in an old woman. As part of the work-up on the fracture service, she had her vitamin D level measured—undetectable. No surprise for an Oregonian, especially the institutionalized elderly who do not get out in the sun, preferring to drive around the city at 20 miles an hour no matter that the posted speed limit.

Vitamin D is required for bone metabolism, so association with hip fracture is no surprise. What is interesting is that Vitamin D is also an important adjunct of the immune system, and there is growing evidence that deficiencies in vitamin D increase infection risk and severity.

Vitamin D deficiency is associated with reactivation of TB, developing TB for the first time, viral upper respiratory infections, pneumonia, and bacterial infections in atopic dermatitis. Variations in vitamin D receptors (polymorphisms) are also associated with upper respiratory tract infections and TB.

Studies of the mechanisms by which vitamin D is used by the immune system and the interplay of the vitamin with risks for infection in their infancy. How much a lack of vitamin D is associated with post-operative hip infections, I cannot say. But I bet it is a factor, and a future paper for someone.

There was a little bit of sun today. I thought about taking off my shirt to get a dose of sun and boost my vitamin D levels. Nope. Wasn't worth making other people sick. We are just getting over the Norovirus outbreak. I'll eat ice cream instead.

Rationalization

Laaksi, I., et al., An association of serum vitamin D concentrations < 40 nmol/L with acute respiratory tract infection in young Finnish men. Am J Clin Nutr, 2007. 86(3): p. 714-7.

Sita-Lumsden, A., et al., Reactivation of tuberculosis and vitamin D deficiency: the contribution of diet and exposure to sunlight. Thorax, 2007. 62(11): p. 1003-7.

Mesquita Kde, C., A.C. Igreja, and I.M. Costa, Atopic dermatitis and vitamin D: facts and controversies. An Bras Dermatol, 2013. 88(6): p. 945-53.

....

What and Why

*W*HAT they have is easy. The culture or the serology or the syndrome often gives the diagnosis.

But *why?* Why do people get infections? Often it seems to be bad luck—wrong time, wrong place. Sometimes it's the patients. There is great variability in the human immune system. Yours is not the same as mine. Some people are born with more ability to respond to infections, others less so. Clinically, I have only the most primitive assays at my disposal to evaluate the immune system, but I wager than in another 10 or 15 years I will have far more sophisticated genetic tests to determine why a patient has an infection.

I did have two "why?"s answered this week.

One patient, who presented with pneumococcal meningitis, turned out to have an IgM deficiency. Not common at all—I cannot find that IgM is specifically associated with pneumococcal meningitis—but it is the first class of antibody to come on-line for infection, so I am crediting IgM deficiency for his relatively slow response to therapy.

The other diagnosis is more common. A patient with recurrent sinopulmonary infections, sore throats, and "catches everything." A common complaint of patients.

Turns out this patient has an antibody deficiency as well: Total IgG, IgG subtypes 2 and 4, and IgA levels are half normal. While absolute antibody levels correlate poorly with infection, it seems reasonable to ascribe her recurrent minor infections to her low antibody levels.

Antibody deficiencies are probably more common than is realized by most clinicians.

Data on 127,000 patients from the Rochester Epidemiology Project found 158 primary immunodeficiency cases over the 31-year study period.

B cell defects accounted for 78% of the cases. B cells make antibodies, so these defects led to deficiencies in one or more antibody types. They saw a variety of deficiencies, all divided about equally. One group was deficiencies in one of the four subclasses of IgG. Another group was deficiency in IgA, the antibodies found on mucosal surfaces. A very unfortunate group of patients had general hypogammaglobulinemia, where levels of all antibody types (IgG A through E) were low. Such patients usually have infections starting from infancy. A fourth group had miscellaneous defects leading to B cell dysfunction.

The overall rate of immunodeficiency seen was 10.3 per 100,000—more common than tuberculosis.

The clinical hint is recurrent infections of any kind.

Anyone who presents by my clinic with recurrent infections gets antibody levels and IgG subtypes measured as part of the evaluation, and I hit pay dirt a couple of times a year.

Rationalization

Joshi, A.Y., et al., Incidence and temporal trends of primary immunodeficiency: a population-based cohort study. Mayo Clin Proc, 2009. 84(1): p. 16-22.

Oksenhendler, E., et al., Infections in 252 patients with common variable immunodeficiency. Clin Infect Dis, 2008. 46(10): p. 1547-54.

Why Why Why

SUMMER time and the living is easy. Except if you have bacteremic pneumococcal pneumonia. It is a bad disease, and people feel mighty poorly when they have it.

That was today's patient, who had a classic upper respiratory infection, then cough, then rigors and fevers and a marked increase in the cough with chest pain. He had "e" to "a" changes on exam, which is always a fun finding. This is when you ask a patient to pronounce a long "e" while listening to the lungs with a stethoscope. If the lung is consolidated by infection or fibrosis, the "e" will sound like an "a." This sign, along with fever and cough, is indicative of pneumonia.

Bring on he magic that is a beta-lactam, and the patient got all better. Except. Why? Why does a 30-ish year-old, otherwise healthy human get streptococcal bacteremia?

One. HIV. Nope.

Two. Immunoglobulin issues.

Always a worry. In older adults I always check for multiple myeloma or other related malignancies in any bacteremic pneumococcal disease, and I hit paydirt a couple of times a year. Pneumococcus in the blood equals serum protein electrophoresis (a test for globulins).

The patient's IgG levels were low. IgG1 and IgG3 are mostly

against protein antigens, and IgG2 is mostly against carbohydrates, so maybe she had an IgG2 deficiency; levels are pending.

Three. This one I didn't know: Pregnancy, which is an issue in this patient. Pregnant women have an increased risk for many infections, including *S. pneumoniae*. The rate of pneumococcal bacteremia is markedly higher among pregnant women, homeless persons, and those in prison. So if you go to jail, do not get pregnant. And have a place to live, although I suppose jail could be considered home.

Fortunately I rarely have to see infected pregnant patients. Although pregnancy is a weird immunosuppressive state, in the U.S. odd infections are not a common issue.

Rationalization

Shariatzadeh, M.R., et al., Bacteremic pneumococcal pneumonia: a prospective study in Edmonton and neighboring municipalities. Medicine (Baltimore), 2005. 84(3): p. 147-61

Postscript

Immunoglobulin levels were normal.

Staring me in the face Part 1

THE patient had been in and out of the hospital three times this month with fevers, intermittent confusion, up and down renal dysfunction, pancytopenia, platelets down to a tenth of normal (30K) and a rash that looked possibly like a drug rash. The last time she presented, it looked as if she might have a necrotizing fasciitis in the leg, but incision and drainage showed only hematoma, probably from her coumadin.

Because she was a transplant patient on cyclosporin and prednisone, I kept looking for an infection and could not find one.

Exam, review of systems, cultures, x-rays, and bone marrow biopsies were all negative, and tests for every opportunistic infection I could think of were negative. Yet the patient was sick and getting sicker.

Medicine is hard. Really hard. Patients get sick and the diagnosis can be frustratingly, aggravatingly elusive. Sometimes I wake up in the middle of the night with a diagnosis, sometimes a diagnosis comes as I am driving home, but where they come from I do not know.

Today I had what I will call, for a lack of better term, my Aha moment. After failing miserably for weeks to get a diagnosis, today it bubbled up from some unknown place, all the information falling into place like a perfect Tetris game. I was looking at all the labs and exams and I said...

When I came up with the diagnosis everyone said at the same time, "Of course that's what it is. It couldn't be anything else."

What did I say?

I'll let you know on the next page....

Care to take a swing at it?

Staring me in the face Part Deux

BINGO. She had a case of bingo.

TTP from cyclosporin. Took a month to figure it out. TTP is short for thrombotic thrombocytopenic purpura.

When evaluating a patient, especially a complicated patient, you start from what is sometimes called the hinge point.

The hinge point is the symptom or lab finding or clinical feature that you think is the most important. In the case of this patient, it was the fact she was a liver transplantrecipient-—that is, an immunocompromised patient—with a fever. She never really developed the purpura that would have served as the hinge point of developing a diagnosis of TTP. I thought maybe the lack of purpura was due to the coumadin the patient was on for a prior pulmonary embolism, but hematology assured me I am wrong. How dare they.

When patients do not have the key finding that makes one think of a disease, the diagnosis can be delayed.

What is really annoying is how day after day I would look at all the data and see no pattern, no diagnosis. It is frustrating to have a sick patient, know there is something evil going on, and not be able to put your finger on it. Then, once I though of TTP, that is all I could see in the same information. It is like staring at an optical illusion for days and not seeing the pattern and then, once the skull is seen instead of the lady at the mirror, all you can see is the skull. ARRRGGGHHHHHHH.

TTP is unusual. The CDC says there are only 1200 cases a year, and this would be the second case I have seen in 25 years, so I suppose I should cut myself some slack. But once you see the diagnosis, with the 20-20 vision of hindsight, it seems so obvious. It was staring me in the face.

Leaks

Figuring out what the patient has is often easy in I.D. Something grows from a fluid that should not have bacteria in it. In this case, it was *S. pneumoniae* in both the blood and the spinal fluid of a 25 year old. Easy enough: bacteremia with meningitis.

The hard part is why. "Why? Why, why, why, why, why? Luck! Blind, stupid, simple, doo-dah, clueless luck!" (that is a quote from a Batman movie. Tommy Lee Jones as Two-Face) Usually the patient has bad luck, but that is not a very satisfying answer to the question.

There are well known risk factors for developing *S. pneumoniae* bacteremia in the adult, the big two being HIV and something wrong with immunoglobulins. In my world the latter usually means a hematologic cancer like multiple myeloma or Waldenstrom's macroglobulinemia, an indolent form of B-cell lymphoma. Anytime I have a patient with *S. pneumoniae* in the blood, especially someone who shouldn't (i.e. a non smoker/drinker) I check for HIV and do a serum protein electrophoresis for globulins. More often than not I hit paydirt.

However, in this case neither of these risk factors were probably going to be the reason, as the patient was too young.

One of the curiosities of meningitis is that if there is a leak of cerebrospinal fluid (CSF) somewhere, the etiology of any meningitis that develops is usually *S. pneumoniae*. This meningitis also tends to recur, always with the same organism. One would think that if your spinal fluid was leaking into your nose or throat that your would get meningitis from the common organisms of that part of the body, but the answer to the question "What is the cause of recurrent *S. pneumoniae* bacterial meningitis?" is "CSF leak." Remember that. Not that I have any inside information, but it could be a bored question.

Finding CSF leaks is both hard and easy. Easy as the patient often has a sweet (yes, people taste their snot), clear, chronic runny nose from one nostril and a history of head trauma.

Years ago, trying to dodge a sprinkler one evening, I ducked right into the back of a metal chair and split my head open. Ever since I have had a chronic left-sided nasal drainage. Or have I? Am I just paranoid doctor? Can you see me through my iSight camera? You can, can't you? Spies everywhere, out to get me... Thank you, I will take my Thorazine now.

Hard in that the leak can be tiny, and finding and fixing it is technically difficult. One patient, when he was told that to fix his leak they had to pop off his skull, lift his brain, and stuff the hole with something to block the leak (the neurosurgeon didn't use quite these words) the patient said no way, they are not doing that to him, and he has now had 7 cases of bacterial meningitis (He now works as a president of GM). And that is not the record. The problem is each episode leaves him a little more brain damaged and less able to make a rational decision; it's hard to change your mind when it has been damaged.

The case in question had a history of head trauma of the worst kind: a gunshot wound to the head a decade ago. It looked like the buckshot may have eroded though the bone, leaving a tunnel from the infected sinus to the brain. A good reason to develop meningitis, and a hard one to fix. She should be seeing a surgeon soon, but in the meantime I made sure she got both of the *S. pneumoniae* vaccines, as that is her best bet for prevention of recurrence.

Rationalization

Paudyal, B.P., Twelve episodes of meningitis in the same patient!
Kathmandu Univ Med J (KUMJ), 2007. 5(2): p. 243-6.

....

Red lips, bloody nose, septic knee

THAT's today's patient. He had a long history of a bloody
nose for the 7 decades of his life and he had red dots at the
vermilion border of his lips. And spiders. Not the arachnid, Mr.
Parker.

And now he had a knee with rubor, dolor, calor, tumor. The
knee was tapped and found to be filled with pus, and the fluid
grew methicillin sensitive *S. aureus*.

It is odd when I read an article in a journal and see a case
shortly thereafter. I suppose if I never read, I would never see
anything new. The reading causes new cases to appear; I am convinced of the cause and effect.

Patient has Osler-Weber-Rendu syndrome, now called Os-
ler-Rendu-Weber, I do not know why they changed the name order since I was a medical student. And the *Clinical Infectious Diseases* article calls it Rendu-Osler, poor Weber is aced out. Osler
better watch his back. OWR is congenital form of arteriovenous
malformations (AVMs), and wouldn't you know it, patients with
the syndrome get infections: brain abscesses and infected joints.

*"Thirty two patients experienced 45 extracerebral severe infec-
tions. Extracerebral infections accounted for 45 (67%) of all 67
severe infections. They included septicemia (9 infections [13.4%]),
arthritis and osteomyelitis (6 [8.9%]), skin infection (abscesses
and erysipelas; 6 [8.9%]), muscular abscesses (5 [7.4%]), spondyl-
odiskitis (4 [6.3%]), hepatic abscesses (5 [7.4%]), and other severe
infections (endocarditis, pneumoniae, pyelonephritis, tuberculosis,
rickettsiose, and acute appendicitis with peritonitis; 10 [15%]).
S. aureus was identified in 14 cases , 1 case of septicemia was
due to Enterococcus faecalis and Pseudomonas aeruginosa (after
a urinary infection), and 2 cases of muscular abscesses were due*

to Streptococcus species and Pseudomonas aeruginosa (in one case) and to Streptococcus viridans and anaerobes (in the other)."

The presumed pathogenesis is that noses often get colonized with staph, and in OWR the prolonged nosebleeds allow staph to gain access to the bloodstream and then spread elsewhere. Brain abscesses occur because pulmonary AVMs allow bacteria to bypass the 'filter' of the lungs and lodge in the brain.

The joints? Got me. There are evidently articular involvements with OWR, but I can't find details on the interwebs and the PubMed references have no abstracts.

What is amazing is how often and how long these patients can bleed from their noses: days and months.

Man, this is one group that wants to keep the index finger as far from the nose as possible.

Rationalization

Dupuis-Girod, S., et al., Hemorrhagic hereditary telangiectasia (Rendu-Osler disease) and infectious diseases: an underestimated association. Clin Infect Dis, 2007. 44(6): p. 841-5.

....

Rash Decisions

THE call was to see a non-Hodgkin's Lymphoma patient on the second round of chemo.

While neutropenic, he developed numerous red nodules all over his body while he was recovering from his neutropenia. As always, they had him on granulocyte colony-stimulating factor (G-CSF) to help his white blood cells return.

The worry when a neutropenic has "red bump disease," as I like to call it, is that it could be a manifestation of a disseminated infection—especially a mold of some sort. So, although he was afebrile, he had two of the lesions on the leg biopsied.

All of the lesions faded except the two on his legs at the biopsy site, which developed painful ulcers with necrotic edges and surrounding redness and edema. His WBC shot to six times normal—60K—presumably from the G-CSF. He did not develop a fever and looked otherwise OK.

The biopsy was negative for mold and showed vasculitis/panniculitis.

I think the patient has *pyoderma gangrenosum*. Dermatology always has such gross names.

It looked like pyoderma (do a Google image search if you want to get an idea what they look like), but the patient did not have a reason for the disease, or so I thought. The "usual" underlying conditions for this uncommon disease include ulcerative colitis, Crohn's disease, rheumatoid arthritis, and myelocytic leukemia.

The interesting thing about pyoderma is that if you operate on it or biopsy it, the lesion gets worse with increased pain and ulceration, and that is what happened to that patient.

PubMed (the consultant's secret weapon) to the rescue, as always.

There are a smattering of cases of pyoderma associated with lymphoma. Here is the cool part: it is associated with the long acting G-CSF, Neulasta, which he was on.

There are a whopping two other reported cases. So here is a third case to languish in obscurity.

Rationalization

Miall, F.M., et al., Pyoderma gangrenosum complicating pegylated granulocyte colony-stimulating factor in Hodgkin lymphoma. Br J Haematol, 2006. 132(1): p. 115-6.

White, L.E., et al., Pyoderma gangrenosum related to a new granulocyte colony-stimulating factor. Skinmed, 2006. 5(2): p. 96-8.

....

True True Related

Laboratory results on a Whipple's patient came back today. Whipple's disease is a rare infection caused by *Tropheryma whippelii*, an actinomycete, a distant relative of *Mycobacterium avium*. Although it's usually thought of as a gastrointestinal illness, it is a systemic infection that is fatal if not treated, and which can affect every organ, including the brain. Most often the symptoms are weight loss, diarrhea, and joint pain.

The patient today had no measurable vitamin D. Interesting. Whipple's is associated with malabsorption, but the patient had no weight loss or other symptoms associated with malabsorption.

Makes one (me being that one) wonder about cause and effect. Malabsorption from Whipple's could lead to a decrease in the vitamin D levels-—or perhaps the low vitamin D helped to put him at risk for the disease. Otherwise, how he might have picked up this rare infection (less than one in a million per year) is a mystery. Whipple's is associated with the human leukocyte anti-gen B27 (HLA-B27) haplotype and the HLA alleles DRB1*13 and DQB1*06 but I tested him and he didn't have any of these genetic factors

Vitamin D deficiency increases the risk for a variety of infections, so perhaps it causes susceptibility to Whipple's as well. PubMed suggests no one else has ever looked.

The other issue is where does the Whipple's bacillus come from? It is environmental, but if you think your job has its downsides, consider this study.

"Whipple's disease is a systemic disorder in which a gram-positive rod-shaped bacterium is constantly present in infected tissues. After numerous unsuccessful attempts to culture this bacterium, it was eventually characterized by 16S rRNA gene analysis to be a member of the actinomycetes. The name Tropheryma whippelii was proposed. Until now, the bacterium has only been found in infected human tissues, but there is no evidence for human-to-human transmission. Here we report the detection of DNA specific for the Whipple's disease bacterium in 25 of 38 wastewater samples from five different sewage treatment plants in the area of Heidelberg, Germany. These findings provide the first evidence that T. whippelii occurs in the environment, within a polymicrobial community. This is in accordance with the phylogenetic relationship of this bacterium as well as with known epidemiological aspects of Whipple's disease. Our data argue for an environmental source for infection with the Whipple's disease bacterium."

And you think your job is bad.

Rationalization

Maiwald, M., et al., Environmental occurrence of the Whipple's disease bacterium (Tropheryma whippelii). Appl Environ Microbiol, 1998. 64(2): p. 760-2.

....

Fever on the fifth day

THE following is opinion with no references. So take it with a grain of salt substitute.

Today's patient had a big abscess that was percutaneously drained, and a few hours later he spiked a fever. So he got more antibiotics piled on. Eh. Not that he needed them. Antibiotics are NOT antipyretics. Remember, give Tylenol for a fever, give antibiotics to kill bacteria. Not the same thing.

Abscesses are not amenable to cure without draining. In the abscess the organisms are not growing, and when they are not growing they cannot be killed. Almost all of our antibiotics kill organisms as they divide. Kind of mean, really—who wants to be killed during reproduction? (BTW: I am currently reading Mary Roach's *Bonk*, hilarious, which is what brought the prior thought to mind).

When you drain an abscess, the organisms start dividing, and when they divide, you kill them.

When bacteria die, they dump endotoxin into the blood, which leads to an inflammatory response and, vwa-la, people have a fever.

The febrile response is what you should expect shortly after draining any abscess.

Speaking, or writing, of fever, what about what I call the 5-day fever? Not a fever that lasts for five days, but the fever that is seen on about day five of hospitalization.

People come in with a fever/infection and get better, then about the fifth hospital day they have a single fever.

Back in the old days, in the pre-antibiotic era, people would have a "crisis," a high fever and clinical worsening, during pneumococcal pneumonia and either live or die. The crisis marked the onset of the IgM response, needed for efficient killing of encapsulated organisms. The crisis would occur about day 10 of illness.

Here is what I wonder about: most of these fevers occur around day 10 of the infection, often day 5 or so of hospitalization. I think this fever marks the onset of the IgM response to whatever is ailing the patient; hence the fever.

If someone wants to do the study to prove this, feel free. Just mention me in the acknowledgements as the genius behind the study.

Hey. Look at my cool case

I LOVE noon report. The residents often present cool non-I.D. cases (yes, surprisingly there are cool cases that are not infectious in nature. Whoda thunk it?).

Today they had a case of a young man with a huge stomach, inflated with gas. The patient had what's called intestinal malrotation, where the intestines don't rotate themselves properly during fetal development. The large intestine is located to the left of the abdomen, and its origin (the cecum) and the appendix float freely in the upper abdomen instead of being attached to the lower abdominal wall. As with this patient, people can live and develop normally with this condition, but complications can occur. Abnormal tissue called "Ladd's bands" can attach the cecum to the duodenum and create a blockage. The intestine can also twist on its own blood supply, cutting off its circulation; this is called volvulus. This unfortunate soul had a complete volvulus of the entire small intestine. The CT scan, when scrolled though, looked just like the gut was being sucked down a whirlpool—hence the "whirlpool sign."

It reminds me there needs to be a journal entitled *Hey, Look at My Cool Case.*

Recently I had a youngish (now that I'm 52, what used to be elderly is now youngish) guy who had a day of intractable vomiting, probably food poisoning.

At the end of the vomit marathon he reached up to wipe the sweat from his forehead, only to find pus draining from his scalp.

25 years ago he had seizure surgery (say THAT five times as fast as you can, worse than toy boat) and he had a chunk of plastic in place of his skull. The pus was draining from the most anterior part of the plastic.

He had had no trauma, and CT showed infection over the plastic, confirmed at surgery when it was debrided and the flap removed.

There are the occasional *Staphylococcus* or *P. acnes* infections that can fester for years. But this particular plastic head flap didn't grow those organisms.

It grew *Streptococcus pneumoniae,* of all things.

I thought maybe the bacteria had leaked in from the frontal sinus, bursting through with the increased pressure from the vomiting, but CT and neurosurgery all attested to the integrity of his sinus. I so wanted this to be a Potts puffy tumor (chronic frontal sinusitis) because I like to pop my p's, but that was a dead-end diagnosis. He also had no immune defect that I could find.

So he received a course of antibiotics for a flap infection.

*Streptococcus pneumonia*e is a distinctly odd species to cause cellulitis in adults—it can cause periorbital cellulitis in kids—and has never been reported to cause a flap infection.

So. Hey. Look at my cool case.

May be that could have been the name of the book.

Rationalization

Garcia-Lechuz, J.M., et al., Streptococcus pneumoniae skin and soft tissue infections: characterization of causative strains and clinical illness. Eur J Clin Microbiol Infect Dis, 2007. 26(4): p. 247-53.

Parada, J.P. and J.N. Maslow, Clinical syndromes associated with adult pneumococcal cellulitis. Scand J Infect Dis, 2000. 32(2): p. 133-6.

Old OI's Return

<sarcasm>

I.D. is a depressing field.

They keep figuring out ways to decrease infections. Best practice bundles have almost wiped out hospital-acquired infections at all my institutions. Colony stimulating factors have made prolonged neutropenia and its resultant infections almost a thing of the past. Thanks to HAART, HIV related opportunistic infections have become rarities. I am tempted to stand at a street corner with a sign that says "Will do I.D. for food" or "Why Lie? I want to treat an infection."

Thank goodness for the likes of Jenny McCarthy. At least the pediatric I.D. docs will get to see some of the almost extinct vaccine-preventable illnesses. Sadly, I will not benefit much from a plague of measles or pertussis. Most of my patients are already immune.

</sarcasm>

Ahh, but thank goodness for Rituxan and its ilk. It just takes the edge off of immune competence and results in patients with the immunological function of a moderate AIDS patient. Rituxan is an antibody that kills off CD20 cells that predominate in NHL (non-Hodgkins lymphoma, nothing can target the National Hockey League). If you combine the immunosuppression of lymphoma with the immunosuppression of Rituxan, you get the <sarcasm> Infectious Disease Recovery Act </sarcasm>.

The patient today had NHL treated with Rituxan and came in with seizures. Her brain filled with too numerous to count (not really, if I took my time I could probably count the hundreds of small white matter lesions scattered through out the MRI) something-or-others.

What are they? The two impressive features were 1) the lack of mental status changes, b) the lack of mass effect on the MRI and iii) the mostly normal lumbar puncture, with just a titch of elevation in the protein. And my inability to count.

It is probably PML (progressive multifocal leukoencephalopathy), brought on by the JC virus. The JC virus, or John Cunningham virus (named after Richie's Uncle, who discovered it in the Fonz; it was why he jumped the shark) will reactivate in patients who receive Rituxan for rheumatologic diseases, or occasionally in NHL, to cause PML. The JC virus directly kills the oligodendrocytes—the cells in the brain and spinal cord that make the myelin that insulates your nerves, the cells that make you. So your brain melts, and you go with it. It is a horrible disease. I was glad to see it go.

I used to see PML all the time in AIDS patients, but I have not seen a case this century. The treatment is to reverse the immunosuppression, and since she is done with her chemotherapy, I hope she will get better with time.

And remember, if you or someone you know received Rituxan treatment and suffered serious side effects, you need to consult our dedicated and experienced defective-drug attorneys immediately. You could be entitled to compensation for your pain and suffering, but if you hesitate, the statute of limitations in your state could end your case before it has a chance to begin. Let us help you get the justice you deserve. I wish that was <sarcasm></sarcasm>.

Rationalization

Yokoyama, H., et al., Progressive multifocal leukoencephalopathy in a patient with B-cell lymphoma during rituximab-containing chemotherapy: case report and review of the literature. Int J Hematol, 2008. 88(4): p. 443-7.

....

Time flies like an arrow, fruit flies like a banana

I WAS searching for information on PubMed this morning and let out a big sigh. It occurred to me that the first time I searched for this topic was 27 years ago as a fourth-year medical student on my infectious disease rotation, when I had to talk about warfarin and endocarditis. Did not have no ECHO back in my day. We had to diagnose endocarditis with history and physical. And we didn't have those highfalutin' third generation cephalosporins neither. Men were real men, doctors were real doctors and small furry creatures from alpha centauri were REAL small furry creatures from alpha centauri. But where does the time go?

I had a patient over the weekend who presented with acute back pain after lifting her walker and was admitted for intractable pain. MRI showed maybe an epidural abscess, maybe a discitis, but not that impressive. She was on immunosuppressive therapy for newly diagnosed myasthenia gravis, an autoimmune disorder that causes muscle weakness by blocking receptors at the neuro-muscular junction. I was less than thrilled by the exam (no spinal tenderness) and the MRI failed to convince me that she had an infection.

But we got blood cultures.

And wouldn't you know? All the cultures were positive 24 hours apart for an enterococcus. My motto: frequently in error, never in doubt. Proven wrong again by the cultures.

The *sine qua non* of endocarditis is sustained bacteremia, so ECHO or no, she will need to be treated for endocarditis. It turned out she was also on anti-coagulants (warfarin) for history of pulmonary embolism. Since vegetations are mostly clot, I keep wondering if prior use of warfarin will lead to false negative ECHOs, since patients on warfarin can't form clot. No one has done that study yet. There's a paper for a budding cardiologist. That's how cardiologists reproduce. Budding.

Interestingly, while warfarin makes endocarditis worse (the vegetations shower emboli), prior use of anitplatelet agents improves outcomes.

"There was a trend for lower mortality among patients started on antiplatelet drugs after admission (AOR 0.29, 95% CI 0.08-1.13). The effect of aspirin on mortality was much the same in patients who received 325 or 80 mg daily. Chronic antiplatelet therapy was not associated with a significantly lower risk of major embolism"

Here is a pearl: aminoglycosides block transmission at the

neuromuscular junction, so I may make her myasthenia worse with the gentamicin.

Yes, some of us still use gentamicin. But I have given up on theophylline. I am making progress.

Rationalization

Anavekar, N.S., et al., Impact of prior antiplatelet therapy on risk of embolism in infective endocarditis. Clin Infect Dis, 2007. 44(9): p. 1180-6.

Liu, C. and F. Hu, Investigation on the mechanism of exacerbation of myasthenia gravis by aminoglycoside antibiotics in mouse model. J Huazhong Univ Sci Technolog Med Sci, 2005. 25(3): p. 294-6.

Pepin, J., et al., Chronic antiplatelet therapy and mortality among patients with infective endocarditis. Clin Microbiol Infect, 2009. 15(2): p. 193-9.

Sine qua non part deux

SINE qua non, Latin for 'that without which it could not be'.

Sustained bacteremia is the *sine qua non* of endocarditis, or to be picky, an endovasular infection. As a rule, only infections in the vascular tree (endocarditis, infected aneurysms, septic thrombophlebitis, etc.) give positive blood cultures day after day.

So in the right patient, no matter what the studies—like some crappy negative transthoracic echocardiogram (TTE)—if the blood cultures are positive day after day, it has to be an endovascular infection. By the way, ever let a negative TTE exclude endocarditis. TTEs are usually only useful if positive for endocarditis.

The patient is admitted with 6 weeks of fevers, chills, night sweats, failure to thrive, malaise, and a prosthetic valve. He was seen in the ER and blood cultures were positive, so he was called back in and the repeat blood cultures were positive again.

Prosthetic valve endocarditis is not that unusual, occurring in about 0.8% of patients per year, at least those with a prosthetic valve. It is more unusual to get a prosthetic valve infection in a patient without a prosthetic valve.

But the blood grew a gram negative rod. Maybe. After several days the lab could not identify it, so they sent it on.

It was *Aeromonas*. No, wait, maybe a *Neisseria* of some sort, but still not fer sure. But at least I have sensitivities on the organism. I may not know what it is, but at least I can try to kill it.

Where did the *Neisseria* come from? *Neisseria* are normal oral flora. He had had some dental work several months before and took the usual prophylactic antibiotic, not like it really works. The clinical data to support antibiotic prophylaxis is nonexistent at best, but I would do it, as prophylactic antibiotics are the standard of care.

There are a whopping 7 cases of *Neisseria* reported as a cause of prosthetic valve endocarditis, several of which were cured with medical therapy. There was one case of *N. meningitidis* and one of *N. gonorrhoeae*, proving yet again you must be careful to whom you give your heart.

The patient began improving on a third generation cephlosporin and an aminoglycoside, so I am cautiously optimistic. But I am not optimistically cautious. That's a one-way street.

Rationalization

Oliver, R., et al., Antibiotics for the prophylaxis of bacterial endocarditis in dentistry. Cochrane Database Syst Rev, 2008(4): p. CD003813

Infections Destroys All

HALF a lifetime of taking care of infectious diseases and I am still impressed with what acute infections can do.

Allegedly normal young male, had fevers and was seen in the ER and gots a course of antibiotics without a diagnosis. You know he was going to get worse. He did. Fevers, stiff neck, altered mental status, he comes back to the ER.

WBC 25,000 in the blood, about five times normal. White blood cells in his cerebral spinal fluid, as well, with a count of 900 where there shouldn't be any. He had a purpuric rash on his soles and conjunctivae.

Meningococcus? He was admitted to the ICU as meningitis and given lots o' antibiotics.

Next day he had a new loud diastolic murmur and all his blood cultures had gram positive cocci in clusters.

ECHO showed a bicuspid aortic valve with a large vegetation and a 1.5 cm abscess in the heart. TEE shows the abscess extending up into the aorta.

All in just two days. Abscesses in the heart are bad, usually incurable with antibiotics and one of the few locations where I cannot get interventional radiology to stick a needle. Something about trying to hit a moving target—if you ask me they are just a bunch of wimps.

He had a surgical repair and survived. The operative report described extensive abscess in the heart and and aorta; the aorta had to be reconstructed. I am SO glad I am not a surgeon. It is all methicillin resistant *Staphylococcus aureus*.

Talking with the patient pre-op, I learned that he had had a festering splinter on his finger for a week (how much time before?). It is not the first time I have seen catastrophic endocarditis in a patient with unsuspected bicuspid aortic valve. Bicuspid valves do not tolerate the stress of infection well at all, with abscess formation and rapid valve decompensation common. This is a common cardiac malformation—about 1-2% of the population has a biscuspid rather than tricuspid aortic valve—but is associated with a variety of complications.

10% or so of ascending aortic dissections have underlying bicuspid valve, and the abnormality is associated with cystic medial necrosis of the aorta. Which may be why bicuspid aortic valve endocarditis seems to form abscesses with endocarditis with such frequency.

Rationalization

Braverman, A.C., et al., The bicuspid aortic valve. Curr Probl Cardiol, 2005. 30(9): p. 470-522.

ALL IN YOUR HEAD: MENTAL ILLNESS MEETS ID

Gross. A true story

My children love stories about work, especially gross stories, and the grosser the better.

The schedule said my next patient had parasites. Always a bad sign if you practice in Portland, Oregon. The great Pacific Northwest is parasite-free and, unless the patient had been traveling abroad lately, the patient was likely to be crazy, or, at a minimum, uninformed. There are other diagnoses on the schedule that give one pause: Lyme, fatigue, and chronic *Candida*. You know in advance that the chance of a good doctor-patient interaction is slim.

As I walked into the room, the smell of garlic was overpowering. Sitting there was a slightly disheveled elderly man who continually ate raw garlic cloves while we talked, one after another, as if they were jelly beans. At least that is how I eat jelly beans. In the small, overly warm exam room the smell was intense. I like garlic. When I cook, I always triple the amount of garlic; one of my favorite recipes is chicken with 40 cloves of garlic. I though there could never be too much garlic. Wrong.

Talking with the patient revealed that parasites floated in the air and would land on his skin, burrow in, then travel through his body and finally come out his nose. Yes, his nose. You may guess where this is going.

I asked how he knew they were parasites, and he said he pulled them out of his nose. It was the garlic that kept the parasites at bay, forcing them to escape out his nose.

I asked, hesitantly, if he had a sample of the parasite, and he produced a large brown jar that rattled when he shook it. He unscrewed the lid and dumped about two cups of dried boogers onto the exam table.

To my credit I neither screamed nor puked. I explained to him that he did not have parasites and why. He did not believe me and left with his jar of dried parasites.

I can eat garlic now, and enjoy it, but for a long while the smell of garlic made my stomach churn.

The patient had delusions of parasitosis, not an uncommon problem for infectious disease doctors. Most doctors, when confronted with these patients, do not have enough background in parasitology to recognize that these "parasites" have a life cycle that makes no sense. When examined under the microscope, the parasites always look like clothing threads or non-specific organic detritus. So they send them to me, both the patients and the pseudo-parasites. The treatment is antipsychotics, which I have never had a patient agree to take—it's even more challenging to get them to see a psychiatrist. There is no doubt the disease causes suffering, but getting the patient treated is problematic.

The current popular incarnation of this syndrome is Morgellons disease, first named in 2002. It manifests as skin rashes with crawling sensations and intense itching, with the belief that parasites or fibers emerge from the sores. Although clusters of the "disease" have been reported in a few Southwestern states, it is simply a manifestation of an *idée fixe,* one that sure looks like delusions of parasitosis to these bifocaled eyes.

Occasionally it is not a delusional state that brings a patient in with a parasite, but someone who is misinterpreting the data. I had a patient who thought he had passed a worm, but it was just an earthworm that had fallen out of his pants and into the toilet; he had been working in the garden and was much relieved to know that he was not infected with worms. At least not earthworms.

Is Insanity Infectious?

EVERY couple of years I get a consult as to whether or not the etiology of someone's insanity is infectious or not.

It is a previously healthy person who, with no personal or family psychiatric history, has a psychotic break, either becoming schizophrenic or manic. The patient does not respond as expected to medications or has an atypical presentation, and a spinal tap is abnormal, suggesting a meningitis of some sort, so the docs call me.

Is insanity infectious? Maybe. Stupidity sure is. Insanity is multifactorial in etiology, like heart disease, so it is hard to tease out infection as a cause. There has been a suggestion for years that some mental illness is due to infections. Part of the problem with neurology is that practitioners do not have good access to the diseased organ. When in doubt you can always biopsy a liver or a lung or a bone marrow. In neurology, the cranium tends to get in the way and removing even small bits of brain is not a good idea. It is a popular myth that people only use 10% of their brains (sometimes it seems less), but I would hate for the neurosurgeon to inadvertently remove third grade.

Anecdotally, I have seen a few infections present as new-onset insanity. One guy was admitted naked and catatonic. Screening chest X-ray showed large potato-shaped lymph nodes in the chest, then he had an abnormal spinal tap l and was found to have neuro-sarcoidosis. His psychosis melted away with steroids.

Neurosyphilis, rare, can also show up as mental illness. In my practice it has been primarily in elderly widows whose husbands brought more home from the war than medals and memorabilia.

Cat Scratch Disease (*Bartonella henselae*) can present as an agitated psychosis followed by coma for a few days. One case I had awoke from his three-day coma, went home after a ten-day uninsured hospitalization, and killed his girlfriend's cats. I wonder if they are still together.

Other diseases are problematic: Toxoplasma can cause behavioral changes in mice, making them less fearful of cats so they are eaten and the parasite can complete its life cycle in the cat. Can it cause mental illness in normal people? Maybe.

Perinatal infections are linked with the development of schizophrenia, especially if the infection occurs in the first trimester. But which virus—CMV? Influenza? Something as yet undiscovered? Many viruses have been associated with schizophrenia. And is there a genetic predisposition? Probably.

Maybe it's a post-infectious disease. Post-streptococcal diseases include chorea, a movement disorder, and there has been some data to suggest strep infections can lead to OCD as well.

There is also epidemiologic data to suggest that schizophrenia is associated with the Borna virus, which is associated with a range of neurologic symptoms in a variety of animals. And it leads to "Borna again" puns in the literature which are now too numerous to count.

Dr. David Gilbert has said for years that the etiology of all diseases is either genetic, wear and tear, or infectious, and I am strongly drawn to this idea.

My consult this week? Acute psychosis in a young woman and a spinal tap/brain MRI that could be infectious. Evaluation so far is negative for infection, which always makes the case harder. It is nice to find an infection you can treat, but the sad truth is that the brain doesn't do all that well with even minor trauma. The thought that a loved one's insanity could be an infection gives the often false hope the person will get better. Most of them don't. I hate that.

Rationalization

Melinda Wenner, Infected with Insanity: Could Microbes Cause Mental Illness? Scientific American, April/May 2008. http://www.scientificamerican.com/article/infected-with-insanity/

Crazy MRSA: A Biochemical Curiosity

THE voices in my head are different than most people's. Mine tell me how wonderful I am, and who am I to disagree? The antipsychotics were never of much help; they made my lips smack too much.

Maybe I will need to get back on my thioridazine (Mellaril), an old school antipsychotic, as the drug—at least in a test tube—has a curious effect on *S. aureus* methicillin resistance: it reverses methicillin resistance.

Methicillin was the first anti-staphylococcal beta-lactam and not surprisingly, the first anti-staphylococcal antibiotic to which *S. aureus* became resistant. Use it and lose it. But that is why it is called MRSA, and not ORSA or NRSA, the other anti-staphylococcal penicillins being oxacillin and nafcillin.

Thioridazine decreases the production of the resistance-mediating PBP-2a (see "Incurable") by decreasing the transcription of the mecA gene.

> *"Transcription of mecA was reduced with increasing concentrations of thioridazine in the presence of a fixed amount of oxacillin. Furthermore, the protein level of PBP2a was reduced when bacteria were treated with the combination of oxacillin and thioridazine."*

Thioridazine decreases mRNA levels of the beta-lactamase gene. Whether this is useful is not known, but the effect does occur at drug levels that are relevant for anti-psychotics. It just might be worth suppressing the voices, which tell me such good things, to treat an MRSA.

Rationalization

Klitgaard, J.K., et al., Reversal of methicillin resistance in Staphylococcus aureus by thioridazine. J Antimicrob Chemother, 2008. 62(6): p. 1215-21.

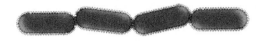

QUACKS

Virus R Me

I'M sick today. One would think that I wouldn't get ill, given my job. My eldest had a cold, and now he has passed it on to me. Sore throat, whopping headache, no legs when I try to bound up the steps. At least I do not have a stuffy nose and can still taste my food. I would bet on an enteroviral infection, and imagine if I had a spinal tap, it would be slightly positive.

I am unlikely to ever get a spinal tap as I am DNR (do not resuscitate), DNI (intubate), DNF (Foley), DNRT (rectal tube), and DNST (spinal tap).

It is the enteroviral season. I just hope I am not going to be the index case for West Nile here in Portland. As of 9/12/08 we still haven't had the epidemic that has been four years in coming.

The worst of the illness is the foggy brain, the neurons firing like they are immersed in molasses. Slow on the uptake, words hard to find, can't understand what is going on around me. I need the same brain surgery as Charlie Gordon, otherwise I will be writing the platform at the Republican National Convention.

The worst is, there is not a damn thing to do about it but suffer. There are treatments for colds, but they are usually worse than the disease. And I know that while NSAIDS can take away the headache, the inflammatory response I am having is important. Most studies that have looked at the treatment of fevers and acute viral infections have demonstrated that treating the fever makes the illness last longer, and the last thing I want is this illness to bleed into the weekend.

So I suffer in silence, unless you no not consider this story silence.

So, rather than be original, in honor of my viral infection I will republish an essay I used to have on the Quackcast (http://edgy-doc.com) site so it can continue to live:

Deconstructing Airborne: How to recognize medical nonsense.

Medicine is complicated. It is estimated that it takes a decade of training before anyone can truly be expert in a field. You probably do not have ten years to spend getting to know the ins and outs of medicine. How, then, to recognize when a medical therapy is legitimate, questionable, or total garbage?

There are some rules of thumb (although I think they would be rules of thumbs, since I count on the thumbs) that are reliable indicators that the medical intervention you are being asked to spend your hard-earned money on is worthless. Airborne is a popular 'cold remedy' that by some accounts sells 100 million dollars a year of product. Using Airborne as an example, let's go through these rules of thumb (1).

Rule 1. The therapy pitches the claim directly to the media.

Given the glut of direct-to-consumer advertising by "legitimate" pharmaceutical companies, this may be a wee bit difficult to use as a criterion. I will also mention in passing that I am one of those zealots who think that big Pharma reps and their advertising represent the biggest impediment to good medical practice currently going, and that the medical literature is replete with good evidence of the pernicious evil that occurs when physicians interact with drug reps. Good doctors practice good medicine, but to have good doctors practice bad medicine requires an expensive dinner at a steakhouse with a cute rep. I have not taken so much as a pen in twenty years, so my opinions are pure as Oregon rain.

With prescription pharmaceuticals, you can quickly discover if the indication is backed by legitimate scientific studies: look it up in the Physicians' Desk Reference (the PDR). Every drug indication in the PDR has been studied and approved by the FDA.

Not so with the directly marketed products. Thanks to Congress, herbal supplements and vitamins are under NO requirement to have proven safety and efficacy data against any disease or condition. None. As long as they have the disclaimer (The Quack Miranda) to the effect that "These statements have not been evaluated by the Food and Drug Administration. This product is not intended to diagnose, treat, cure, or prevent any disease." These words are taken from the Airborne box (2) where they are in teeny tiny letters that I can't see unless I take off my bifocals and squint.

Read the box and the advertising. If they have the above words or something similar, it's garbage. By law they can say anything they want as long as they include this disclaimer. It's no different from a shaving commercial that suggests the use of the particular razor will get you a partially clad supermodel rubbing you cheek with the back of her hand. You know that is not true. I mean, you do, don't you? These products are no different. If it looks too good to be true, then it probably is.

Real, effective medications are backed by randomized, placebo-controlled clinical studies published in peer reviewed medical journals and the results are in the PDR.

Rule 2. The discoverer says that a powerful establishment is trying to suppress his or her work.

While the makers of Airborne do not make this claim, at the monthly secret meeting of the Medicine Subcommittee of the Tri-Lateral commission, we work hard to suppress the information that the ingredients in Airborne are effective. Just do a Google search on the ingredients of Airborne. It is safe to say we are failing miserably.

It is often said that big Pharma suppresses data on the effectiveness of herbal preparations and will not do the studies because when clinical trials prove the efficacy of these supplements, people will use the cheap supplements instead of expensive pharmaceuticals. Unfortunately, many of these supplement companies are owned by big Pharma, so they win either way, and, at $7 for 8 tablets, I am not so certain that Airborne is all that inexpensive.

Rule 3. The scientific effect involved is always at the very limit of detection.

Evidence to support Airborne? I quote from the website:

"Each ingredient in the Airborne formula has been repeatedly documented in published studies to contribute to a strong, healthy immune system."

This is true in the same way I am related to the Queen of England. I am. But it will take a whole lot of death before the crown devolves on to my head.

Only by the world's largest stretch of the imagination can it be said the ingredients in Airborne have been repeatedly documented in published studies to contribute to a strong, healthy immune system. Try it yourself. Enter the ingredients of Airborne into PubMed and search the medical literature. Be impressed with what you do not find.

"Additionally, we conducted a study in 2003 that showed Airborne had a marked effect on reducing the duration of symptoms. Our Medical Advisory Board members are currently formulating a study that in addition to the studies in the literature, will further support Airborne's immune boosting properties."

I assume the last sentence was not meant for humorous effect, but I laugh out loud every time I read it. Which is it? Does it boost immune function? Or does it reduce duration of symptoms? Ain't the same thing.

The key words are "contribute to a strong, healthy immune system." What does that mean? Zip. Zilch. Nil. Nada. Nothing. That is a meaningless assertion. Immune boosting. Healthy immune system.

This whole concept of boosting the immune system baffles me. The immune system not a biceps that you can build up by lifting weights or taking steroids. It's an amazingly complex series of interacting proteins and cells. There is no meaningful way to measure the immune system in a normal person, much less boost it.

Normal people have normal immune systems, and as long as you have a reasonable diet and exercise, there is no way to boost it.

But the statement on the box is so vague and sounds so good and beneficial, it doesn't matter that it cannot be disproved. It could be argued that many severe vitamin deficiencies lead to poor immune function, so, yes, the vitamin and minerals in Airborne are good for the immune system, in the very basic and generic way taking a multivitamin is good for the immune system IF you have a vitamin deficiency. But they are not saying that the Vitamin C is being used to treat scurvy or that they are treating other deficiency states.

It's like oxygen. Breathing strengthens the immune system. Don't breathe for 10 minutes and your immune system will weaken. I am surprised they don't put the oxygen in the bottle as part of the immune boosting ingredients. Given them time.

You cannot find the study the company touts that specifically proves Airborne is effective. According to ABC news, "GNG [the people who did the study to prove Airborne's efficacy] is actually a two-man operation started up just to do the Airborne study. There was no clinic, no scientists and no doctors. The man who ran things said he had lots of clinical trial experience. He added that he had a degree from Indiana University, but the school says he never graduated."

What is in Airborne? Vitamins, herbal extracts, and amino acids that do not do anything to prevent or treat a cold. Echinacea and Vitamin C, the most commonly touted cold remedies, do not work when tested in careful clinical studies.. Sorry. The data is in and Vitamin C and Echinacea do not do diddly.

Looking at the list on the package, only Zinc has been effective in decreasing cold symptoms—and then as a lozenge sucked every two hours, not as an effervescent tablet. Zinc is their gateway drug. As long as these products contain zinc, they can say something to the effect that the active ingredient has been proven in clinical trials to decrease cold symptoms and not be called liars. Most of these cold remedies have zinc in one form or another. At best, it is like taking a very expensive and not very complete multivitamin.

Rule 4. Evidence for a discovery is anecdotal.

I hear it all the time—"I thought I had a cold coming on, I took 'fill in the blank,' and I did not get a cold." Or the flu. I am just glad people don't use this reasoning in choosing contraception. Or, given the population of the planet, maybe they do.

People love anecdotes, especially if they come from someone like, oh, I don't know, Oprah. Remember. The plural of anecdote is anecdotes, not data. Memory is faulty and biased. Just remember the argument you had in the car with your spouse over that abominable behavior at the last party you attended. Who had the correct memory? (Duh. My wife). We remember hits, not misses, we remember events that confirm our bias and ignore the contradictory, and we grossly underestimate the role of chance. Combine this with the emphasis we put on the stories of others, and you can see why anecdotes are worthless for judging efficacy of medical interventions.

I always tell the residents that the three most dangerous words in medicine, especially when applied to treatments, are 'in my experience.' The problem with anecdotes in medicine is they suggest a causality where none exists.

Causality is a difficult thing to prove, although I will confess I have a pair of special shoes. I take care of infections all day. Ever since I bought the pair of shoes I wear to work each day, I do not remember getting an infection. In fact, when I was getting ready for work this morning I thought I was getting a cold, but after I put on my Rockports, my symptoms faded. You would probably dismiss my claim that my shoes prevent infection. Apply that skepticism to all forms of medical claims. My shoes are no different from any other form of questionable medicine: beware of faulty causality.

Humans love anecdotes. A single story for most people is far more impressive that the best clinical trial ever published. Even though "40,000 customers contact (Airborne) every year," that is meaningless to support the claim that Airborne works. What separates humans from other animals is selfdelusion. 40,000 times zero is zero.

Rule 5. The discoverer says a belief is credible because it has endured for centuries.

This is especially true of traditional Chinese medicine. People used it for thousands of years, it must be effective. Never mind that the life expectancy for the Chinese was less than 40 years until, in part, the use of Western medicine at the beginning of the 20th century.

Airborne contains a hodgepodge of Chinese herbs used for the most part for a variety of infectious diseases. Most have never been tested rigorously or, in the case of echinacea, definitively shown to not work.

There is little from 2000 years ago, or 200 years ago, or even 20 years ago that I would use today. I would not wear 2000-year-old clothes, travel in 2000-year-old vehicles, use 2000-year-old heating, grow food with 2000-year-old farming techniques. Why use 2000-year-old medical therapies? Unless, of course, I want to get sick and die. Our ancestors were invariably wrong about a lot of things since they did not use the scientific method to understand the world. And they died young as a result.

But I feel good in knowing that the herb Chinese Videx in Airborne has been used for 2500 years for PMS. That's a cold, all right. Just like PMS.

Rule 6. The discoverer has worked in isolation.

Many forms of quackery were invented out of whole cloth by one goofball (I know, an *ad hominem* attack. If the shoe fits...). Examples include Hanneman and homeopathy or D.D. Palmer and chiropractic. And their systems, like the word of God, are never questioned or altered, despite data that may or may not modify or contradict them.

In the case of Airborne, it was "created by a second grade teacher." A teacher, and a second grade teacher at that. While we don't necessarily support them financially, teachers have a certain cachet in this country, and those that take care of our young children are thought of especially highly. If it had been created by a community college creative writing professor, would you have been as impressed?

Americans do love the idea the lone inventor, toiling away in the basement before becoming rich with the pet rock or MS-DOS.

Certainly when I think of cutting edge health care research, I think do not think of the NIH or big Pharma—I think second grade teacher. Especially since US students are ranked 17th and falling in science when compared to the rest of the world. I suppose that those who have the most exposure to snotty noses are those most expert in avoiding and treating them. Experience in an area does not mean expertise otherwise by the same reasoning I should own a brewery.

Rule 7. The discoverer must propose new laws of nature to explain an observation.

This is common to all of quackery: they all violate what is known about chemistry, physiology, anatomy, and physics. Either 500 years of scientific progress is right OR alternative medicine represents insights into the nature of the universe that surpass all we have learned to date. The alt med proponents are either self-deluded buffoons or future Nobel Prize winners. Guess what I think.

Besides boosting the immune system, here are some words to watch for that guarantee the speaker is a quack: any reference to energy of any kind, whether it be blockage, flowing, vibrating, harmonic, holistic. They all sound good. They all mean squat. Energy is not this vague, shimmery cloud that can be tapped into. Energy is a defined attribute of physical systems: the ability to do work.

Beware of any therapy that maps the entire body on to one area: the iris, the foot, bumps on the head. I saw an ad in the Gadget universe catalog where all of the acupuncture sites are actually located in the hand. Makes it easier to apply therapy, I suppose, but I get worried now whenever I clap.

Natural: Infections are natural. Death is natural. Natural is neither good nor bad. But like organic, it sounds good.

Above all, beware of anyone who suggests the therapeutic effects are due to quantum mechanics, especially if they mention quantum entanglement to explain their nonsense. They are blowing smoke up your Heisenberg. Quantum mechanics is a surefire way to intimidate and overwhelm and is never an answer for systems bigger than an electron. I was a physics major in college and have spent my time with the concepts of quantum mechanics. It doesn't apply to the world you and I see and hear.

So those are the seven ways, with some examples, to recognize quackery and worthless medications. The rules are widely applicable to all kinds of hokum. Apply as needed.

Rationalization

1. Modified from Robert Park, The Seven Warning Signs of Bogus Science, Quackwatch. http://www.quackwatch.com/01QuackeryRelatedTopics/signs.html

2. From the Airborne box.

Infectious Body Art

WHAT marks me as an old geezer is that I do not understand hip-hop. Or visible underwear. Or goatees. Or those hideous rectangular glasses that seem to be *de rigueur*, but make everyone who wears them look dorky without adding style. And body art. I am deep into mid-life, and perhaps I should acquire one of the above as part of my midlife crisis. I'm thinking a bar code on my forehead. I am due.

Of course, given my body, there is no art short of a large bag that could improve my aesthetics, and older guys like me can only look lame with a tattoo or a diamond stud in a body part. But maybe a ponytail...

When I was a resident, tattoos were a sure sign of psychopathology. Only ex-prisoners and sailors had tattoos. And only the lobe of the ear was pierced. Now a days everyone under 30 has a tat and all parts of the body are open to piercing. And they open up people all sorts of unexpected and interesting infections.

Hepatitis from tattoo parlors is old hat and, thankfully, uncommon with good technique. But given the fine coating of bacteria we all have, and the fact that body surfaces cannot be sterilized, just be made very very very clean, seeing the odd bacterial infection from piercing and tattoos is expected.

I have seen two people lose an ear from getting the upper part of the ear pierced. Mark Anthony went on to do body art, I suppose. The lobe is made of fat, but the upper ear is cartilage and if bacteria reach the cartilage with a piercing, they rip through the ear faster than antibiotics can keep up. Both *Staphylococcus*, from the patient's skin, and *Pseudomonas*, from the ice and water sometimes used for anesthetic and cleaning, are the common bacteria. Plastic surgeons can make a new ear for you later using a piece of rib cartilage, but the van Gogh look, even if temporary, is so 19th century.

There are also, not unsurprisingly, local infections and abscesses depending on where the piercing was done. The belly button is the residual of the umbilical cord. In some people there is a residual cyst from the umbilical cord, called a urachal cyst. I had a patient who had a huge belly button abscess as a complication of the ring passing through the unsuspected urachal cyst. The abscess needed to be surgically removed and, in the process, she lost her belly button. It is my understanding she later had one reconstructed, but for a period of time was unable to practice omphaloskepsis.

The most worrisome infection from piercing is endocarditis, which is an infection of the heart valves. Endocarditis is not a trivial disease, 100% fatal if not treated, and it is not unusual for the disease have significant morbidity—including strokes and valve replacement.

Not unsurprisingly body art has a low, but real, chance of leading to endocarditis.

"In all, 22 specific cases of IE spanning 1991–2007 have been reported that were associated with piercing the tongue (seven), ear lobes (six), navel (five), lip (one), nose (one), and nipple (one), and reported in one heavily tattooed person; other general IE cases have also been mentioned. Twelve cases were in females, and one patient died; nine of these individuals had CHD (congenital

heart disease). Twenty-one cases have been published in the 10 years from 1997-2007."

There are probably more case reports out there, as cases tend to be underreported because it is a pain to write them up. I am always amazed at how the little things, the seemingly inconsequential choices we make, can lead to infectious disasters. Yesterday it was a dog in the lap, today a piercing. Dem dare bugs are always waiting to kill us, dontcha know.

One of the cooler blogs is Street Anatomy, where there is a nice collection of tattoos that reflect the underlying anatomy. It would be particularly appropriate if someone with the tattoo of a heart got a heart infection as a consequence. I like that kind of symmetry. Not that I would wish such a disease on anyone. I guess I'll have to come up with an alternative for my mid-life crisis. Perhaps I'll start a blog...

Rationalization

Armstrong, M.L., S. DeBoer, and F. Cetta, Infective endocarditis after body art: a review of the literature and concerns. J Adolesc Health, 2008. 43(3): p. 217-25.

Measles: Where is MY angry mob?

In my world there are facts and practices that are so ingrained, such a major part of the underlying structure of Infectious Disease, that challenging them can only be viewed as jaw-dropping ridiculousness.

If you are a physicist, you take relativity as a given.

Chemists, I suppose, take atomic theory as a given.

In medicine, anatomy is a constant.

In infectious disease, germs cause disease. Duh. To fight the diseases there are two options: antibiotics and the immune system. Of the two, the immune system is far superior, and without a good immune system all the antibiotics in the world will not stop you from dying of infection, as AIDS and cancer chemotherapy have proven with depressing regularity.

The best use of the immune system is to have preexisting immunity-—from, say, a vaccine—so when exposed to an infection, you do not get it.. The efficacy of vaccines is, to an I.D. doctor, beyond question.

They work. Vaccines, along with nutrition and flush toilets, are why we all get to live to our 80s and we do not have to have 9 children in the hope that one or two will survive to adultery.

Take measles, a nasty disease.

In the not-so-good old days there were 400,000 cases a year in the US, with 400 deaths. Even today there are 25 to 30 million children infected each year in the world, and measles kills 345,000.

Vaccine efficacy is 90-95%. I have seen exactly one case of measles in 25 years or so of Infectious Disease, and it was imported into the US (yet another failure of border patrol).

The vaccine is safe, with little in the way of side effects: not autism, allergic reaction in one in a million.

In 2000 measles was declared eliminated in the US. Gone. No more local disease.

Crap.

I make a living from infections and their complications, and the elimination of measles represents yet another vanished income opportunity. You think Fanny Mae has issues, try being an I.D. doc. Damn you, vaccines. Where is MY bailout?

But good news is always around the corner. There is a group of people who think vaccines, cause autism, despite voluminous data to the contrary. And they have a small, but vocal, following. People like me rely on science and reason to make medical decisions—pesky things like facts and data and clinical studies.

Those who support the Infectious Disease Employment Act, i.e. the anti-vaccination folks, have a different way to determine the proper course of medical interventions: the angry mob. Actress Amanda Peet is one of my heroes—she is a spokesperson for Every Child By Two, a vaccine awareness nonprofit, and has called parents who don't vaccinate their children "parasites." As a result she has drawn the ire of Jenny McCarthy, who doesn't make much attempt to conceal her tactics."...[T]here is an angry mob on my side, and I like the fact that I can say she is completely wrong," says the actress and model whose son's autism has made her a rallying point for anti-vaxxers.

We all know the ongoing benefits to society brought about by angry mobs. Ask Dr. Frankenstein. Angry mobs worked well for him.

I am thinking that this might be a workable approach for The National Center for Complementary and Alternative Medicine (NCCAM). After millions spent investigating SCAMs, they have yet to discover a use for these modalities using the scientific method. Perhaps, instead, they should use the 'angry mob' as the way to validate homeopathy, acupuncture etc.

Thanks to religious exemptions and anti-vaccine wackaloons, we have had a small resurgence of measles this year. Not much. Only 131 cases, of which 91% were in kids who were not vaccinated. It is a small beginning. But I am hopeful. If Jenny could just be against flush toilets...

Rationalization

CDC, Update: measles—United States, January-July 2008. MMWR Morb Mortal Wkly Rep, 2008. 57(33): p. 893-6.

UNICEF measles site: http://www.unicef.org/immunization/index_measles.html

Michael Destries, Jenny McCarthy Strikes Back At Amanda Peet On Child Vaccinations, Ecorazzi (September 30, 2008). http://www.ecorazzi.com/2008/09/30/jenny-mccarthy-strikes-back-at-amanda-peet-over-child-vaccinations/

Warning: there was some sarcasm in the above chapter that may go unnoticed by some readers.

Oprah wants your children dead and I am moving

WELL, Oprah really doesn't want your children to die. At least I do not think so. But one wonders. If you spend anytime at all in the antivax world then you are aware of Jenny McCarthy, who believes, despite all the evidence to the contrary, that vaccines are dangerous and cause autism. She has even go so far as stating in her *Time* interview that

"I do believe sadly it's going to take some diseases coming back to realize that we need to change and develop vaccines that are safe. If the vaccine companies are not listening to us, it's their f___ing fault that the diseases are coming back. They're making a product that's s___. If you give us a safe vaccine, we'll use it. It shouldn't be polio versus autism."

It isn't. Holy False Dichotomy, Batman. Vaccines are safe. The diseases they prevent are bad. Real bad. We do not want them back.

Time does not approve of 'uck' or 'hit' but has no problem giving antivax wackaloons space.

But the wise and powerful O. has hired Ms McCarthy for, perhaps, a talk show where she can take her vaccine delusions to an even wider audience. And kids will die. And, in the end, Oprah will need to be added to the Jenny McCarthy body count.

"Everyone look under your seats. Everyone here gets a child dead from pertussis."

When it comes to healthcare, and woo, Oprah is a goof; there is a nice evaluation over at Newsweek. Go to her website and let her know that indirectly killing babies by supporting antivaccine nonsense is a bad idea. Let her know it will make her fat. But let her know.

Rationalization

Jeffrey Kluger, Jenny McCarthy on Autism and Vaccines, Time magazine, Wednesday, April 1, 2009.

Good News in Bleak Times

B EING an I.D. doc is not all roses and champagne. Not that the two go together. Work used to be busier. There used to be nosocomial infections and ventilator associated pneumonias, but thanks to applying infection control procedures at my hospitals, I have ICUs that have gone for over a year without a ventilator associated pneumonia. Damn. My kids are reaching college age.

New medications for transplant patients and recombinant granulocyte colony-stimulating factor have made infections in cancer and transplant patients a relative rarity.

Don't get me started on AIDS. Thanks to HAART and prophylactic antibiotics, we can go for years without seeing an opportunistic infection. I haven't seen a cerebral toxoplasma or cytomegalovirus retinitis this century. Oh, for the bad old days.

I was sliding into a funk about the grim future in infectious diseases when good news arrived out of the United Kingdom.

Measles is increasing. In some areas one in four children have not had a measles-mumps-rubella vaccine, and they are at risk for measles as herd immunity wanes.

Studies estimate that England could see 30,000 to 100,000 measles cases. They will probably only see a tenth that many, but I can dream, can I not? My dreams are not as noble as Dr. King's. The only downside is that the problem is in England and in children. It is a good start, but I need an outbreak in US adults. I need a really bad epidemic of something, anything, infectious. Flu would be good, but it seems to be a relatively benign flu season so far.

The BBC credits the debunked vaccine-autism link, made popular by Dr Wakefield in his now discredited paper, as the reason for the poor vaccination rate.

I hope that the anti-vaccine crew continues their good work in America and we have a plague or two here.

It is said that the anti-vaccine crowd do not want children to get diseases, suffer, and occasionally die from vaccine-related diseases. I am sure that tobacco farmers don't want their end users to get lung cancer, that handgun manufacturers are against children accidentally shooting themselves, and that alcohol producers don't want people to develop cirrhosis. It just happens to be the end result of what they are selling.

The Green our Vaccine folks say they just want safer vaccines. What they will get are measles outbreaks and maybe mumps and rubella as well, with all the concomitant morbidity and mortality these diseases, and others, have to offer. It just happens to be the end result of what they are selling. The only thing that will be green will be the grass on the graves of those who died of preventable infections.

Rationalization

Fergus Walsh, Measles cases surge to new high, BBC News, Friday, November 28, 2008. http://news.bbc.co.uk/2/hi/health/7753210.stm

Hypnagogic Rat Hole

As you may have gathered, I have in interest not only in infectious diseases, but in the area of quackery and also what is generally considered skepticism. I have read about hypnagogia, where there is a waking dream. And I actually had one last night. I usually detest hearing about dreams.

ROMEO

I had a dream last night.

MERCUTIO

So did I.

ROMEO

Well, what was your dream?

MERCUTIO

My dream told me that dreamers often lie.

That sums it up for me. But last night I woke up to see a white, tall, thin glowing person at the foot of the bed looking at me, and I could not move or talk. My first though was, Shit, who is in the room? Then I realized, I am having a hypnagogic dream. Cool. It looked like like an alien or a ghost and it had me paralyzed. Then I really woke up and it went away.

I can really see after last night how someone could think he had seen a space alien if they did not know what hypnogogia was. It sure looked like the real deal, but I had read too may Skeptical Inquirers I suppose, and my rational brain took over far too fast.

No infectious disease pearls today; instead I had to prepare a talk . Back to pus tomorrow, unless it really was an alien and it comes back tonight to get me. I am not sanguine that space aliens sterilize those anal probes between uses. There have been outbreaks associated with colonics:

"Persons who were given colonic irrigation immediately after a person with bloody diarrhea received it were at the highest risk for the development of amebiasis. Tests of the colonic-irrigation machine after routine cleaning showed heavy contamination with fecal coliform bacteria."

—and that would alienate me.

Rationalization

Istre, G.R., et al., An outbreak of amebiasis spread by colonic irrigation at a chiropractic clinic. N Engl J Med, 1982. 307(6): p. 339-42.

....

All the way to the bank

As the cognoscenti are aware, I also pontificate, er, blog, over at Science Based Medicine, where the issue from the anti-vaccine wackaloons are discussed at length. The need to defend vaccines has always stuck me as odd. It is like defending clean water or fresh air.

Of course, I have a variety of vested interests in promoting vaccines.

First, as I have mentioned in the past, is the opportunity to inject the new version (6.66 I believe) of tracking bots that are ATP-powered. Much better and longer-lasting than the old bots, they can pinpoint your location far better than those cell phone tracers.

But more important is all the money we doctors make from vaccines.

The anti-vaccine wackaloons often mention that it is the loads of cash we docs bring in from vaccinating people that keeps the vaccines coming. I was looking over my IRS forms for the last several years to tally up all the money I have made from vaccines and it was, um, carry the zero, add those column up and it's, yeah. Nothing. I didn't make dime one from giving any vaccines last year. I went around the hospital giving flu vaccines, but I made the mistake of doing it for free because I think it is important that people get vaccinated. Silly me. Not only did I not charge exorbitant fees for vaccinating my colleagues, they are not going to get sick and pass the flu to their patients. Crap. I could really make some money from a good flu outbreak, seeing as how I only get paid for seeing sick people.

Of course, it could be argued that I am in the thrall of the evil medical-industrial complex, and I am only serving my masters by promoting vaccines.

Lets tally up all the money I have received from Big Pharma in the last 25 years: again, carry the zero, add the columns from 1985 to present and the sum is, yeah, zero. I don't do drug companies. Never talk to the reps, never take their food or pens or hospitality. I usually refer to them as lying bastards, and for some reason I am not been asked to participate in their speakers' bureau. I wonder why Big Pharma does not advertise on my podcasts or website.

I am an adult I.D. doc (meaning I take care of adults, not that I act like one. You are only young once, but you can be immature all your life, that's my motto). It is the pediatricians who make the bling from vaccines. The excessive vaccine schedule that weakens the immune system and causes all sorts of evil in children exists to make pediatricians wealthy. Heartless bastards. It's the childreeeennnnnnn.

Turns out vaccines are not so lucrative after all.

It costs docs about $1500 dollars to purchase the vaccines. Given reimbursement, sometimes docs can't cover the cost of the vaccine, much less pay to keep the doors open. It costs somewhere around $100 an hour or more to run a medical office.

How much to docs make giving a vaccine?

"The net yield per dose ——calculated as the reimbursement minus price paid ——averaged from $2.90 for the Haemophilus influenzae type b vaccine PedvaxHIB to $24.34 for Pediarix. Across practices, the range of net yields varied from $10 for one vaccine to $90 for another. For the heptavalent pneumococcal conjugate vaccine alone, some practices had a positive net yield of up to almost $39.00 per dose whereas 11% had a negative net yield for the vaccine."

As a result, some practices are not purchasing the more expensive vaccines and others are considering no longer offering vaccination. That's good news for me. Less vaccination may lead to a plague of some sort. Now that will make me some cash.

Rationalization

Berman, S., Is our vaccine system at risk for a future financial "meltdown?". Pediatrics, 2008. 122(6): p. 1372-3.

Freed, G.L., A.E. Cowan, and S.J. Clark, Primary care physician perspectives on reimbursement for childhood immunizations. Pediatrics, 2008. 122(6): p. 1319-24.

Freed, G.L., et al., Variation in provider vaccine purchase prices and payer reimbursement. Pediatrics, 2008. 122(6): p. 1325-31.

....

Water is wet, fire is hot, media is biased

Captain Renault: I'm shocked, shocked to find that gambling is going on in here!

[a croupier hands Renault a pile of money]

Croupier: *Your winnings, sir.*

Captain Renault: *[sotto voce] Oh, thank you very much.*

[aloud]

Captain Renault: *Everybody out at once!*

~ Casablanca

My local newspaper, the Oregonian, usually gets some details wrong on their stories about infectious diseases. One wonders how I can believe the veracity of the rest of the information reported in our fine daily.

The other issue is bias in reporting. It is certainly an issue in clinical trials, as the outcome is in part determined by who pays for the study. If the study is funded completely by a pharmaceutical company, it is much more likely to be favorable to the study drug than if the funding is independent. You have to know who is paying for the study to accurately judge the result.

I am always wary of bias in the medical literature, which is part of the reason why I have had no interactions and have accepted no gifts from pharmaceutical companies during my entire career. Well, not entirely true. A few years ago the Unasyn rep sent me a Fleet enema with his company sticker on it. I still display it proudly on my desk.

Unfortunately, the media is not good at reporting the potential sources of bias in clinical studies.

A recent *JAMA* study looked at 306 news articles from a variety of sources and found:

42% did not mention if there was pharmaceutical company funding;

67% referred to the study drugs by their brand names more than half the time;

most did not have written policies to address these issues.

The problem? Given that the funding source introduces (probably unconscious) bias into any study, you have to discount at least part of the results based on who is paying for it. It is a curiosity that even in studies where the results do not reach statistical significance between two study drugs, the non-significant data almost always look better for the study drug. If the potential source of bias is not reported—and, more importantly, the bias explained—consumers are not given important information to help evaluate a drug and its purported efficacy.

When I evaluate a study and see that the funding is all from one company or that the investigators are drug company whores (I mean speakers), I discount the result by a fudge factor: 10 —20%, with no data to back me up. But it seems about right.

As to brand names versus generic, I am a bit more skeptical as to any adverse effect for consumers, although I do make the housestaff speak only generic. Some patients do think that generic medications are not as good as brand name medication, but that is not true. A drug is a drug is a drug. Brand names are just more expensive. And the price? I realize that bringing drugs to market is very expensive and that they need to make back their R&D and make a nice profit as well. That is the American way. But so often the price of unique drugs appears to be set more on what the market will bear rather than what is reasonable, as if I know what reasonable is. And I need to make some pun about a bear market and just can't do it.

Bias is ubiquitous in medical studies, but fortunately physicians are immune to its effects and easily recognize when they are being manipulated. HAHAHAHAHAHAHAHAHAHAHA-HAHAHA.

God, I am funny.

Rationalization

Hochman, M., et al., News media coverage of medication research: reporting pharmaceutical company funding and use of generic medication names. JAMA, 2008. 300(13): p. 1544-50.

Dead Parrot Sketch

PEOPLE are always stranger than I can possibly imagine. In medicine we get to see doozies, and one of things that makes being a doc fun and interesting is that I get to see all kinds of people, from crazy street people to presidents of banks, but I do not have to go home and have dinner with them.

When you have spent a quarter of a century in medicine, and in particular Infectious Disease, you become comfortable believing that infectious diseases are due to germs. There are lots of different germs, and they cause a variety of diseases. Group A streptococci cause cellulitis, *P. falciparum* causes malaria, and HIV causes AIDS.

HIV has been a particularly interesting one because I have watched it from the beginning. The first cases of HIV were reported in the MMWR in 1981, when I was in my second year of medical school. By the time I was a resident I was seeing cases of young gay men dying of some sort of disease, but what it was and how it killed them was a mystery. Then virologists discovered what was at first called HTLV then HIV. We knew what was killing our patients but we couldn't do squat to prevent it. Then there were some roller-coaster years as new HIV medications were developed that worked for a short period of time, failed, and then the inevitable death.

Over the last 25 years we have gone from a 9 month life expectancy to, in many patients, an almost normal life expectancy due to the application of a remarkable understanding of the physiology of the human immunodeficiency virus and the development of highly active anti-retroviral therapy (HAART). It has been an astounding change.

This week I saw one of my HIV patients who presented in 1999 dying of AIDS with a CD4 T-cell count of 90, *Pneumocystis carinii* pneumonia, and an HIV viral load of 300,000. Now his virus is suppressed, his immune system is normal, and he has a productive, happy life.

It is immensely satisfying to know he has a good chance of

outliving me.

It is why I find the HIV deniers so baffling. Christine Maggiore died last week of untreated AIDS. She was one of the leaders of the HIV deniers and she so believed that HIV did not cause AIDS that she evidently let her daughter acquire and die of AIDS.

It is sad and odd. The information that supports HIV/AIDS is enormous, with almost 194,000 references on HIV in PubMed as of today. When I read the web sites of those who deny HIV as the cause of AIDS, it is like reading papers from bizarro world, with a twisted alternative understanding of what I would call the real world. The willful disregard of reality is mind boggling, akin to denying gravity or the inability to breathe under water, then behaving accordingly. And dying. I am reminded of a Monty Python bit, where one of the characters refuses to recognize reality, be it the Black Knight (it's only a flesh wound) or a pet shop owner. More of Monty Python meets the Twilight Zone, really, given the outcome.

You unlock this door with the key of imagination. Beyond it is another dimension —a dimension of sound, a dimension of sight, a dimension of mind. You're moving into a land of both shadow and substance, of things and ideas. You've just crossed over into the Twilight Zone. Submitted for your consideration, a parrot dies of AIDS.

Dead Parrot Sketch

The cast:

MR. PRALINE

John Cleese

HIV Denier

Michael Palin

The sketch:

A customer enters a pet shop.

Mr. Praline: 'Ello, I wish to register a complaint.

(The owner does not respond).

Mr. Praline: 'Ello, Miss?

HIV Denier: What do you mean "miss"?

Mr. Praline: I'm sorry, I have a cold. I wish to make a complaint!

HIV Denier: We're closin' for lunch.

Mr. Praline: Never mind that, my lad. I wish to complain about this parrot what I purchased not half an hour ago from this very boutique.

HIV Denier: Oh yes, the, uh, the Norwegian Blue...What's, uh... What's wrong with it?

Mr. Praline: I'll tell you what's wrong with it, my lad. 'E's dead from HIV, that's what's wrong with it!

HIV Denier: No, no, 'e's uh,...he's resting.

Mr. Praline: Look, matey, I know a dead parrot when I see one, and I'm looking at one right now.

HIV Denier: No no he's not dead, he's, he's restin'! Remarkable bird, the Norwegian Blue, idn'it, ay? Beautiful plumage!

Mr. Praline: The plumage don't enter into it. It's stone dead from HIV.

HIV Denier: Nononono, no, no! 'E's resting!

Mr. Praline: All right then, if he's restin', I'll wake him up! (shouting at the cage) 'Ello, Mister Polly Parrot! I've got a lovely fresh cuttle fish for you if you show...

(HIV Denier hits the cage)

HIV Denier: There, he moved!

Mr. Praline: No, he didn't, that was you hitting the cage!

HIV Denier: I never!!

Mr. Praline: Yes, you did!

HIV Denier: I never, never did anything...

Mr. Praline: (yelling and hitting the cage repeatedly) 'ELLO POLLY!!!!! Testing! Testing! Testing! Testing! This is your nine o'clock alarm call!

(Takes parrot out of the cage and thumps its head on the counter. Throws it up in the air and watches it plummet to the floor).

Mr. Praline: Now that's what I call a dead parrot.

HIV Denier: No, no.....No, 'e's stunned!

Mr. Praline: STUNNED?!?

HIV Denier: Yeah! You stunned him, just as he was wakin' up! Norwegian Blues stun easily, major.

Mr. Praline: Um...now look...now look, mate, I've definitely 'ad enough of this. That parrot is definitely deceased, and when I purchased it not 'alf an hour ago, you assured me that its total lack of movement was due to it bein' tired and shagged out following a prolonged squawk. Turns out e 'as AIDS.

HIV Denier: Well, he's...he's, ah...probably pining for the fjords.

Mr. Praline: PININ' for the FJORDS?!?!?!? What kind of talk is that?, look, why did he fall flat on his back the moment I got 'im home?

HIV Denier: The Norwegian Blue prefers keepin' on its back! Remarkable bird, id'nit, squire? Lovely plumage!

Mr. Praline: Look, I took the liberty of examining that parrot when I got it home, and I discovered the only reason that it had been sitting on its perch in the first place was that it had been NAILED there.

(pause)

HIV Denier: Well, o'course it was nailed there! If I hadn't nailed that bird down, it would have nuzzled up to those bars, bent 'em apart with its beak, and VOOM! Feeweeweewee!

Mr. Praline: "VOOM"?!? Mate, this bird wouldn't "voom" if you put four million volts through it! 'E's bleedin' demised!

HIV Denier: No no! 'E's pining!

Mr. Praline: 'E's not pinin'! 'E's got AIDS E's passed on! This parrot is no more! He has ceased to be! 'E's expired and gone to meet 'is maker! 'E's a stiff! Bereft of life, 'e rests in peace! If you hadn't nailed 'im to the perch 'e'd be pushing up the daisies! 'Is metabolic processes are now 'istory! 'E's off the twig! 'E's kicked the bucket, 'e's shuffled off 'is mortal coil, run down the curtain and joined the bleedin' choir invisibile!! THIS IS AN EX—HIV INFECTED PARROT!!

(pause)

HIV Denier: Well, I'd better replace it, then. (he takes a quick peek behind the counter) Sorry squire, I've had a look 'round the back of the shop, and uh, we're right out of parrots.

Mr. Praline: I see. I see, I get the picture.

HIV Denier: I got a slug.

(pause)

Mr. Praline: Pray, does it talk?

HIV Denier: Nnnnot really.

Mr. Praline: WELL IT'S HARDLY A BLOODY REPLACE-

MENT, IS IT?!!???!!?

HIV Denier: N–no, I guess not. (gets ashamed, looks at his feet)

Mr. Praline: Well.

(pause)

HIV Denier: (quietly) D'you.... d'you want to come back to my place?

Mr. Praline: (looks around) Yeah, all right, sure.

And I bet they didn't use a condom.

....

Second to none

HEALTH care in the US is second to none. Probably because we are 29th.

"Among 33 industrialized nations, the United States is tied with Hungary, Malta, Poland and Slovakia with a death rate of nearly 5 per 1,000 babies, according to a new report. Latvia's rate is 6 per 1,000."

USA. USA. USA.

It's not just infant mortality. A fifth of US citizens do not have health care insurance, and if you do not have insurance you should avoid the opportunity to get sick. The nice thing about the US health care 'system' is that I get to take care all sorts of illnesses that people in advanced societies, those who actually work together to help each other, do not get an opportunity to see.

Untreated hypertension, untreated diabetes, untreated syphilis, progressive HIV, advanced tuberculosis.

Because some people do not have health care insurance and live from paycheck to paycheck, they let their health slide, sometimes ending up with advanced disease, sometimes dying. People die every now and then because they can't afford heath care, often of infections. I sometimes want to put on the death certificate for cause of death: uninsured and too proud to seek care.

I don't have to travel back in time or go to third world countries to see diseases that should be of purely historical interest in an advanced society.

Like today. Patient with an infected hip fracture who is insane and who did not seek health care.

In the olden times, when there were no antibiotics or surgery, patients with bone infections developed large masses of scar tissue around the infected fracture, which subsequently calcified. A mass of calcium two or three times the size of the normal bone would end up surrounding the fracture. That is what my patient had: a huge, calcified callus over the fracture. It is rare to see this response in the 21st century since we can treat infections and fractures. At least if you have sanity and money. If you lack one or both, you get the rare opportunity to develop findings that were common in the 19th century.

Serologies

D IAGNOSING infectious diseases with serology is sketchy. Infections will lead to an antibody response and, by measuring the type of antibody and the increase in the titer of antibodies and what bacterial structures have caused an antibody response, you may be able to identify an infection with something you cannot grow.

The problem is that serologies are unreliable.

Patients may make antibody that you cannot measure.

Patients may not make antibody to the infection.

Patients may have a positive test, but it is cross-reacting to another organism, resulting in a false positive test. HIV is screened with an ELISA test, which has a high false positive rate because there are similar viruses (viri? Plural like Elvis?) that are not pathogenic but which cause a similar reaction on a blood test. You have to confirm the HIV diagnosis with a Western blot (there is a Southern blot, but back in the day when I did these blots in the lab, there were no Eastern or Northern blots. Things have changed; all the points of the compass current have a blot. But I am but mad when I blot north-north-west: when the blot is southerly I know a hawk from a handsaw), which is less sensitive but more specific.

If you live in an area where a disease does not exist—like Lyme in Portland, Oregon—then a positive Lyme test is more likely to be a false positive than a true positive. You have to interpret the test in the context of the patient's symptoms. Making a diagnosis based on serologies alone is stupid.

Then there is the issue of labs that, because of a loophole in the rules, can run home grown tests that have not been approved by the FDA or validated. These labs are are self-fulfilling prophecies, specializing in worthless tests, and naturopaths and their ilk send multiple serologies for diseases for which patients have no risk or reason to have. And the tests almost always come back positive, but that is probably confirmation bias, as the patients then come to me only when the tests are positive. I lost confidence in one lab when they sent me a picture of *Babesia* with a big arrow pointing to a platelet clump.

Lyme is particularly problematic. I saw a patient today who has no good exposure history for Lyme and a symptom complex that is not consistent with Lyme, but the Lyme serology was sent by the naturopath, to —I am too chicken to mention it, as the US has 30% of the world's lawyers-—Labs and it was positive. As it always is.

I remember that one of these labshad a test for Lyme that was positive in everyone tested, and they concluded that everyone had Lyme, not that the test was worthless. I cannot find the reference.

I have two rules of thumb (rule of thumbs?).

2) Use serologies to confirm what you think the diagnosis is based on the history.

1) If the serology doesn't support the clinical diagnosis, it is probably the serology that is wrong.

Live Blood

Most of my consults come from other doctors: the patient has an odd infection and the doc wants my involvement.

It is less common to get see a patient in consultation at the patient's request. Usually these are "hand holding" consults where the primary doctor has it under control, but the patient wants expert confirmation from a second opinion.

Doctor: "I'm afraid you are crazy."

Patient: "I want a second opinion."

Doctor: "OK. You are ugly, too."

The outpatient today was billed as a bloodstream infection. So I immediately start thinking as I walked to the room: Staph? Strep? Endocarditis? Something exotic and travel-related? Most patients with bloodstream infections are ill and in the hospital; bacteremia is not a subtle clinical problem. The list of the patient's medications contained no antibiotics, so it appears that if he does have an infection he either has not yet been treated, which would be odd, or he has finished treatment.

In the room is a healthy-appearing young human with a thick sheath of papers that do not look like standard lab reports.

After routine introductions, I ask my standard, "What can I do for you?"

"I have a bloodstream infection."

He doesn't look ill to me. "What kind? How was it diagnosed?"

"Well, I was having problems and since I don't have insurance, I went to a naturopath who ran a bunch of tests. One of them was live blood analysis. They take a drop of blood and put it under a microscope, and they can see your immune system attacking infections in your bloodstream. He showed them to me. He wanted to give me a colon detox treatment, but I thought I would see a real doctor first."

Damn.

He had a copy of the photograph of his live blood analysis. I asked him to point out the infections. He couldn't. Neither could I.

A review of his symptoms and a few physical exam findings later revealed no infectious diseases, but a moderate case of asthma and some allergies to account for his symptoms.

I rarely get a referral from quacks, er, naturopaths and chiropractors. I wonder why. After I told the patient that live blood analysis is total crap (the word I used) I do not think I will see patients from that ND again. ND is short for 'Not a Doctor'.

"Live blood analysis" is one of those forms of quackery where real and imaginary medicine overlap. There are a smattering of diseases, non-infectious and infectious, that can be diagnosed on a blood smear: leukemia, some forms of anemia. For infections to be seen, you usually have to use stains specific to certain organisms, such as malaria or leptospirosis. The vast majority of infections do no show up in a smear of unstained blood.

Why is that? It's a simple matter of concentration. If you can see one organism per high power field on a light microscope you have 100,000 bacteria per milliliter. In infected persons that degree of bacteria in the blood leads to what we call "rapid death." Standard culture methods can detect on the order of 1 organism/mL, which is a typical concentration seen in most types of bacteremia. In streptococcal endocarditis, for example, blood concentrations are usually 1-30 bacteria/mL. With Gram negative septicemia in children, counts can be as high as 1000/mL—but even then, well below the sensitivity of a smear.

There is also the issue that bacteria are very small, only about a micrometer in diameter, and it takes some skill to be able to distinguish them from artifacts. I perused some sample web sites of live blood analysis practitioners and they were a remarkable trip into nonsense and incompetence. They were identifying the usual dirt and debris that appear on slides as pathogens.

My favorite is

"Fibrous Thallus. Indicates a nationalization of garbage, like bacteria, yeast/fungus, mould, and their acid wastes and acid crystals lying in a dormant/inactive state. The diet is too high in protein, carbohydrate (sugar), and junk food, experimentation with recreational drugs and/or use of prescription drugs."

It reminded me of the ancients who would sacrifice an animal and examine its entrails for auguries of the future. Live blood analysis is a high-tech equivalent.

Total crap.

The patient also had a collection of his labs in a bound notebook from his DC/NP with an explanation of each lab. For his CO_2, which was normal, there was the comment "Normal. Keep breathing healthy." As if he had a choice.

He paid hundreds of dollars for nonsense and didn't even get his asthma diagnosed correctly.

At least he avoided the detox colonic.

Rationalization

Quackwatch: http://www.quackwatch.com/01QuackeryRelatedTopics/Tests/livecell.html

....

Overlap

I WEAR multiple hats, mostly to cover the bald spot on my head. As I am sure you know, besides being an I.D. doc and babbling away in these essays, I have an interest in medical woo—or Supplements, and Complementary and Alternative Medicine (SCAMs).

Although I ask my patients if they see a quack, er, I mean alternative (alternative to what, effective therapy?) providers, it is rare that my patients see anything beyond a chiropractor for low back pain.

Occasionally they see a naturopath, and their care is limited to herbs. I thought I had heard it all until my patient with chronic sinusitis told me her naturopath told her to wear wet socks to bed. As the socks dry, the evaporating moisture draws the fluid out of the sinusitis and out the feet. She thought it sounded hinky, and did not do it.

I lost my composure and burst out laughing. I could not believe this was the real deal. It is. From the Swanz Naturopathy web site:

"Wet Socks —a must have hydrotherapy treatment"

This sounds much more difficult to implement than it actually is. Most people worry about sleep quality, but then report that their sleep actually improves with the wet socks. It is an old folk remedy, tested and true. It is great for colds, sinus infections, sore throats, ear infections, coughs, and much more. I have personally used it to support healing in the legs after a sprained ankle. I know first hand how effective the treatment can be for infections and when sick, I am often discouraged that I did not put the wet socks on a day earlier and potentially avoid the later symptoms of the infection. It is great for kids. Surprisingly, they typically don't complain about having cold wet socks put on their feet.

Supplies:

1 pair white cotton socks

1 pair thick wool socks —as close to 100% wool as you have

Directions:

1. Wet cotton socks and soak them completely with cold water. Be sure to wring the socks out thoroughly so they do not drip. If you desire, place wet socks in the freezer for 3 to 5 minutes (do not freeze if using this treatment on children).

2. While cotton socks are chilling, warm your feet. This is very important to increase the efficacy of the treatment. Warming can be accomplished by soaking your feet in warm water for at least 5-10 minutes, massaging the feet vigorously, using a heating pad, etc.

3. Dry the feet off completely.

4. Place cold wet socks on feet. Cover with thick wool socks. Go directly to bed. Avoid getting chilled.

5. Keep the socks on overnight. The cotton socks should be dry in the morning.

This treatment works by forcing an increase in circulation down through the legs at night to dry the socks from the inside. The increased circulation supports drainage in the sinuses and throat at night while you sleep. Typically during the night our circulation throughout the body is very stagnant. Wet socks changes that normal dynamic. It works. Try it sooner than later."

The author of this won an award for naturopathic excellence. Really.

Another site suggests it as a cold remedy and concludes "The next morning your cold will be gone. Congratulations! If you feel sniffles by the end of the day, perform the procedure each night until you feel relief."

Well, duh. Treat a self-limited disease every day and eventually it will get better.

Bastyr (Not how I would spell it) University says

"The body reacts to the cold socks by increasing blood circulation, which also stimulates the immune system. You have to rev up the immune system, so it's ready for battle against the affliction or condition.

This treatment acts to reflexively increase the circulation and decrease congestion in the upper respiratory passages, head and throat. It also has a sedating action, and many patients report that they sleep much better during the treatment. The treatment is also effective for pain relief and increases the healing response during acute infections. The wet sock treatment is used in conjunction with other modalities to treat inflammation, infection or soreness of the throat, headaches, migraines, nasal congestion, upper respiratory infections, coughs, bronchitis and sinus infections."

This is an institution of 'higher' learnin'. Is it any wonder I have no respect for their teachings?

Some humor writes itself. You just can't make this stuff up. And in Oregon they have prescriptive privileges.

Rationalization

http://swanznaturopathy.blogspot.ca/

http://www.bastyrcenter.org/content/view/197

SYMPTOMS AND SIGNS: DIAGNOSTIC HINTS

780.6

You can tell what doctors do for a living by the ICD-9 codes they have memorized.

780.6. Fever. My personal favorite.

There is a code for everything. Weightlessness is 994.9 (this is a repeat; could replace). Decapitation (by guillotine): E978. There, I suppose, in case Marat returns from the dead. Ready for a zombie French revolution? 666 is postpartum hemorrhage. Draw your own conclusions. A code for everything except my most common diagnosis: I don't know.

I don't know is my most frequent conclusion. For every great diagnosis I make, I have 100 shoulder shrugs. It is the least satisfactory answer for the patient and not billable. At least I always have 780.6 to fall back on.

Today was yet another shrug of the shoulders (I do it with Gallic exaggeration). Elderly female with fevers, chills, sweats. No focal symptoms on exam, on labs, on review of systems, or on x-rays.

Pan cultures (including cultures of the wine flagon and goat hooves) all negative.

Probably viral, but the look from patient and daughter when I said 'Probably viral' was one of 'Can you get me a real doctor who knows what they are doing?'

Part of the problem is that fevers in the elderly are often the only manifestation of serious underlying medical problems.

I remember back when I was an intern I had an elderly woman admitted to me in the middle of the night with just a fever. I thought, in the immortal words of Betty Davis, what a dump. As I wheeled her to her room (at the county hospital we did transportation at night if we wanted the patients expedited to their rooms) she dropped her pressure and almost coded. She grew Enterococcus in her blood that next day. That's when I learned that fever in the elderly can be significant.

However, I can't find a reason for the fever in the current patient, so I am betting that it is a self-limited nothing. I have a routine with patients under these circumstances: I tell them that in medicine we are good at diagnosing serious, life-threatening or -injuring illnesses that we can treat, but are no good at putting a name on the self-limited, ultimately trivial illnesses that are not life threatening or injuring, just life inconveniencing. So, I reassure them, it is good that we do not have an answer.

Most of the time patients understand and appreciate that explanation.

This time the daughter looked at me like I was too stupid for words.

Oh well. As long as the patient gets better.

Rationalization

Gur, H., et al., Unexplained fever in the ED: analysis of 139 patients. Am J Emerg Med, 2003. 21(3): p. 230-5.

Marco, C.A., et al., Fever in geriatric emergency patients: clinical features associated with serious illness. Ann Emerg Med, 1995. 26(1): p. 18-24.

Postscript

She got better.

....

Calor?

A Winner, The Open Laboratory, 2008.

M Y normal temperature is 97, so 98.6 is a fever for me."
I hear a version of this phrase at least once a week. But is it true? What is normal body temperature?

98.6. A Boy Band? Average IQ of the Bush administration? The marking on a mercury thermometer? You remember mercury thermometers? No? Back in the day we had thermometers that used mercury and had a red mark at 98.6, and if your temperature went above the red mark, you got to stay home from school. We loved to crack thermometers open and play with the mercury, which may explain why I have a passing resemblance to the Mad Hatter.

Let's go back in time.

In 1868 Carl Reinhold August Wunderlich published "Das Verhalten der Eigenwärme in Krankenheiten" (The Course of Temperature in Diseases). Wunderlich gave "37 °C (98.6 °F) special significance with respect to normal body temperature," based on a million observations in about 25,000 people. He found a mean of 98.6 °F without an electronic calculator to aid in the calculation. Only those living in the Victorian age were devoted enough to spend that kind of time calculating the average of a million numbers. Wunderlich gave 38 °C (100.4 °F) as the upper limit of the normal range, so a temperature greater than 100.4 was the first quantitative definition of a fever.

Tests conducted with one of Wunderlich's thermometers demonstrated they were mis-calibrated by as much as 1.4 to 2.2 °C (2.6 to 4.0 °F) higher than today's instruments. Therefore 98.6 is based on data collected with inaccurate thermometers.

So what is normal temperature?

A study in 1992 measured 700 oral temperatures in 148 healthy men and women between the ages of 18 and 40, using modern thermometers. There was a range of temperatures from 35.6 °C (96.0 °F) to 38.2 °C (100.8 °F):

—a mean of 36.8 ± 0.4 °C (98.2 ± 0.7 °F).

—a median of 36.8 °C (98.2 °F).

—a mode of 36.7 °C (98.0 °F).

Mean, median, mode. Does that take you back? I had to look them up to help my son with his math homework. But it is 98.2, not 98.6, that is the average temperature.

The mean temperature varies during the day: lowest at 6 a.m. (about a degree below the mean) and highest at 4 to 6 p.m (about a degree above the mean). Like a stopped clock being right twice a day, people are 98.6 twice a day: once on the way up and once on the way down.

The important exception is ovulating females, who are above the mean, or warm, in the early morning. People use this fact, called the rhythm method, as a form of birth control. The medical term for these people is "parents."

Women had a slightly higher (women are hotter than men?) average oral temperature than men (men are cooler than women?): 36.9 °C (98.4 °F) versus 36.7 °C (98.1 °F). Black subjects had a slightly higher mean temperature but slightly lower diurnal oscillations compared with white subjects: (36.8 °C (98.2 °F) versus 36.7 °C (98.1 °F) and 0.51 °C (0.93 °F) versus 0.61 °C (1.09 °F), respectively. These differences approached, but did not quite reach, statistical significance. Oral temperature recordings of smokers did not differ significantly from those of nonsmokers.

So what's a fever? Depends on the time of day.

"Fever is most appropriately defined as an early-morning temperature of 37.2 °C (99.0 °F) or greater OR a temperature of 37.8 °C (100 °F) or greater at any time during the day."

The other way to judge a fever is to have my wife hold her hand against your forehead. At least where the children are concerned, she says it is more reliable than the thermometer.

This is of practical importance since I see a couple of patients a year with the diagnosis of fever of unknown origin who, it turns out, took their temperature at 4 in the afternoon. By golly, it was 99.9, as it was on each subsequent day. Normal temperature is 98.6. They have a fever. Patients can get thousands of dollars wasted on the work-up of their nonexistent fever.

"Normal temperature is 98.6" is a medical myth.

Rationalization

Mackowiak, P.A., S.S. Wasserman, and M.M. Levine, A critical appraisal of 98.6 degrees F, the upper limit of the normal body temperature, and other legacies of Carl Reinhold August Wunderlich. JAMA, 1992. 268(12): p. 1578-80.

....

Drug Fever

All the glitters is not gold

All who wander are not lost

All who are febrile are not infected.

—ancient Elvis saying.

FEVER, fever, fever. 780.6.

Why does the patient have a fever?

This week, one of the patients had a fever due to drugs. She came in infected, the infection resolved, the white count decreased, she felt better and, after a period of time, the fever returned. Routine work-up was negative so they called me.

I didn't find any infection to account for either, so I looked at the drug list. Could it be drug fever? Vancomycin and Zosyn were the only drugs to worry about.

When do you worry about drug fever? First of all, what is drug fever? A patient has a fever and is on a drug. Hence the name. There are other hints. Continuous fever, where it temperature does not fall to normal, is an inconsistent finding. Eosinophilia is another. It can be any drug, any time, first dose or the hundredth.

You have to play the odds: antibiotics are common causes, and vancomycin—which, due to MRSA, I have had to use by the bucketful—seems a very common cause, as are beta-lactams and sulfa. Of the unimportant (i.e. non-antibiotics)drugs, H2 blockers and anti-seizure drugs lead the list.

In the end you have to stop the drug and see if the fever goes away, usually in about four half-lives of the drug. The only way to prove it is drug fever is to re-challenge which, since it is not an allergic reaction, you can do safely. This is rarely needed; the few times I've seen a re-challenge occur is when there is a change of housestaff and they inadvertently restart the medication. Oops.

For the patient in this anecdote, her fever curve drifted down over 48 hours after I stopped the antibiotics. Probably the vancomycin. He shoots. He scores. No fever for 48 hours—then, just to piss me off, she has a fever. Just one, which doesn't recur. It was a mustache on the Mona Lisa of my diagnosis.

Rationalization

Johnson, D.H. and B.A. Cunha, Drug fever. Infect Dis Clin North Am, 1996. 10(1): p. 85-91.

Potato, Potatoe

THERE is an ongoing 'discussion' in my family of what is better: rice or potatoes. I am a rice fan, my wife prefers potatoes. Mashed, fried, boiled or baked, she likes her hot potatoes.

And that brings us to the clinical sign of the "hot potato voice."

What is it about old-time doctors and their urge to describe everything after one food or another? Makes eating less enjoyable.

Today's patient had fever, a bad sore throat, and was toxic-appearing with a marked left shift—meaning that there were immature neutrophils in the blood smear, a sign of infection or leukemia. There was also a soft, deeper than usual, whispery voice, the "hot potato voice," so called because it sounds like the patients are talking with a hot potato in their mouths. This is a sign of peritonsillar abscess or cellulitis.

And sure enough, the CT scan showed two early tonsillar abscesses and peritonsillar inflammation. Though the magic of antibiotics, the patient is getting better.

However. Let's see a show of hands: everyone who has listened to someone talk with a mouth full of hot potato. I thought so. Nobody.

Is the peculiar way of talking with a peritonsillar abscess really like talking with a hot potato in your mouth? There is no question in medicine that is not worth a study. Dr M.F. Bhutta compared the speech of people with tonsillitis to those with a hot potato in their mouths, and the sounds were different:

The study, "Hot Potato Voice in Peritonsillitis: A Misnomer," appeared in the *Journal of Voice*.

"Voice changes are a well-recognised symptom in patients suffering from peritonsillitis," it says. "The voice is said to be thick and muffled, and is described as a 'hot potato voice,' because it is believed to resemble the voice of someone with a hot potato in [their] mouth. There have been few studies analyzing ... the voice changes in tonsillitis or peritonsillitis and none that have compared these changes with those that occur with a hot potato in the oral cavity."

To remedy this lack of knowledge, the three doctors recruited two sets of volunteers. The first group comprised 10 hospital patients whose suffering related to their tonsils. Each volunteer pronounced three particular vowel sounds, which the doctors recorded and subsequently analyzed using special software.

The second group were 10 healthy hospital staffers, "with each of these participants placing a British new potato of approximately 50 grams in their oral cavity, warmed by microwave to a 'hot,' but not uncomfortable, temperature."

The doctors detected unmistakable differences. The unique sound of someone burdened with an actual potato, they explain, "is related to interference with the anterior tongue function from the physical presence of the potato."

There are obvious flaws in the study. The potato should have been an Idaho baker, not an English new potato. Wrong thermodynamics. Part of the reason people with tonsillitis talk that way is to decrease the pain they have when talking. The potato should have been HOT, not hot. It should hurt.

They need to repeat the study, or use hot pizza instead.

Baboon butts and hot potatoes, this book has it all.

Rationalization

Marc Abrahams, Why voice change study is a hot potato, The Guardian, Tuesday, 13 January 2009.

Bhutta, M.F., G.A. Worley, and M.L. Harries, "Hot potato voice" in peritonsillitis: a misnomer. J Voice, 2006. 20(4): p. 616-22.

....

The Secret

SOMETIMES you suspect the diagnosis as soon as you walk in the room.

The patient was billed as chronic cough with an elevated white count. Why?

He was thin and tanned, the latter odd for Oregon at this time of the year. What was striking was his clubbed fingers. The most impressive I have seen in years.

I took the history: a slight non-productive cough, 10-pound weight loss, his long bones have been aching for a couple of months. Two pack a day smoker for years.

Labs showed an elevated white count—14,000 to 16, 000, about three times what's expected—but otherwise normal. His chest x-ray was OK.

His exam was negative except for the clubbing and muscle wasting. He said his fingers had always been that way. There is such thing as congenital clubbing, but no way is this is congenital, although I hoped so. I went looking for the cancer that should have been there.

The CT scan showed a 4-centimeter mass—some sort of cancer—in his mediastinum, right behind his heart where it could not be seen on chest x-ray. The clubbing was the hint.

"Of patients with idiopathic pulmonary fibrosis, 65% have clinical digital clubbing. In these patients, an increased occurrence has been shown in patients with higher grades of smooth muscle proliferation in the lungs.

Clubbing has been reported in 29% of patients with lung cancer and is observed more commonly in patients with non-small cell lung carcinoma (35%) than in patients with small cell lung carcinoma (4%). Digital clubbing was reported in 38% of patients with Crohn disease, 15% of patients with ulcerative colitis, and 8% of patients with proctitis. Clubbing was observed in up to one third of Ugandan patients with pulmonary tuberculosis.)"

The long-bone pain is probably pulmonary osteopathy, an unusual cause of bone pain resulting from inflammation of the long bones due to underlying severe pulmonary disease. All his symptoms were from his cancer, which will be biopsied later in the week.

The reason I recognized this case is that I compulsively go to noon report, where the residents present interesting cases as unknowns and the Chief of Medicine, Dr. Jones, discusses the cases with input from the house staff.

Not five days earlier they had presented a similar case and Dr. Jones finished by saying, "Some people say it is a waste of time teaching these rare physical findings, but you never know when one will walk into clinic."

And sure enough, there was a case in the office less than a week later. Weird. Or can you say confirmation bias? Sure, I thought you could.

I am disinclined towards the supernatural, but it is spooky how often you hear about a good case or read about something new, and you see a similar case a week or two later. I always wonder how many similar cases I have missed over the years because I did not know about the disease. It is why I try to say "I have never diagnosed a case" rather than "I have never seen a case." I wonder how many I have seen and not known it. The Secret is true. Just by knowing about a disease, the universe delivers it up to you. The Secret doesn't create health and wealth; it creates cancer, infection and death. A much more interesting, if awful, result.

Rationalization

Stone, O.J. and J.D. Maberry, Spoon Nails and Clubbing. Review and Possible Structural Mechanisms. Tex Med, 1965. 61: p. 620-7.

Leukocytosis

THE patient was initially admitted with urosepsis. After developing multi-organ system failure, she required three days of blood pressure support that kept her alive—if somewhat cool and mottled in her extremities due to the clamp-down of her arteries from the pressors used to keep her blood pressure from plummeting in septic shock.

Norepinephrine (brand name Levophed) makes the toes blue and cold, especially in patients with underlying vascular disease. Worse than dopamine. When you need levophed patients often do not make it—it was levophed, leave 'em dead.

She slowly improved and was weaned off her pressors and then, four days into her hospitalization, she got a fever for a day and her WBC jumped to 29,000—almost three times normal.

New infection? Undrained abscess? Complication of her bacteremia?

The work-up was negative for all of the above. Here is what I bet was happening.

It is not that unusual to see patients bump their white count and get a fever after prolonged hypotension. More often than sepsis, I occasionally get called to see a patient with a fever and leukocytosis after coronary artery bypass surgery (CABG). While on the bypass pump, patients are relatively hypotensive for an hour or so, and they have a decreased blood flow to the abdominal organs.

I think what happens is that hypotension leads to tissue damage, and then the reperfusion results in a flood of white blood cells into the tissues to clean up the dead meat. The result is a brief inflammatory response with a fever and an increase in the white count.

This is an extrapolation from studies that demonstrate that reperfusion of the heart is associated with a fever. There are a variety of animal models that show that reperfusion of heart or lung or liver leads to fever and leukocytosis. Ischemic colitis and pancreatitis are also occasionally seen after CABG, both of which are causes of fever.

I tend to see this syndrome more in people who have underlying vascular disease or risk factors for underlying vascular disease: diabetes and hypertension. I can't prove it, unfortunately, for like diarrhea, the diagnosis is made by a process of elimination. At least one fact and one bad pun per post. That's my goal.

If there is an article on post-sepsis/hypotension leukocytosis that is not infectious, I can't find it.

Feel free to do the study, just make me the lead author. Call it Crislip's syndrome.

We did nothing and she got better. It is the importance of time wounding all heels, or something to that effect. As an intern, it is don't just stand there, do something. As an attending, it is don't just do something, stand there. And as my wife can attest, I am excellent at doing nothing.

Rationalization

Ascione, R., et al., Splanchnic organ injury during coronary surgery with or without cardiopulmonary bypass: a randomized, controlled trial. Ann Thorac Surg, 2006. 81(1): p. 97-103.

Ben-Dor, I., et al., Body temperature - a marker of infarct size in the era of early reperfusion. Cardiology, 2005. 103(4): p. 169-73.

Yoshida, K., et al., Gastrointestinal complications in patients undergoing coronary artery bypass grafting. Ann Thorac Cardiovasc Surg, 2005. 11(1): p. 25-8.

....

Hyperhidrosis, or Sweating with the I.D. doc

THERE are symptoms that, by themselves, are difficult to evaluate. The hardest is sweats.

Night sweats occur frequently and may be a sign of infections: endocarditis is the leading infectious reason in the West. However, any infection can cause a drenching sweat, usually to break a fever. The standard pattern is a rigor, then a fever, then a sweat to break the fever.

The patient today never had a fever, just 6 years of occasional drenching sweats that occurred out of nowhere, anytime day or night, and had no other associated symptoms. Over the last two months the symptoms crescendoed to occur 5 to 10 times a day.

The patient sweated enough to raise his blood urea nitrogen and creatinine levels from simple dehydration (yep). That's a lot of water loss. It's almost like the Axe deodorant commercials that have been on during the NBA playoffs.

Go, Orlando. Sorry. I am in Portland. I can never, ever root for L.A. for any reason. But I digress.

No other symptoms. The referring docs looked for infections, collagen vascular disease, and neuroendocrine causes and came up with nothing.

The patient had an extensive travel history to the lands of Chagas, Old and New World *Leishmania*, and malaria, but there was nothing to suggest these diseases were present. *P. malariae* has been known to become symptomatic decades after the patient leaves an endemic area, but usually with fevers and chills as well as sweats.

But it seemed a real stretch that these sweats were infectious, especially as they had been going on for 6 years. If the sweats were not due to fevers, not due to infections, and not due to collagen vascular disease or Hodgkins, then what were they?

I thought maybe it was autonomic dysfunction. Autonomic hyperreflexia, or dysreflexia (AD), is most common in spinal cord injuries, though can occur with other central nervous system lesions as well. It is a result of impaired feedback from the brain to the spinal cord to shut down an autonomic response, so that any minor irritant, such as a crease in clothing, can lead to out of control sweating and sometimes raised blood pressure. It so happened that my patient had carried the diagnosis of multiple sclerosis for 15 years, although no other symptoms of MS since the diagnosis.

PubMed is not that helpful for other case reports of sweats and MS: one of decreased sweating, one of unilateral sweating, but nowhere can I find out-of-control sweating as the only symptom of MS. Thermoregulatory issues are common in the disease, but are mostly reported to raise the sweating threshold. Autonomic dysfunction appears common, but studies have looked mostly at blood pressure changes as a symptom.

However, the MS sites have many testimonials of patients with MS and hyperhydrosis. The plural of anecdote is anecdotes, not data. And the pleural of empyema is... never mind.

So maybe MS is the reason for the sweats. But I hate a diagnosis that is made by exclusion.

Go, Magic.

Rationalization

Baker, D.G., Multiple sclerosis and thermoregulatory dysfunction. J Appl Physiol (1985), 2002. 92(5): p. 1779-80.

....

Hyperventilation

RESPIRATORY rate of 35 to 40 in my meningitis patient—almost twice normal. No fever, white count improving, no cardiac or pulmonary reasons for the increased respirations. Repeat CT scanning shows no brainstem herniation or basal ganglia stroke.

Why the increased respiratory rate?

One hint from PubMed:

"We present the case of a 57 year old man who developed a B-cell lymphoma which involved his lymph nodes, liver, spleen, bone marrow, and peripheral blood. Shortly after attaining a complete remission with chemotherapy, the patient developed profound hyperventilation with no apparent cardiac or pulmonary cause. After one month, the patient developed a 7th nerve palsy and a subsequent work-up demonstrated that he had lymphomatous meningitis. The hyperventilation resolved completely with intrathecal chemotherapy, although the patient eventually died of widely disseminated lymphoma."

Whether a similar issue occurs with bacterial meningitis, I cannot say. Endotoxin can lead to hyperventilation by a variety of mechanisms, both central and peripheral. Few diseases dump endotoxin into the body like meningococcus, so perhaps I can postulate that a flood of CNS endotoxin was driving his respiratory rate by, oh, evil humors.

I found this as well. I would have thought the opposite was true, as I think of meningococcus as endotoxin production central:

> *"Endotoxin is liberated following antibiotic killing of Gram-negative rods, and antibiotics may differ in this respect. Although the amount of filterable endotoxin has also been reported to increase following antibiotic killing of meningococci, it is unknown how this influences the host response. We investigated the influence of three antibiotics on levels of free endotoxin in culture medium and cytokine production in whole blood ex vivo during killing of four strains of meningococci. Bacterial killing was significantly more efficient with penicillin or ceftriaxone than with chloramphenicol, and free endotoxin levels were lower after exposure to antibiotics as compared with no treatment (ANOVA, P < 0.001). Endotoxin levels were lowest after exposure to chloramphenicol. In three of the four strains exposure to antibiotics resulted in considerably lower cytokine levels (ANOVA, P < 0.001), and TNF-alpha levels were significantly lower after exposure to penicillin or ceftriaxone than after chloramphenicol treatment. Only in the strain that induced the lowest levels of TNF-alpha were cytokine levels comparable for untreated and treated samples. We conclude that fear of excessive endotoxin release or cytokine production caused by effective antibiotics is not justified in the treatment of meningococcal infections."*

The heck.

Rationalization

Karp, G. and K. Nahum, Hyperventilation as the initial manifestation of lymphomatous meningitis. J Neurooncol, 1992. 13(2): p. 173-5.

Prins, J.M., et al., No increase in endotoxin release during antibiotic killing of meningococci. J Antimicrob Chemother, 1997. 39(1): p. 13-8.

MISCELLANY

....

ECHO echo echo

I AM a grouchy old fart and and have the AARP card to prove it. Get off my lawn, punk. I have been a Mac user from day one and still have a functioning 128K original Mac. Dark Castle, anyone? But this upgrade to Snow Leopard has pissed away a day. Argh. So much not working right. Double argh. Every time I have upgraded in the past everything has worked better, not worse. Triple Argh.

I am old enough to have treated many an endocarditis without benefit of echocardiography. Really. There was once a time when we did not have an ECHO and had to rely on physical and, most importantly, positive blood cultures for an organism that esd huh;? known to cause endocarditis. I also walked to the hospital, uphill and barefoot in the snow and made my own penicillin from mould that grew on old bread and coffee grounds.

These days there is a shift in how medicine is done. Back in the day, we were trained to do things a step at a time and wait for results before moving on to the next test. However, that would lead to a prolonged length of stay and the real cost, I am told, is keeping people in the hospital. As a result, it seems that every possible test is done on every patient to reach a diagnosis as fast as possible.

So as result, if you have someone with a risk for endocarditis, you do not wait for the blood cultures to come back positive to order an ECHO to 'rule out endocarditis.' Sometimes, even if they do not have a risk for endocarditis, an ECHO may be ordered. If I had my way I would never allow an ECHO that had the indication 'rule out endocarditis.'

The problem is that an ECHO in the absence of the classic findings of endocarditis, like, say, positive blood cultures and emboli, is of little utility and is more likely to have a false rather than a true positive. If your pretest probability of a disease is low, the chance that a test is a true positive is low.

Like today. Patient had end stage liver disease and came in septic. ECHO, to rule out endocarditis, showed a possible abnormality. Blood cultures grew *E. coli* and the patient responded rapidly to therapy. There have been, since 1909, 36 cases of native valve endocarditis reported in the literature due to *E. coli*. Given the maybe 250,000 cases of *E. coli* bacteremia in the US each year, the odds that the questionable goober on the valve was due to infection from *E. coli was* neither clinically nor statistically likely. The patient went on to a TEE, which showed a sclerotic valve. No endocarditis. No surprise.

Endocarditis is still a mostly clinical diagnosis, based on sustained positive blood cultures, exam and risks. The ECHO never need be done to 'rule out' endocarditis.

> *"Thus echocardiography is useful in confirming the clinical diagnosis of infective endocarditis, but only rarely detects vegetations in patients who lack the characteristic clinical features of endocarditis, regardless of whether they have positive negative blood cultures."*

A waste of time and money, both of which are better spent on ID docs.

Rationalization

Micol, R., et al., Escherichia coli native valve endocarditis. Clin Microbiol Infect, 2006. 12(5): p. 401-3.

Donaldson, R.M., et al., The role of echocardiography in suspected bacterial endocarditis. Eur Heart J, 1984. 5 Suppl C: p. 53-7.

....

Zombies

I AM tired. I moved 1345 pounds of pea gravel from Home Depot to the car to the back yard. Why my wife cannot decorate with styrofoam, I do not know, but my new rule is that if the sack of rocks weighs more than my age, I am not lifting it.

Last night I finished World War Z: An Oral History of the

Zombie War by Max Brooks. If you like that sort of thing, and I do, it is a fun read. What, you may ask, does a book about zombies have to do with Infectious Disease? Dude. Everything as something to do with infectious disease. I.D. is the Kevin Bacon of connectedness.

Infections, of course, have done more to change the world than most people realize. If you pay any attention to the history of world, you quickly notice it is also the history of infections. Plagues of all kinds have continually swept though the world and killed enormous numbers of humans. Up to two thirds of Europe died of a plague in the middle ages. The 1918-1919 flu pandemic killed about two percent of the world's population. That flu pandemic was a bird flu strain, and if history repeats itself, 2% of 7 billion is a lot of people.

In WWZ, the zombie plague is spread by the bite of a zombie. It infects the bitten, who die and then are reanimated as zombies that eat the living; they can only be killed by having their brains destroyed. Typical zombie fare, but the story takes place after a zombie pandemic that almost annihilates the human race and is told from the perspective of the survivors.

As an I.D. doc, you could substitute flu, or smallpox, or bubonic plague and see the book as a metaphor for the effects of a world wide contagion. The world is primed for a huge pandemic. We were lucky that SARS was not very infectious and that it came to a county with a first-class health care system, namely Canada, and not to one with a second rate system such as-—Oh, I don't know, the US. Large populations with widespread travel would make it easy for a plague to rapidly spread across the world. The 1918 pandemic swept the world before air travel. If you have ever wandered the rat warrens of Chicago O'Hare, you can imagine what would happen if some lunatic terrorist decided to infect himself and wandered the airport. How quickly one vector could infect huge numbers of people.

I.D. docs do worry about pandemics. So do those in public health, who also have to consider what would happen to the economy if half the workforce didn't come to work one day due to an influenza or zombie pandemic. It has the potential to be a real nightmare.

One of the better chapters of *WWZ* from a medical point of view (as opposed to the creepy zombie army attacking and eating your innards point of view) is early in the book. A character named Breckenridge Scott who made a fortune selling a fake zombie cure called Phalanx, is interviewed Heis the archetype of every purveyor of supplements in the U.S., from Airborne to Enzyte, and the whole chapter is worth reading.

A good horror novel, or any other work of fiction, needs to stand on its own. This book is a fun, creepy read. A great piece of fiction has a broader understanding of the human condition, and read as a possible example of any post plague existence, *WWZ* works at the higher level as well.

Read it for fun, read it to be creeped out, read it to look at how our world could react to a global catastrophe of, oh, climate change and the resulting spread of many forms of zombies, er, I mean, infections.

Mmmmmmmmmmmm. Brains.

All those in favor

BACTERIA communicate with each other. Really. They send each other information that subsequently changes their behavior.

It called Twitter, no, quorum sensing, and has probably been present in bacteria for a billion years. It's called "quorum" sensing because the bacteria and yeast communicate with each other when the colony reaches a critical number of bacteria. They then alter their metabolism, make some virulence factors. or start to form biofilms in response to communications with each other.

"Hey, there are a awful lot is us here! Let's eat a little less, build us a home and invade the host."

There are at least a half dozen quorum-sensing systems in pathogenic bacteria, depending on the species, and others in non-pathogenic organisms.

Bacteria communicate with each other using small molecules and peptides, some of which suppress other strains of the same species to gain a local advantage in a disease.

Not only do bacteria communicate with each other, they may communicate with other colonies of organisms, other bacterial species, and even with host cells. The strain of *S. aureus* that gets there the firstest with the mostest prevents other *S. aureus* from thriving. Not only do the fittest survive, the fittest prevent the weaker from growing. I bet this system helps accelerate pathogenicity.

Some bacteria can sense host molecules like endorphin or epinephrine, and in response alter the production of their virulence factors to enhance infection. On the other hand, host enzymes can degrade bacterial quorum-sensing molecules to prevent the bacteria from plotting and taking you over.

Back and forth they chatter and we try and jam the communications. The Cold War writ small.

I used to think I was hearing voices. I wasn't. It's the bacteria in and on me. Talking. Planning. Conspiring. There are out to get us, you know. In the end they will. Eat, drink and be merry, for tomorrow you will be bacterial dinner.

Rationalization

Sifri, C.D., Healthcare epidemiology: quorum sensing: bacteria talk sense. Clin Infect Dis, 2008. 47(8): p. 1070-6.

....

Incompletely Inured

YESTERDAY, Sunday, was a busy day, that in no way had anything what so ever to do with Infectious Disease. Hard to believe that I could spend an entire day and not see something that was related to infections. I guess I wasn't looking hard enough to notice some germ or other. Monday, back to work, and no shortage of infections.

Acute care medicine gets you used to all sorts of human conditions. Four of the six senses (I am psychic) are stimulated, often unpleasantly, during rounds—fortunately, taste is spared. We all get good at switching off those parts of the brain that lead to a less than professional response to the various sights, sounds and odors that flood the hospital. Patients do not want to see their provider puking.

Sometimes you will walk onto a ward and the distinctive tang of melena (bloody diarrhea) will hit the first nerve. You inhale deeply and with appreciation: it is the fragrance of internal medicine; you are home, in your element, the hospital. Ahhhh.

Today there were two sensory assaults I have not experienced for many years.

The first was wet gangrene in a diabetic foot. The smell of putrefying flesh when it is still attached to the patient is distinctive. You know the microbiology of the infection instantly, as only the combination of anaerobes plus aerobes in dead tissue makes that smell. There are people who have done olfactory studies to elucidate the microbiology of stench, sometimes using technology in lieu of their own noses. It is probably *Bacteroides* spp. that accounts for most of the infectious funk, but the research is curiously minimal, and what chemical(s) cause the smell I cannot find. It is probably a complex mélange, like a good red wine. The treatment, like with most anaerobic infections, is surgical rather than antibiotics. I have become good a keeping my expression calm, not wrinkling my nose to the acrid smell coming from the foot of the bed or the foot in the bed. The patients probably think I have Parkinson's. That Dr. Crislip is so unexpressive.

The other I still cannot deal with, even after twenty-five years. When someone with acute pneumonia gives one of those deep, hacking, wet coughs and brings up a large specimen, expels it into a tissue, and offers it to me to examine, I lose it. It still brings on my gag reflex better than a bottle of ipecac. As a medical student I had mentioned to my attending that I had an issue with sputum production and he was kind enough to provide, as my final in the history and physical class, a patient with tri-lobar pneumonia who coughed up his body weight in green sputum while I did my final exam. Tears literally ran down my face as I (successfully) tried not to vomit. I passed. And not out.

Today was a little easier. The patient horked up a big wet loogie and offered it to me. I long ago learned to avert my eyes, stare in the middle distance, and politely decline the offer, explaining that sputum is one of my peccadilloes and that the patient probably did not want to examine my last meal in exchange. The patients have always understood and seem to appreciate my honesty. Or they are too kind to call me a wimp.

The respiratory therapists and the nurses derive no end of pleasure from my inability to deal with pulmonary secretions, enjoying the occasional opportunity to display a juicy sputum specimen to me. As an I.D. doc, they tell me, I should be comfortable with all things pus, including sputum. I always tell them that as an infectious disease doc, pus is a theoretical construct (and my vanity license plate). Others collect it for me, the lab analyzes it, and I determine what to do with it. I want to keep it that way.

Rationalization

Bowler, P.G., B.J. Davies, and S.A. Jones, Microbial involvement in chronic wound malodour. J Wound Care, 1999. 8(5): p. 216-8.

Brook, I. and E.H. Frazier, Clinical and microbiological features of necrotizing fasciitis. J Clin Microbiol, 1995. 33(9): p. 2382-7.

Yamada, Y., et al., Association of odor from infected root canal analyzed by an electronic nose with isolated bacteria. J Endod, 2007. 33(9): p. 1106-9.

Osteo, Cancer and Insurance

HEALTHCARE in the US is second to none. Because we are 17th. Or worse. The patient this week was a laborer and never had health insurance. Ever.

Over 15 years ago he developed a pimple on this shoulder. He doctored it himself. Over the next decade and a half it progressed to the point where he had a dinner-plate-sized defect over his shoulder. You could see his humerus, his clavicle, and his whole shoulder joint, all of which was infected, at the bottom of an enormous soft tissue divot.

His plain x-ray was great/awful. All the bones of this shoulder were mottled and looked as though a rat had been gnawing on them. Very chronic osteomyelitis.

Even more impressive were the huge amounts of heterotopic bone. He had more calcium in the soft tissues of his arm than he did in the bone. Heterotopic bone is bone deposition in soft tissues and is only seen in chronic, untreated osteomyelitis of years duration. It used to be seen in the pre-antibiotic era, but is extremely rare where people have access to good health care.

Like not here. When asked, he said the reason he never had it cared for is that he did not want to incur the cost. It was healthcare or food and rent. He chose to eat. Now the only chance of cure is to amputate his arm and the upper chest. Not a good outcome.

The odd thing was how this process ate away all the soft tissues of his shoulder. It looked like a hyaena had been having at go at his shoulder. Chronic osteomyelitis is not usually so destructive, more often having recurrent sinus tracts and drainage.

Years ago, back last century, I wore an onion on my belt.... which was the style at the time...you couldn't get those white ones, you could only get those big yellow ones ... , there was a case of a patient who let his—Basal cell? Squamous cell? I cannot quite remember which—eat away his entire abdominal wall, skin and fat, leaving the underlying muscle exposed.

I was amazed at the amount of soft tissue destruction, and wondered if it started as an underlying skin cancer.

Alternatively, chronic osteomyelitis is associated with various cancers of the draining sinus tract. For you eponym mavins, it is called Marjolin's ulcer.

To quote from the reference below:

"A Marjolin ulcer, is identified as a squamous cell carcinoma that develops in post–traumatic scars and chronic wounds. It has been well documented that it was first described by Jean Nicholas Marjolin in 1828, and then Hawkins reported in 1835 a case of

squamous cell carcinoma that appeared to have originated from a site of chronic osteomyelitis. Although well described, squamous cell carcinoma consistent with the diagnosis of a Marjolin's type is an uncommon entity. Its incidence ranges from 0.23% to 1.7% . Cases of chronic osteomyelitis that may develop into squamous cell carcinoma have an incidence range of 0.2;.7% . It most often occurs in Caucasian males, age range 18 -40 years. The average reported duration of osteomyelitis before the development of the squamous cell carcinoma is 27-30 years, but ranges from 18 to 72 years. Mean latency period is 30.5 years."

I like the fact the mean latency period can be longer than the ages of the patients who develop the disease. Probably some sort of time travel involved.

Squamous cell carcinomas are not the only cancers associated with osteomyelitis: all the cell lines in the skin have resulted in at least one case report.

Rationalization

Ogawa, B., et al., Marjolin's ulcer arising at the elbow: a case report and literature review. Hand (N Y), 2006. 1(2): p. 89-93.

Follow up

The patient was found to have basal cell carcinoma in all the biopsies: skin and bone. Fifteen years or so of letting a malignancy slowly eat away his shoulder. He eventually had has arm and chest wall removed at another hospital and was lost to follow-up.

Whoa.

I have seen some impressively destructive cancers ignored by patients over the years. I remember (25 years in medicine gives me the right to tell stories. And I have my AARP card, so I can complain about anything, anytime. Get off my lawn and turn off that damn hip-hop) when I was a medical student doing my ER rotation a guy came in with a hemoglobin of 5, about one-third normal. He was feeling light-headed (the patient, not me). So I did the usually excessive medical student history and review of systems and found nothing, then on exam found a cancer the size and shape of a large mushroom on his back, oozing blood. A biopsy showed it was melanoma, the deadliest form of skin cancer. He totally dismissed it when I asked him about it. "Oh," he said, "that's nothing."

As our former President said, denial is more than a river in Syria.

As those who work with me know, there is no part of medicine I enjoy more than making an unlikely diagnosis. I do feel a tad guilty exulting in being right, as it usually means someone also has a terrible illness.

All the best cases are someone else's tragedy.

Rationalization

Falagas, M.E. and P.I. Vergidis, Narrative review: diseases that masquerade as infectious cellulitis. Ann Intern Med, 2005. 142(1): p. 47-55.

....

Bacterial Boogers

I REALLY do not remember why I went to medical school. What delusion I was suffering under at the time that made me pick medicine, I do not know. I occasionally talk to premeds and they are so clueless about the practice of medicine. Maybe I am a doc because my Dad is a doc; beware of role models.

Don't get me wrong. I love what I do. I have the best gig in the city, the sole I.D. doc (if I were in South Korean doc, I would be the Seoul I.D. doc) at 4 hospitals, I get to see all the cool cases and rarely do I get called to see something dull. I get all the clinical gold and little of the pyrite.

It is a nice part of the job that I meet nice people (It's nice to be nice to the nice —Frank Burns, MD) and help get them better. But it is not what gets me up in the dark to head off to work. What I enjoy more than anything else is figuring things out. I love to call the diagnosis before the confirming tests. I know I know I know. Arrogant self-centered bastard who uses his publications to trumpet his clinical triumphs. But it is fun to get the diagnosis before the confirmatory tests.

I am more often wrong than right, but no one ever remembers when you are wrong, because in medicine you are always wrong. Babe Ruth also lead the league in strike outs.

A 65-year-old diabetic female on dialysis had a cardiac arrest. She survived (obviously, else why would I see her? I have had one post mortem consult in my career, but usually those are reserved for the pathologist). She was febrile and her blood cultures grew *Enterococcus* and *Klebsiella*. Review of symptoms revealed a month or two of sweats, she had right upper quadrant pain and her transaminases were three times the normal level, suggesting liver damage of some kind.

Diabetics plus *Klebsiella* equals liver abscess. Simple math. Why, I wonder, is the English math plural, maths? They have such a singular way of talking.

But not just any *Klebsiella*, there is a strain that started in Taiwan and is hypermucoviscous. Ugh. What does this mean? It means it's like snot on a plate, and the hypermucous probably inhibits the ability of white blood cells to kill the beast. It also makes it more likely to cause eye and brain infections. Snot bad. Bacterial snot worse.

So the CT scan did show what looks to be a liver abscess or a liver tumor or both; as always there were confounding factors that obscured the diagnosis until we could do a liver biopsy.

Unfortunately (for me, not for her), the *Klebsiella* was not the hypermucous strain, just a regular old *Klebsiella*.

I'll give me half credit.

Rationalization

Chung, D.R., et al., Evidence for clonal dissemination of the serotype K1 Klebsiella pneumoniae strain causing invasive liver abscesses in Korea. J Clin Microbiol, 2008. 46(12): p. 4061-3.

Keynan, Y., et al., Pyogenic liver abscess caused by hypermucoviscous Klebsiella pneumoniae. Scand J Infect Dis, 2007. 39(9): p. 828-30.

Kim, J.K., et al., Risk factor analysis of invasive liver abscess caused by the K1 serotype Klebsiella pneumoniae. Eur J Clin Microbiol Infect Dis, 2009. 28(1): p. 109-11.

....

My liver quiver

My liver quivers.

~ Bob Marley

Rearrange your liver to the silent mental grace.

~ Yes.

THE liver is not well represented in popular music. Send in better lyrics if you know any.

The liver, however, is well represented in infectious disease. Today was a liver abscess, bacterial, from a diverticular abscess.

Most liver abscesses are due to some sort of biliary disease, and it is odd to see one due to colonic disease in this century. It was a more common cause in the old days, before CAT scans and antibiotics.

This patient had a risk factor that lead to his liver abscesses: he was single.

He had symptoms for over two months of a diverticular abscess, and he kept expecting it to go away.

The first question I often ask a patient is some version of, "What brings you to the hospital?"

Often in men it is some variation of, "My wife/girlfriend made me."

(BTW: anyone who answers "My car" is instantly eligible for physician-assisted suicide, as is anyone who says "My fingers" in response to the question "How do you feel?" Be original, puh leaze).

Not having a girlfriend to make him come to the hospital, he let it fester. Fester. That's a great word. I did not realize that Uncles Fester from the Addams Family had an odd name until well into medical school.

We older XYs would probably not survive to senescence except for the XXs 'making' us go to the hospital.

The other curiosity of the liver abscess is he had time to develop a thrombus in his portal vein. His was bland, but occasionally these are infected thrombi (therefore the pleural of Elvis is Elvi). In my experience (the most dangerous words in medicine) I do not see many portal or hepatic vein thrombi, despite what the references say. Perhaps they have a hospital filled with single men.

Rationalization

Lee, K.H., et al., Hepatic attenuation differences associated with obstruction of the portal or hepatic veins in patients with hepatic abscess. AJR Am J Roentgenol, 2005. 185(4): p. 1015-23.

....

Infected Infarctions

HEPATOCELLULAR carcinomas are bad. Often you can't cut them out, and they are not particularly responsive to chemotherapy. They are preventable, since many hepatomas are due to chronic hepatitis B, and are found in hepcats. The consult today was an elderly female from SE Asia with a lifetime of chronic hepatitis B and now a mass in her liver.

What they do to kill these tumors is cut off their blood supply, and they do that mechanically: stuff the hepatic artery that feeds the tumor with beads and gelfoam, the artery clots off, and the tumor dies. It works, but is not without its potential problems—like bacterial seeding of the dead liver and a subsequent pockets of pus.

She had had several days of fevers, chills, fatigue and, after admission, E. coli in the blood. A CT scan looking for the source of the E. coli demonstrated that the tumor, which had been embolized about a month ago, now had a pocket of gas in it. The liver is downstream from the colon, which is filled with hundreds of species of bacteria in the feces . Sometimes the bacteria relax, turn off their minds, and float downstream and lodge in the liver. Tomorrow never knows when that will happen. (Are the beatles lyrics too obscure?)

Only way to get gas in the dead tumor is if something is making gas, and, as my 12-year-old likes to demonstrate loudly, to be alive is to make gas. While one worries about gas gangrene when you find gas in tissues the end by-product of all metabolism is gas, and every organism, from anaerobes to E. coli to Candida, can make gas. The worst gas-forming infection I have ever seen, at least in terms of quantity of gas made, was a Staphylococcus aureus infection that looked like a seltzer bottle had been released into the patient's muscles.

Infected infarctions are also problematic to treat, as the dead tissue is a huge foreign body with no antibiotic penetration, so they tend to respond poorly to drainage and antibiotics. I am not optimistic that I can cure the infection.

Rationalization

Jansen, M.C., et al., Adverse effects of radiofrequency ablation of liver tumours in the Netherlands. Br J Surg, 2005. 92(10): p. 1248-54.

Postscript

No follow-up. Patient had a change in insurance which led to a change in hospital systems.

....

Incidentaloma

TECHNOLOGY becomes increasingly inexpensive and available. I hear that there is now an ultrasound probe that uses your iPhone as the screen. I am sitting in the parking lot at the mall, with my netbook in my lap as my children look for a Mother's Day present, writing this.

And the anesthesiologists have transesophageal echocardiograms (TEE) and they can check out cardiac function any time they please, and this time they pleased.

The patient had a chronic foot infection that needed debridement, and in the OR the anesthesiologists slipped that old probe down the esophagus and there was the heart, beating away nicely and there was that aortic valve and, hey, what the..?

A vegetation.

Really. I looked at the ECHO and it sure looked like a veggy to me: a 6 mm clot on the tip on the aortic valve, flopping in and out.

Once I got to talk to him and examine him, I found that he had no constitutional symptoms, no murmur, no emboli, and no lab findings of endocarditis. Nothing to suggest endocarditis except a really abnormal TEE.

Blood cultures were negative, but he was on antibiotics for the foot infection.

Classically, an incidentaloma is an adrenal mass found on CT when you were not expecting it.

It does not typically refer to a vegetation on a valve, but I have been called twice this year about unexpected clots on valves. The other was a 1.4 cm aortic vegetation that was found on a routine ECHO obtained for other reasons.

So what is it? Treated endocarditis? Partially treated endocarditis? Culture-negative endocarditis? Murantic endocarditis (sterile vegetations from a hypercoagulable state)? A really really really odd tumor on the valve? I don't know. Only way to know with certainty is to cut it out, and that hardly seems worth it. The heart is one of the few place I can't get my interventional radiologists to biopsy. Go figure.

If the cultures remain negative, I will send of all the serologies that in 20 years have yet to strike paydirt. In the end he may have to be treated for culture negative endocarditis; safe is better than sorry.

Rationalization

Vancollie, O., E. Rombaut, and J. Donckier, Cardiac incidentaloma. Ann Cardiol Angeiol (Paris), 2001. 50(6): p. 316-8.

Houpikian, P. and D. Raoult, Blood culture-negative endocarditis in a reference center: etiologic diagnosis of 348 cases. Medicine (Baltimore), 2005. 84(3): p. 162-73.

Postscript

Patient never had a diagnosis and the endocarditis was a cure, if one can cure a disease you are not certain someone really had.

....

True, true and probably unrelated

MY latest patient was a middle-aged female who, months and months ago, presented with endocarditis from viridans strep. She had the usual therapy and, as best I could tell, was a cure.

Several weeks after therapy ended she developed pain in her left hip, and on MRI was found to have inflammation of the left pelvic girdle muscles. No fevers, no increase in the creatine kinase that would indicate muscle injury, no increased white count. The reading on the MRI was myositis—maybe, maybe not, pyomyositis. That is, she had inflamed muscle, but we didn't know if this muscle had pus in it.

She improved on clindamycin, a macrolide antibiotic given because she was allergic to penicillin. Then she relapsed after a 4-week course. MRI showed more of the same, so she was then placed on a longer course of clindamycin. And, after 6 months, she was finally pain free and the MRI showed it was all better.

I know. Probably should have done a biopsy. During the prolonged clindamycin she was also diagnosed with scleroderma, an autoimmune disease characterized by an overproduction of collagen.

Now the plot really thickened.

Two weeks or so off the clindamycin and the pain, but nothing else, came back.

Why?

There is a myositis/scleroderma overlap, as there is with all rheumatologic syndromes. Everything overlaps in rheumatology. So maybe this is relapsing myositis from scleroderma. But why the apparent response to the clindamycin?

Here is where I go off the deep end. I sure hope there is some water in there.

I used to think that the clinical significance of the immuno-modulatory effects of macrolides were a heap of fetid dingoes' kidneys.

However, there have been two clinical studies and one animal study to show survival benefit of macrolides even when the organism is resistant to the clindamycin, probably from the immunomodulatory effects of the antibiotics rather than any antibacterial effect. They are ever-so -slightly immunosuppressive. Since what people die from in sepsis is an excessive inflammatory response (if you say cytokine storm, I will slap you upside the head. Long story), if you can take the edge off the inflammation, you may take an edge off the death rates.

So maybe, maybe the effects on the myositis are due to the immunomodulatory effects of the clindamycin on the myositis/scleroderma. Just wee bit o' immune suppression from the clindamycin, and the myositis improves. Stop the macrolide and the myositis returns. Or not. I can find nothing on PubMed to support my hypothesis. But as I am sure you are aware by now, I don't let those pesky facts get in the way of a good story.

But it is a curious association. Probably nothing, no causality, but if there is, it is to be called the Crislip effect. I want something named after me before I die, and it is not the glove breaking on the prostate exam.

I am repeating the MRI and, if positive, will get a muscle biopsy. I will let you know.

Rationalization

Spyridaki, A., et al., Effect of clarithromycin in inflammatory markers of patients with ventilator-associated pneumonia and sepsis caused by Gram-negative bacteria: results from a randomized clinical study. Antimicrob Agents Chemother, 2012. 56(7): p. 3819-25.

van der Eerden, M.M. and W.G. Boersma, Impact of macrolide therapy on mortality in severe sepsis caused by pneumonia. Eur Respir J, 2009. 34(2): p. 521.

Karlstrom, A., et al., Treatment with protein synthesis inhibitors improves outcomes of secondary bacterial pneumonia after influenza. J Infect Dis, 2009. 199(3): p. 311-9.

Postscript

The MRI was negative, I did not give clindamycin and she improved.

....

A Cold

I TOOK my Echinacea, I took my vitamin C, I took my Airborne, I took my zinc, and I boosted by immune system with Dannon. And I still got a cold today. Stuffy, runny, scratchy, I am a living NyQuil commercial. So I spent my day wearing a mask. Everyone said I looked better.

As usual, I saw lots of cases that I could not, and maybe never will, figure out.

Like the 45-year-old with a history of asthma, maybe acute pneumonia on chest x-ray,but some lung nodules showed up on the CT scan. The patient was febrile, and a creatinine of 5 mg/dL—about five times normal, suggesting renal dysfunction of some kind

The weird thing was the proptosis. Both of her eyes were bugging out. It could be Graves' disease, common things commonly being common. Tautologies being taut? Doesn't work, but I tried. Blame the endogenous interferon.

But.

If it turns out she does have an pulmonary-renal syndrome, then maybe the proptosis was a manifestations of Wegener's, as I learned today thanks to the magic of PubMed. It would tie it all together nicely.

Ask me in a week, I will let you know if the anti-neutrophil cytoplasmic antibody test is positive.

Rationalization

Haynes, B.F., et al., The ocular manifestations of Wegener's granulomatosis. Fifteen years experience and review of the literature. Am J Med, 1977. 63(1): p. 131-41.

Postscript
And it wasn't Wegener's, it was Graves' hyperthyroidism.

....

Warts

O NE of the many infrequently mentioned benefits of working in a hospital is the people you work with. Good, smart people tend to go into healthcare. One of the ongoing pleasures of work is the docs and nurses and social workers and nutritionists and techs, and I am sure if I try to make an inclusive list I will forget a group, so I will say etc etc and etc.

As a result of long association, people seem comfortable curbsiding me with their infectious disease issues. Like yesterday I got to see a wart. A big wart that was inflamed and annoying to its owner.

How, I was asked, do I treat it?

Compound W works, and you could have it burned off with liquid nitrogen, but given its location on the hand I wouldn't burn it off.

How come if you use cold it is called burning it off?

Got me. Language is funny (both in the ha ha and odd meanings of the word) that way.

Then someone suggested duct tape. Now I know that duct tape is a useful product outside of medicine, but warts?

I was skeptical. Hard to believe, I know.

The theory proffered on the ward was it cuts off oxygen so the wart dies. Didn't seem likely, since the oxygen gets to the wart by way of the blood supply, although a duct tape embolism would work.

So off to PubMed, and oh yeah you betcha, there are 24 references about removing warts with duct tape.

The some studies says it does not work, some studies demonstrate efficacy. I prefer the Tom Sawyer technique

"Why, you take your cat and go and get in the graveyard 'long about midnight when somebody that was wicked has been buried;

and when it's midnight a devil will come, or maybe two or three, but you can't see'em, you can only hear something like the wind, or maybe hear'em talk; and when they're taking that feller away, you heave your cat after'em and say, Devil follow corpse, cat follow devil, warts follow cat, I'm done with ye!"

It hasn't failed me yet. A dead cat is always a plus.

Duct tape? I don't know. Just doesn't seem plausible to me, but more papers than not suggest that it is effective. But I am not treating genital warts with it.

Rationalization

de Haen, M., et al., Efficacy of duct tape vs placebo in the treatment of verruca vulgaris (warts) in primary school children. Arch Pediatr Adolesc Med, 2006. 160(11): p. 1121-5.

Focht, D.R., 3rd, C. Spicer, and M.P. Fairchok, The efficacy of duct tape vs cryotherapy in the treatment of verruca vulgaris (the common wart). Arch Pediatr Adolesc Med, 2002. 156(10): p. 971-4.

Wenner, R., et al., Duct tape for the treatment of common warts in adults: a double-blind randomized controlled trial. Arch Dermatol, 2007. 143(3): p. 309-13.

Keogh-Brown, M.R., et al., To freeze or not to freeze: a cost-effectiveness analysis of wart treatment. Br J Dermatol, 2007. 156(4): p. 687-92.

....

The Misery of a Mystery

I get to work the three day weekend, lucky me. But things are not too bad, a few consults each day, and my kids have reached that age where they prefer to spend time with their friends rather than with their dorky parents.

I had left one hospital today and was on my way to the next when I got called back to the ER to look at a most peculiar case.

For five days he had had bilateral red, swollen very painful ears, both his arms had a rash and he had some anterior chest pain.

Exam? Funny you should ask. Both his ears had rumor, dolor,

calor, tumor, with some subcutaneous ecchymosis but no blisters. The arms looked like a folliculitis, if anything, with crusting. His sternoclavicular joint was tender to palpation.

Labs were OK, the rest of the exam was negative, no past medical history of note. He did not look systemically ill, like patients with a serious infection.

What the hell was it?

If it was Zoster (Shingles), it was bilateral and Zoster is never bilateral, and there were no lesions that looked like Chicken Pox.

Relapsing polychondritis? That would explain the ears and the chest wall tenderness, but not the rash, although the interwebs give a variety of rashes with polychondritis. And he has not relapsed yet.

Cellulitis? Never, ever, bilateral, and why the ears? Does not look like a strep infection, and he is non-toxic.

The one hint, maybe, perhaps, is that he lived on a boat, and 24 hours before the onset he had taken a bath in the Columbia river. Rivers are not the cleanest source of water, even in the Pacific Northwest.

Aeromonas? It could be, especially with the ecchymosis. *Aeromonas* is a fresh water organism that causes a cellulitis, but why the bilateral ears and arm involvement? And I think of *Aeromonas* as a systemic illness with more local tissue damage.

What was it? I'll be damned if I could figure it out. I await cultures with interest.

Rationalization

Ko, W.C., et al., Clinical features and therapeutic implications of 104 episodes of monomicrobial Aeromonas bacteraemia. J Infect, 2000. 40(3): p. 267-73.

Postscript

I never did get a diagnosis. Where is House when you need him?

AFTERWORD

That is it. One year of Puswhispering. I continue to whisper to pus about every other day over at Medscape.com.

And the amazing thing? Something different every post. ID is so cool.

There will be a year two, and a year three, and so on. Until I die or retire, whichever is first.

You know the motto that guides all I do: The world needs more Mark Crislip ™.